HYPERACTIVE CHILDREN
A Handbook for Diagnosis and Treatment

HYPERACTIVE CHILDREN
A Handbook for
Diagnosis and Treatment

RUSSELL A. BARKLEY

The Medical College of Wisconsin and
Milwaukee Children's Hospital

Foreword by Dennis P. Cantwell

THE GUILFORD PRESS

New York   London

©1981 The Guilford Press, New York
A Division of Guilford Publications, Inc.
200 Park Avenue South, New York, N.Y. 10003

Printed in the United States of America

Library of Congress Cataloging in Publication Data
Barkley, Russell A., 1949–
  Hyperactive children.
  Includes bibliographies and index.
  1. Hyperactive child syndrome. 2. Behavior
therapy. I. Title.
RJ506.H9B37   618.92'8589   81–1382
ISBN 0–89862–609–9   AACR2

TO PAT AND STEPHEN

The knowledge we have acquired ought not to resemble a great shop without order, and without an inventory; we ought to know what we possess, and be able to make it serve us in our need.—*Gottfried Leibnitz*

FOREWORD

"Hyperactivity" is one of the most common—if not *the* most common—causes of referral to child psychiatric clinics. Over the years many articles and books have been written about this clinical problem. However, much of this literature has not served to further knowledge about the diagnosis and management of this condition due to confusion in terminology reflecting very different theoretical orientations.

The history of this particular problem in the United States probably dates back to the encephalitis epidemic in 1917–1918. After the epidemic there were a number of children who, after having recovered from their encephalitis, developed a behavior problem characterized by three primary sets of symptoms: hyperactivity, short attention span, and impulsive behavior. For these children the term "brain damage behavior syndrome" was coined, an apt term indeed in this case; these children did have brain damage from their encephalitis, and it was as a result of their encephalitis that their behavior problem developed.

Unfortunately, as Dr. Barkley points out nicely in this book, several "myths" about this disorder began to develop, two of which were as follows: (1) If a child presented with hyperactivity, short attention span, and impulsive behavior, *ipso facto* that meant the child had brain damage. Brain damage would be diagnosed on the basis of this behavioral constellation even in the *absence* of any other objective physical, neurological, or laboratory signs of brain damage. (2) When brain damage did lead to a psychiatric disorder in childhood, it uniformly would lead to the picture of hyperactivity, short attention span, and impulsive behavior. Both of these myths, however, have been dispelled by current research evidence. Nevertheless, the fact that research evidence has proved them wrong has not necessarily led to their diminution in the minds of many in the general public and, in fact, of many professionals.

As our techniques for diagnosing brain damage became more sophisticated, it became obvious that the great majority of children who present with this behavioral constellation have no other signs of brain damage if "brain damage" is used in its literal sense of structural abnormality in the brain. Likewise, we also now know that while children with definite brain damage do, in fact, have a greater likelihood of developing psychiatric disorders than do children in the general population, the nature of their psychiatric disorder is not "unique"—that is, they are just as likely to develop emotional disorders as they are to develop behavior disorders characterized by hyperactivity, short attention span, and impulsivity. The classic Isle of Wight studies of Michael Rutter and his colleagues have demonstrated this fairly conclusively. Thus, a change in terminology began to reflect a change in etiological thinking. The term "brain damage" was replaced by the softer term "minimal brain damage," implying that since this particular behavioral constellation is present, brain damage of a minimal nature must be there even though it cannot be detected by ordinary clinical methods.

Primarily as a result of a major national task force, the term was softened even more to "minimal brain dysfunction," indicating that while damage itself may not be present, central nervous system dysfunction must be present to explain this behavioral constellation. However, to preface a term like "brain dysfunction" with the term "minimal" implies that we can quantify something that we cannot even measure. For if there is a minimal brain dysfunction, there must be a maximal brain dysfunction, and every child could be graded from 0 to 100 according to the degree of brain dysfunction. The current state of the art does not allow such precise measurement and quantification of something as global as brain dysfunction.

More behaviorally oriented terms began to become popular since they did not have any etiological implication. "Hyperactive child," "hyperactive child syndrome," "hyperkinetic syndrome," "hyperactivity," and similar terms began to be used to describe this constellation of behaviors. Unfortunately, even such behaviorally oriented terms lacked precision since hyperactivity could be used, and indeed has been used, to describe motor activity *only* or to describe the entire constellation of hyperactivity, short attention span, and impulsive behavior. Thus it is not surprising that some clinicians and researchers were using the same terms to describe different children and different terms to describe the same children.

With the publication in 1980 of the third edition of the *Diagnostic and Statistical Manual of Mental Disorders* (DSM-III) by the American Psychiatric Association, two significant changes occurred which have both theoretical and practical implications. First, the name of the disorder was changed from Hyperkinetic Reaction of Childhood to Attention Deficit Disorder. This change reflected the current thinking that the motor activity symptoms are clearly not the primary symptoms. As Dr. Barkley points out in the first chapter, the short attention span and impulsivity are considerably more important and are certainly more persistent. Second, operational criteria were specified for this disorder for the first time in any official diagnostic nomenclature. Indeed, DSM-III specifies operational diagnostic criteria for all of the disorders described in the manual. In addition to specifying operational criteria, DSM-III contains an extensive textual description of the essential features, associated features, age of onset, course, complications, predisposing factors, family patterns of illness, and differential diagnosis. While the criteria may have some weaknesses, as outlined by Dr.

Barkley in Chapter 1, they are likely to make the current diagnosis of this disorder a much more standardized procedure.

Hyperactivity as a symptom—that is, excess motor activity—is one that has little predictive validity; it is quite common among children with no psychiatric disorder and occurs as a presenting symptom in children with many different types of psychiatric disorders, including anxiety disorders and psychotic disorders such as infantile autism. It is not surprising that when a disorder is relatively common and relatively ill defined, as hyperactivity has been up until now, a large myth-filled literature on possible etiological factors and treatment modalities will develop. Such is true of this disorder.

Dr. Barkley's book is unique in a variety of ways. First and foremost, it is written primarily for the clinician who deals with hyperactive children and their families on a day-to-day basis. The clinicial description of the disorder emphasizes the myriad of problems that these children present to their teachers, to their families, to their peers, and to themselves. Children with this disorder are best viewed as multihandicapped. The disorder is obviously of multifactorial etiology, and thus no one treatment modality in and of itself is likely to be effective for every child with this disorder. This view is well represented in this book.

The second unique feature of this volume is the amount of attention devoted to significant others in the child's life, particularly the families and the teachers. There is research to suggest that some parents of hyperactive children had similar problems themselves during childhood and that many of them have significant psychopathology in adult life. Moreover, these parents may have greater difficulty managing any child, but have particular difficulty in managing children with attentional problems, impulsivity, etc., because of the unique reciprocal interaction that occurs between any parent and any child. It has been long overlooked in child psychiatric and psychologic research that children probably affect parents as much as parents affect children and that a transactional process goes on in which each modifies the behavior of the other over time. Dr. Barkley describes this process quite nicely.

The third unique aspect is the detailed description of the various evaluation techniques and their role in the treatment of children with this disorder. Generally, information will come from interviews with the parents, interviews with and observations of the child, behavior rating scales, and laboratory measures including psychological tests. In a clear and coherent fashion which would be helpful to clinicians of any theoretical persuasion, Dr. Barkley discusses the utility of these various diagnostic instruments with hyperactive children.

Finally, there is a very admirable discussion of the various types of therapeutic interventions that may or may not be effective with this problem.

Of particular note is the balanced discussion of drug treatment and a clear exposition of the use of a social learning theory approach with parents and with teachers.

This book should be of immense value to all professionals who deal with hyperactive children on a regular basis. While no one clinician will agree with everything that is in the book, it is safe to say that this is the single best source of information about this problem that is likely to be of practical utility to any practicing clinician. Dr. Barkley is to be congratulated for his effort in putting this manual together.

Dennis P. Cantwell, MD

PREFACE

The present volume was designed and written to achieve several purposes. Chief among these was a need to reorder my thinking and clinical approach to the assessment and treatment of hyperactive children after many years of conducting research and clinical practice with these children and their families. This book is also, however, intended to meet the needs of other professionals in their own clinical work with hyperactivity, on which more research has been conducted than on any other childhood psychological disorder currently known. Much of the vast literature that has appeared on this subject to date is primarily aimed at the audience of research and clinical scientists who pursue basic and applied studies with hyperactive children. Yet few of these textbooks can actually serve as a guide to clinicians in the evaluation and treatment of hyperactive children and their families. My intent was therefore to write a text to meet the needs of child psychologists, child psychiatrists, pediatricians, social workers, and others who must provide clinical services to hyperactive children and their families on a frequent, if not a daily, basis. The writing of this clinical text was also brought about by the urging of my professional colleagues as well as of the parents of many hyperactive children with whom I have worked. In presenting more than 200 lectures, speeches, and workshops to various groups of clinical professionals, I have found that many of them remark about the absence of a textbook designed to educate clinicians in specific matters of evaluation and intervention with hyperactive children. These presentations also brought to my attention the myths and misconceptions that abound in clinical lore and practice. That many of these misconceptions have now been dispelled by current research does not prevent their influence in the arena of clinical practice, where scientific findings may take several years to become evident. These misconceptions continue to guide the manner in which families with hyperactive children have been treated by clinical professionals, and they often create either great anguish and guilt for these families, or great expectations of hope where lesser expectations ought to rule. This served to convince me that clinicians require more accurate information and more specific guidelines on the evaluation and treatment of these families.

Obviously, then, the present text is not intended as an exhaustive review of the scientific literature on the subject of hyperactive children, for several books have recently appeared that have nicely accomplished this task.

Although its purpose is to provide a set of guidelines for clinical practice, these are intended only as suggestions that should be molded by the unique aspects of individual cases and by the wisdom gained by clinicians in their experience with psychologically disturbed children and their families. Because the book was not designed as an exhaustive review of the literature, individual research studies receive little attention throughout the volume. Only those findings which appear to be of direct clinical relevance are reported, often without specific reference to the studies from which they come. Readings that are believed to be helpful to clinical practice are listed at the end of each chapter.

The book contains several unique characteristics that, it is hoped, will make it useful to the reader. First, as noted earlier, it is expressly written for a clinical rather than a research audience. Second, the view of hyperactivity taken here seems to be different in many ways from those views espoused by earlier authors. The disorder known as hyperactivity, and more recently called Attention Deficit Disorder, is viewed in this text as a developmental disorder of attention span and rule-governed behavior, or self-control, which arises early in the lives of children, is to some extent cross-situational in nature, exerts some degree of influence over the adult prognosis of the individual, and is to a great extent neurophysiological rather than environmental in origin. Its physical nature, however, does not preclude the effective application of behavioral methods of assessment and treatment for the improvement of the children's welfare and that of their families. Yet, in spite of the possibilities for changing the symptoms of the children to some degree through behavioral or medical methods, this viewpoint does imply that there are currently no known "cures" for hyperactivity. What is required is an approach emphasizing *coping* in the day-to-day care and education of these children, so as to achieve a "best fit" between the children's characteristics and those of their caretakers.

As with any such endeavor, the contributions of others who have been involved directly or indirectly in this project require some acknowledgment. I am first of all indebted to my wife and my son for unselfishly permitting me time away from family activities and responsibilities in order that this volume could be written. Their patience, tolerance with my fits of frustration over the chores of this task, and encouragement to see it to its final completion are genuinely appreciated. I am also beholden to Seymour Weingarten, Editor-in-Chief at The Guilford Press, for his enthusiastic acceptance of the idea for this volume and his nurturance and encouragement throughout its accomplishment. Sincere gratitude should also be expressed to Deanna Andre, Mary Holbrook, Judy Walker, Jennifer Karlsson, Jean Moberg, and Susan Pollard for their assistance in the preparation of the manuscript, and to Judith Grauman for her help in the production of this book. Finally,

I am forever indebted to the hyperactive children and the parents with whom I have worked for the invaluable education they have given me on the nature, evaluation, and treatment of hyperactivity. Their influence is undoubtedly interwoven throughout the information and guidelines contained within this volume.

Russell A. Barkley, PhD
November 1980

CONTENTS

HYPERACTIVE CHILDREN
A Handbook for Diagnosis and Treatment

CHAPTER ONE

CLINICAL DESCRIPTION

The more extensive a man's knowledge of what has been done, the greater will be his power of knowing what to do.—*Benjamin Disraeli*

Hyperactivity is now believed to be the most common problem referred to child guidance clinics in this country. Scientific papers abound on the subject, with many books and special journal issues being devoted to it yearly. Without a doubt, it has become the most widely studied disorder of childhood during the past decade. A number of newspaper and magazine articles on hyperactive children have also appeared within the past few years; many of these articles are inaccurate in their descriptions of the children or of the treatments most likely to be used with them. Where both scientific and public interest is great, many controversies are bound to develop, as they have with this childhood disorder. Disagreements over diagnosis, characteristics, prognosis, and treatment are commonplace, leading to much confusion over the way in which the practicing clinician should approach the management of the disorder. It is the intent of this book to provide such an approach, based upon the most recent research and theoretical writings as well as upon my own clinical experience. Throughout this volume, the terms "hyperactivity," "hyperkinesis," and "Attention Deficit Disorder" will be used interchangeably, despite the fact that some have viewed the first of these terms as merely describing problems in activity level, while the latter two describe syndromes involving other symptoms in addition to overactivity.

This chapter briefly reviews the more commonly accepted findings about the nature, prognosis, and etiologies of hyperactivity, while the majority of the remaining chapters are devoted to more practical and clinical issues and procedures. Suggested readings are provided at the end of this and subsequent chapters for the reader wishing to pursue the research literature more thoroughly.

DEFINITION

Hyperactive children are commonly described as persistently overactive, inattentive, and impulsive, as well as more likely than normal children to have a variety of academic and social problems. Despite this widely held belief, previous efforts at defining the disorder have proven difficult and short-lived.

Given the increasing emphasis in the literature on the disorder, many might believe it is a relatively modern one that did not occur before the 1940s or '50s. Yet reports about hyperactive children can be found as early as the late 1800s and early 1900s, though the problem was given by entirely different labels. While the symptoms of the disorder have not changed much since then, the disorder itself has probably been renamed more than 20 times during the past 80 years. Such labels as "organic driveness," "postencephalitic behavior disorder," "restlessness," "fidgety phils," "conduct disorder," "brain-damaged child," "brain-injured child," "minimal brain damage," "minimal brain dysfunction," "learning disability," "hyperkinesis," and others have been used. Most recently, the American Psychiatric Association has chosen to rename the problem Attention Deficit Disorder (ADD), with or without hyperactivity. The changing labels reflect changing schools of thought on the causes, major symptoms, and treatments of hyperactivity; this most recent label indicates a general consensus among scientists that the major deficiency in hyperactive children consists in their attentional problems—an issue to be discussed in detail later.

The earliest reported papers by Still, Ebaugh, and others at the beginning of the 1900s described restlessness, impulsivity, poor concentration, and overactivity in groups of retarded or severely neurologically impaired children. These early investigators quite rightly ascribed these behavior problems as secondary to obvious neurologic trauma, diseases, or disorders recently experienced by the children. Later, in the 1940s, such writers as Strauss, Lehtinen, and Leviri argued that since the behavior changes followed brain injuries in children, any children showing such hyperactive behaviors must also be brain-injured. This notion was advanced even though the causes for and evidence supporting the brain injuries were not nearly as apparent as in the earlier writings. Nonetheless, the concept appeared to gain favor, despite the fallacy of such a logical syllogism, and it has held great influence over theories and treatments of hyperactivity up to the present time. Michael Rutter (1977) has recently reiterated what many should have recognized all along—that most children suffering brain injuries do *not* develop hyperactivity and that fewer than 5% of hyperactive children have any hard evidence of structural brain damage. This should lay to rest ideas that damage is a prime etiology of hyperactivity, though, as we will see later, this does not mean that more subtle neurologic problems may not be found to create these difficulties in behavior.

Certainly, serious scientific attention to hyperactivity has developed only within the past 20 years. Using a variety of ingenious measurement devices, research in the 1960s focused primarily on the motor activity levels of hyperactive children. Definitions of the disorder reflected this emphasis in proposing that hyperactivity was simply excessive quantities of motor activity that brought children exhibiting such activity into conflict with their environment. Problems with measurement and with operationally defining such a view of hyperactivity probably partially accounted for its abandonment in favor of other views of hyperactivity. At that time, the work of Virginia Douglas and her colleagues at McGill University in Montreal began demonstrating major deficits in attention span in hyperactive children that could be more easily studied than the concept of activity level. In her classic paper presented as the presidential address to the Canadian Psychological Association in 1972, Douglas set forth her belief that the major deficiency of hyperactive children was in their ability to stop, look, and listen—that is, to sustain attention and inhibit impulsive responding as a situation demands. Other scientists replicated the findings of the Montreal group, for the most part, and poor attention span became recognized by many as a paramount problem for hyperactive children. It should also be noted that both Douglas and John Werry (1968) stressed the early onset of the disorder, its relatively pervasive nature, and its chronicity in terms of lasting well into adolescence.

In the late 1970s, however, research from a variety of sources began to suggest that the hyperactive child's problems were more widespread and that they encompassed problems in obedience to rules, self-control, and social conduct, as well as the aforementioned attentional deficits. Susan Campbell at the University of Pittsburgh (1975) reported several studies on the mother-child interactions of hyperactive children that demonstrated that these children are less compliant, more attention-seeking, and more in need of supervision than normal children. These findings were replicated and extended by myself and Charles Cunningham, now of McMaster University Medical Center (1979), in studies that found hyperactive boys to be more negative and noncompliant and to interact less positively with their mothers. In turn, their mothers were more directive and negative, and less responsive to the children's play and interactions. More recent research has shown that similar reactions occur in the manner in which teachers and peers respond to the hyperactive child. Many investigators now believe that the problems in social behavior are the more enduring and lead to social maladjustment in the teenage and young adulthood years.

At the same time, several books began appearing in the lay literature suggesting that hyperactivity was a myth constructed by intolerant parents and teachers against overly exuberant, normal children. While such a notion may have a certain simplistic appeal, it hardly accounts for the many physical, behavioral, and social differences demonstrated between hyperactive and normal children. Although the problems of some of these children may simply reflect adult intolerance, the vast majority of them present problems in social interactions across a variety of situations with many adults and other children; this leads to the inescapable conclusion that there is, in fact, something "wrong" with these children.

Yet, while many scientists clearly recognize the existence of the disorder and seem to agree on its major presenting symptoms, there is no uniformly acceptable definition of the disorder. It is likely that most would endorse the idea that hyperactivity is a chronic, pervasive deficiency in attention span, impulse control, and overactivity that occurs in children of at least average intelligence. However, in a review of more than 200 studies of hyperactive children, I found that more than 70% failed to use any objective or specifiable criteria for diagnosing the children as hyperactive, other than the mere opinion of the author of the study. If scientists are to convince the lay community of the existence of this disorder and the need for scientific study of it, we will first have to operationalize our definition of the disorder and employ objective guidelines in selecting such children for research.

The American Psychiatric Association has specified the criteria used to diagnose ADD, with or without hyperactivity, in the third edition of the *Diagnostic and Statistical Manual of Mental Disorders* (DSM-III) (1980). The APA hopes that this set of criteria will gain widespread acceptance among clinicians and scientists as the criteria for determining hyperactivity in children. The criteria are set forth in Table 1.1 and are much improved over those stated in the DSM-II for what then was referred to as Hyperkinetic Reaction of Childhood.

There are several disadvantages to this definition, however. First, it attempts to draw a distinction between ADD with and ADD without hyperactivity. There is little research to support the need for or desirability of such a distinction. It is probably just as useful simply to label the child as ADD without specifying hyperactivity as present or absent, as it may be likely that a particular child will change from being ADD with hyperactivity to ADD without it as he or she develops into later childhood. The distinction is also of little value in making treatment decisions. Second, the criteria in Table 1.1 do not address the issue of the pervasiveness of the child's problems. Although it is assumed by many that ADD manifests itself in many situations in the child's daily environment, just how pervasive it should be for a clinician to make a diagnosis is unspecified. If the child only shows these ADD symptoms while in public places or with babysitters, is this sufficient for the diagnosis? I doubt it. Third, how serious or deviant must the child's symptoms be to enable the clinician to distinguish them from normal childhood exuberance? The criteria in Table 1.1 require the child to have at least three descriptors in each of the three symptom categories, but we do not know how many normal children would also show these descriptors as well. Some statistical criteria for deviance on these symptoms would be helpful. Fourth, the age of onset of symptoms is specified as 7 years or less, although

TABLE 1.1. Diagnostic Criteria for Attention Deficit Disorder with Hyperactivity

The child displays, for his or her mental and chronological age, signs of developmentally inappropriate inattention, impulsivity, and hyperactivity. The signs must be reported by adults in the child's environment, such as parents and teachers. Because the symptoms are typically variable, they may not be observed directly by the clinician. When the reports of teachers and parents conflict, primary consideration should be given to the teacher reports because of greater familiarity with age-appropriate norms. Symptoms typically worsen in situations that require self-application, as in the classroom. Signs of the disorder may be absent when the child is in a new or a one-to-one situation.

The number of symptoms specified is for children between the ages of 8 and 10, the peak age for referral. In younger children, more severe forms of the symptoms and a greater number of symptoms are usually present. The opposite is true of older children.

A. *Inattention.* At least three of the following:
   1. Often fails to finish things he or she starts.
   2. Often doesn't seem to listen.
   3. Easily distracted.
   4. Has difficulty concentrating on schoolwork or other tasks requiring sustained attention.
   5. Has difficulty sticking to a play activity.
B. *Impulsivity.* At least three of the following:
   1. Often acts before thinking.
   2. Shifts excessively from one activity to another.
   3. Has difficulty organizing work (this not being due to cognitive impairment).
   4. Needs a lot of supervision.
   5. Frequently calls out in class.
   6. Has difficulty awaiting turn in games or group situations.
C. *Hyperactivity.* At least two of the following:
   1. Runs about or climbs on things excessively.
   2. Has difficulty sitting still or fidgets excessively.
   3. Has difficulty staying seated.
   4. Moves about excessively during sleep.
   5. Is always "on the go" or acts as if "driven by a motor."
D. Onset before the age of 7.
E. Duration of at least 6 months.
F. Not due to Schizophrenia, Affective Disorder, or Severe or Profound Mental Retardation.

Note. From the *Diagnostic and Statistical Manual of Mental Disorders* (3rd ed.). Washington, D.C.: American Psychiatric Association, 1980. Copyright 1980 by the American Psychiatric Association. Reprinted by permission.

it is acknowledged that most ADD children would be identified as problems by age 3. The 7-year cutoff is quite liberal (perhaps too much so) and may result in many learning-disabled (LD) children being too easily labeled as ADD. The LD child may develop conduct problems in school after several years of academic failure and probably as a reaction to it. In my and others' opinions, the LD child is not actually hyperactive. Perhaps a better criterion would be to require that the child be identified by the parents as having ADD symptoms by age 6 or before entry into formal elementary school programs (first grade), so as to eliminate this possible confounding of LD children and their reactive conduct problems with more typical ADD children having true developmental hyperactivity. I have used this 6-year cutoff in my own clinic and research programs, with a negligible number of typically hyperactive children (less than 2% of children scoring as deviant on standard rating scales of hyperactivity not meeting this criterion. Virtually all of these children missing the 6-year cutoff were only children of young parents who were uncertain whether the children were in fact deviant until teachers drew it to their attention. Finally, there is no mention of the ways in which one determines whether the child's symptoms are age-inappropriate, other than reliance on parental or teacher report. At the very least, some standardized scale of adult opinion ought to be employed so that some statistical criteria of the child's deviation from same-age norms can be established.

While the reader may wish to employ the DSM-III criteria, I believe them to be too liberal or vague on enough issues in diagnosis that I have instead adopted the following more rigorous definition for my clinical and research use (see Barkley, 1981, in "Suggested Reading"). Obviously, any child meeting these criteria would also meet those of the ADD category in DSM-III; the opposite is not necessarily the case.

Hyperactivity is a developmental disorder of age-appropriate attention span, impulse control, restlessness, and rule-governed behavior that develops in late infancy or early childhood (before age 6), is pervasive in nature, and is not accounted for on the basis of gross neurologic, sensory, or motor impairment, or severe emotional disturbance.

The following criteria are used for the diagnosis:

1. Parental and/or teacher complaints of inattentiveness, impulsivity, and restlessness.

2. Age of onset of problems by 6 years as reported by parents.

3. Deviation from age norms on a standardized parent or teacher rating scale of hyperactive behavior of at least two standard deviations above the mean (98% or higher). For retarded children, the child's score is compared against chronological age norms consistent with the retarded child's mental age.

4. Problem behaviors occurring in 50% of 16 situations discussed with the parent or 12 situations discussed with the teacher (see the Home and School Situations Questionnaires in Chapter 3).

5. Duration of symptoms of at least 12 months.

6. Exclusion of deafness, blindness, or other gross sensory or motor impairment, or severe emotional disturbance (e.g., childhood psychosis).

By definition, these criteria limit the diagnosis to 2% to 3% of the childhood population. The age-of-onset criterion (#2 above) is waived in my clinical practice for those children with acquired neurologic disease or trauma at any age who develop hyperactive symptoms immediately succeeding the trauma or disease. Such children would not be included in my research on developmental hyperactivity, due to the obviously acquired nature of their disorder as distinguished from the idiopathic nature of the symptoms of most hyperactive children. However, if their symptoms persist beyond 1 year in duration, they should be labeled as having "acquired hyperactivity" or "acquired ADD."

PREVALENCE/INCIDENCE

Unless hyperactivity is clearly defined, its true incidence cannot be accurately determined. Based upon varying definitions, some have estimated its occurrence to be as much as 20% of the school-age population, while others say it is no more than 2%. Rema Lapouse and Mary Monk (1958) had teachers evaluate a large sample of school-age children as to the presence of various behavior problems. Their findings revealed that 57% of the boys and 42% of the girls were rated as overactive. Similarly, Werry and Herbert Quay (1971) also surveyed a large population of school children and found that their teachers rated 30% of the boys and 12% of the girls as overactive. In addition, 46% of the boys and 22% of the girls were judged disruptive, while 43% of the boys and 25% of the girls apparently had short attention spans. Restlessness was noted in 49% of the boys and 27% of the girls. Thus, depending on which symptoms of hyperactivity one chooses, as well as the sex of the children involved, prevalence estimates may vary widely. This further suggests that if one is to avoid diagnosing large numbers of children as deviant, the clinician must rely on more than one symptom and on other criteria in addition to symptom presence (e.g., chronicity, pervasiveness).

How, then, are we to distinguish the truly hyperactive child from the quite common rough-and-tumble, active, and inattentive normal child? Some have approached the matter statistically, using child behavior rating scales completed by parents and teachers. As noted, children who score at least two standard deviations above the mean for normal children on these questionnaires are considered hyperactive. One commonly used scale is the Conners Parent Symptom Questionnaire, to be discussed in detail in Chapter 3. Most investigators consider a mean score of 1.5 or higher on the 10 items assessing hyperactivity to be two standard deviations above the normal mean. A similar questionnaire for teachers can also be used.

Using the teacher's questionnaire, Ronald Trites (1979) conducted a survey of 14,083 children in the Ottawa, Canada, schools. Results indicated that if a 1.5 cutoff score were used, 14.3% of the children would have been considered hyperactive. This is far more children than would be expected to be hyperactive if the 1.5 score were indeed two standard deviations above the mean. For this population of children, then, a higher cutoff score would have been needed to limit the label "hyperactivity" more rigorously. These findings also suggest that if only a rating scale is used and if only a teacher's opinion serves as the source of information, then a large percentage of children will be called hyperactive. Clearly, more rigorous criteria for the diagnosis are required than these.

In a different approach to studying the prevalence of hyperactivity, Nadine Lambert and her colleagues (1978) determined what percentage of a group of children was called hyperactive by physicians, teachers, and parents. If the opinion of only one of these people was taken as the criterion, then at least 5% of the children were called hyperactive. However, if the consensus of all three observers was required for making the diagnosis, then only 1% of the children were so labeled. Hence, the prevalence of hyperactivity varies not only as a function of the definition, measures, and statistical cutoff scores to be used, but also as a function of the number of observers needed for agreement on the diagnosis. This suggests that while observers may agree on what symptoms constitute hyperactivity, they do not necessarily agree on which children should be called hyperactive. At this time, most investigators accept a prevalence estimate for hyperactivity of between 3% and 5% of school-age children.

Several other factors seem to affect the prevalence rates of hyperactivity. Through the work of Robert Sprague and Esther Sleator at the University of Illinois at Champaign–Urbana and of C. Keith Conners and his colleagues, now at Washington National Children's Medical Center, cross-cultural studies of prevalence have been conducted. Hyperactivity is often called by other names in other countries, and the percentage of children that present symptoms of hyperactivity using the Conners rating scale varies somewhat across them. This can be seen in Table 1.2, where the percentage of children who would be called hyperactive using the Conners scale ranges from 9% to 22% of boys and 2% to 9% of girls if the typical 1.5 cutoff score is employed.

It has often been reported that England has considerably fewer hyperactive children than the United States. For instance, Rutter and his colleagues (1977) found that only 1.6% of children with psychiatric disorders in the Isle

TABLE 1.2. Percentage of Children Identified as Hyperactive in Four Countries According to Cutoff Score Selected on the Conners Scale

	Boys	Girls
Utilizing a 1.5[a] cutoff yields the following percentages:		
United States (Sprague, Cohen, & Werry, 1974)	9%	2%
Germany (Sprague, Cohen, & Eichlseder, 1977)	12%	5%
Canada (present study)	21%	8%
New Zealand (Werry & Hawthorne, 1976)	22%	9%
Utilizing a 1.8[a] cutoff yields the following percentages:		
Germany	6%	3%
Canada	11%	4%
Utilizing a 2.1[a] cutoff yields the following percentages:		
New Zealand	5%	4%
Canada	7%	2%

Note. From "Prevalence of Hyperactivity" by R. Trites, E. Dugas, and G. Lynch, *Journal of Pediatric Psychology*, 1979, *4*, 179–188. Copyright 1979 by Plenum Publishing Corp. Reprinted by permission. References within table to other sources are detailed within original source.
[a]Reflects scoring on a 0–3 scale.

of Wight survey in England were called hyperactive. This is now recognized, however, as simply reflecting different definitions of the disorder. In the United States, a child presenting with problems of restlessness, poor concentration, and impulsivity would be called hyperactive, while in England these traits would be called "conduct disorder." That the difference in definition is probably the basis for the sharply divergent prevalence figures between these countries was borne out in the Isle of Wight survey. Of those children diagnosed as having psychiatric problems in this survey, 54.4% were restless, 60.8% were fidgety, and 81.8% had poor concentration.

Another factor influencing prevalence appears to be socioeconomic status (SES). Many investigators have reported that not only the incidence of hyperactivity, but the severity of symptoms increases as one descends the scale of SES. This is illustrated in Figure 1.1, taken from the prevalence study by Trites in Ottawa. This demographic three-dimensional graph indicates that rates of hyperactivity vary widely across different sectors of the city. Higher prevalence rates correspond to poorer economic areas of the city, suggesting in some cases that as many as one out of every four children in these areas could be called hyperactive if only the Conners rating scale were used. Several explanations have been offered to account for this variation. One is the generally accepted notion that lower economic groups have poorer pre-, peri-, and postnatal medical care and nutrition. If hyperactivity is related to deviations in function of certain parts of the central nervous system (CNS), this might account for its greater representation

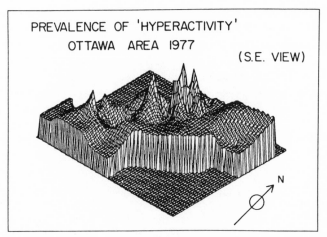

FIGURE 1.1. Prevalence of "hyperactivity" in Ottawa, Canada, 1977; southeast view. (From "Prevalence of Hyperactivity in Ottawa, Canada" by R. Trites. In R. Trites (Ed.), *Hyperactivity in Children.* Baltimore: University Park Press, 1979. Copyright 1979 by University Park Press. Reprinted by permission.)

among income groups at greater risk of difficulties in CNS functioning. Second, lower-income groups are also more likely to be experiencing family instability and parental psychiatric problems, both of which might create or exacerbate hyperactivity in the children born to such families. A third possible explanation is that lower-SES groups tend to be less educated and perhaps less well-informed regarding normal child development and effective child behavior management methods. Related to this may be the fact that lower-SES groups have fewer resources available to them for coping with child behavior problems and are less likely to utilize those that may be available. Finally, the notion of social drift may apply to this situation. That is, it does not matter to which SES group one originally belongs, since those who have trouble adapting to society will drift into a lower-SES group. The more maladaptive the disorder, the greater the downward drift. If there is also a hereditary predisposition to the disorder, then more children with the disorder will be procreated in the lower classes to which the original individual descended. All of these explanations probably account to some degree for the greater prevalence of hyperactivity in the lower-SES groups.

A further variable known to covary with prevalence estimates of hyperactivity is the sex of children. As noted by many investigators, hyperactivity occurs more often among boys than girls. While the sex ratio has been reported to range anywhere from 3:1 to 9:1, a generally accepted figure is 6:1 in favor of males. Again, several hypotheses have been advanced to account for this observation. It should be noted, however, that males are more likely than females to experience a variety of psychiatric and psychological problems, and the greater male preponderance of hyperactivity among males may simply be one further example of this. One hypothesis is that hyperactivity is a sex-linked inherited disorder occurring predominantly in the male side of the child's family. Although current research supports the notion of a greater prevalence of conduct disorders and other psychiatric problems in male relatives of the hyperactive child, increased psychiatric problems also occur in female relatives. A greater occurrence of hysteria, hypochondriasis, and depression has been reported in female relatives of the child, compared to relatives of normal children or adoptive parents of adopted hyperactive children. Other researchers have suggested that cultural factors may predispose more males than females toward hyperactivity. This view is based on the fact that males are generally permitted to be more active, restless, and rough-and-tumble in this culture than are females, in whom such behavior is deemed inappropriate. On closer inspection, however, such a view would suggest that males would be less likely to be labeled hyperactive, since, given equal rates of hyperactive behavior in a male and a female, the female's behavior would be less tolerated and more likely to result in a psychiatric referral. A different explanation suggests that since males are more likely to experience pre-, peri-, and postnatal complications, they are more likely to present with psychiatric disorders stemming from such insults, such as learning disabilities, mental retardation, psychosis, and hyperactivity. While such an explanation of the "biological instability of maleness" is at first glance appealing, the causal link between pregnancy and obstetrical complications and these disorders remains to be established. The greater association of such complications with certain psychiatric and developmental problems suggests only a relationship, not a causal direction.

A related issue is the question of whether the incidence of hyperactivity is increasing. Some writers suggest that it is, probably as a result of increasing environmental pollutants, family dissolution, permissive child-rearing practices, and poor nutritional habits. Others intimate that more sophisticated medical technology and treatments, as well as more rigorous life-saving attempts applied to neonates with life-threatening conditions, may be increasing the occurrence of psychiatric and developmental disorders related to the residual deficits of those surviving such conditions. This concept of reproductive risk and casualty was initially set forth by Pasamanick and Knobloch in the 1940s. Finally, the actual occurrence of hyperactivity may not be increasing, while its detection may well be. This may partly stem from earlier and more rigorous preschool screening programs and from greater dissemination of information about the disorder to parents and professionals dealing with children, as well as from greater awareness by adults of developmental and psychiatric conditions in general.

PRIMARY PROBLEMS

Investigators and clinicians generally tend to agree on the primary problems of the hyperactive child. Primary symptoms are those felt to be necessary in order for a clinician to make the diagnosis. One of the central symptoms of hyperactivity already mentioned is inattentiveness. Difficulties in attention can occur in many forms. Children can have trouble orienting to stimuli or fail to detect altogether those stimuli to which they are expected to respond. Or the children may orient and respond to the wrong aspects of a stimulus or to an entirely inappropriate stimulus. Many hyperactive children are felt to have their most significant problems in *sustaining* attention to task-relevant stimuli while inhibiting their responding to stimuli not relevant to the task (i.e., controlling impulses). It is these two aspects of attention that have undergone the most research and have been found to be the most deficient in hyperactive children.

In the home, these difficulties with sustained attention often appear in a child's failure to complete assigned chores, to listen to directions when given, to complete homework assignments, to play for prolonged periods of time without supervision or attention from others, or to watch television for prolonged periods (especially if the show is not particularly appealing to children). At school, problems with attending to the teacher during class lectures and completing assignments during individual work time are also reflections of the child's attentional difficulties. Often, the child is distracted by more interesting items in the class or outside the window, or by what other children may be doing. Many times it appears as if the child's eyes are focused on almost everything except what he or she has been asked to do.

Although clinicians believe that hyperactive children are more active, restless, and energetic than normal children, this has not been demonstrated as reliably as the attentional problems noted above. Using a variety of unique measuring devices and techniques, scientists have attempted to assess wrist and ankle activity, locomotion, total body motion, seat restlessness, task-relevant versus task-irrelevant activity, and many other aspects of activity level. In general, the findings suggest that hyperactive children are not necessarily more active than other children in all situations. It seems that the more restrictive the environment and the more concentration required by the assigned tasks, the more likely it is that differences in activity level will be found, generally in seat restlessness and task-irrelevant types of activity. More recent research has also shown that hyperactive children are likely to display rates of activity closer to normal while in highly novel or unfamiliar situations. As they become accustomed to the setting, however, levels of activity become more excessive—a pattern not seen in normal children under similar circumstances.

Typically, the child's overactivity is more likely to show up in the class-room than at play or at home, as academic classes demand considerably more sustained attention and inhibited activity than these other situations. In the classroom, hyperactive children are often observed to move about in their chairs more, leave their seats more often, wander about the class, manipulate objects that are not part of the assigned task, kick their feet back and forth while seated, and generally behave more restlessly than normal children. At home, similar behaviors may be seen while the child is seated at the table during meals, watching television, lying in bed, seated in public places (e.g., churches, restaurants), or riding in the car. For school-age hyperactive children, homework periods at home may also bring out more restlessness than is usual with normal children.

Impulsivity, or a failure to inhibit responding, has also been reported as a primary problem with hyperactive children. This has typically been shown in studies requiring children to observe a picture and then to choose from among a group of highly similar ones the picture that is identical to the first. Hyperactive children respond more quickly under such circumstances and make more errors in responding. It is believed that this reflects an inability to inhibit responding before studying the test materials thoroughly enough to detect the correct answer. This type of impulsivity shows up in many ways in the natural environment as well. Hyperactive children often do not stop to think about the consequences of their behavior before acting, and they generally make more mistakes in classroom settings, place themselves in generally more dangerous and risky situations, and fail more often to appreciate all aspects of instructions they may be given than normal children do. They are also more likely to respond aggressively (both verbally and physically) when frustrated or emotionally hurt by others, without considering the impact of their statements or actions. Such responding on impulse often leads to their being perceived as both socially and emotionally immature and to their being shunned by other children. Further, they are likely to experience more sanctions, censure, and punishment from others than are normal children.

Although inattention, overactivity, and poor impulse control are the most common symptoms cited by others as primary in hyperactive children, my own work with these children suggests that noncompliance is also a primary problem. The studies supportive of this notion are discussed in detail in the next chapter. Suffice it to say here that my research with Cunningham (see Table 1.3) has revealed that the most commonly used parent rating scales of hyperactivity correlate very highly with noncompliance, while showing no significant relationship with measures of activity level or attention span. Parents therefore seem to be responding to the child's noncompliance in their completion of these scales, and we believe it is this noncompliance that prompts their referral for professional assistance. As will be shown later, many seemingly diverse and unrelated behavior problems in children can be construed as noncompliance, either to direct commands of adults, to rules known through actual experience to govern behav-

TABLE 1.3. Correlations between Rating Scales and Actometer Scores and Objective Measures of the Mother–Child Interactions of Hyperactive Boys

Interaction measures	Conners hyperactivity score	Werry–Weiss–Peters–score	Wrist activity	Ankle activity
Free play				
Mother interacts	−.22	−.44**	−.04	−.04
Mother directs	.44**	.35*	.43**	.44**
Duration of compliance	−.38**	−.70***	−.29	−.38
Child interacts	−.15	−.54**	−.31	−.31
Child compliance percent	−.42**	−.57**	.22	.29
Child's competing behavior	.19	.46**	.53**	.60***
Child plays independently	.08	.24	.11	.02
Mother controls play	.48**	.20	.23	.30
Task setting				
Mother interacts	−.15	−.65***	−.03	−.12
Mother directs	.35*	.49**	.12	.19
Duration of compliance	−.31	−.16	−.27	−.23
Child interacts	−.51**	−.61**	−.02	−.08
Child's compliance percent	−.08	−.13	−.29	−.44**
Child's competing behavior	.32	.64***	.19	.38**
Child plays independently	.09	−.40**	.25	.19
Mother controls play	.18	−.02	.21	.16
Activity scores				
Wrist activity	.13	.24		.93***
Ankle activity	.04	.29		

Note. From "The Parent–Child Interactions of Hyperactive Children and Their Modification by Stimulant Drugs" by R. Barkley and C. Cunningham. In R. Knights and D. Bakker (Eds.), *Treatment of Hyperactive and Learning Disordered Children.* Baltimore: University Park Press, 1980. Copyright 1980 by University Park Press. Reprinted by permission.
*$p < .10$.
**$p < .05$.
***$p < .01$.

ior in a situation, or to given rules of conduct and etiquette while interacting with others.

One issue that has been hotly debated in the scientific literature is that of the degree of relationship among the foregoing symptoms. In other words, is there a true syndrome of hyperactivity in which the major symptoms covary, respond uniformly to treatment, and have a single etiology? The issue of etiology will be discussed later in this chapter, but the answer to this question seems to be "no" to all aspects of a syndrome. Numerous studies have attempted to correlate a variety of measures of activity level, attention span, and impulsivity. Their results suggest that these three constructs are not strongly related to each other and therefore do not necessarily covary uniformly in hyperactivity. The conclusion has been that hyperactivity comprises a quite heterogeneous group of children, with some being inattentive, others being overactive, and still others having both symptoms.

Efforts have subsequently been made to subdivide hyperactivity into subgroups hoped to be more homogeneous. One dimension for doing so is the response of the child to stimulant drugs. Research on these drugs reveals that approximately 75% of hyperactive children respond positively to them, while 25% do not. However, despite many studies attempting to find reliable differences in various characteristics between these two groups of children, only the degree of attention span seems to differentiate these groups. That is, responders seem to have poorer attention than nonresponders. This is hardly surprising, since the primary effect of these drugs appears to be on attention span; the "law of initial values"—the further from the mean a person's score on a given measure is, the greater the change on that measure in response to treatment—is thereby reaffirmed. As previously noted, another approach to subclassifying hyperactive children has been taken recently in DSM-III, with the label of ADD, with or without hyperactivity (overactivity). While this distinction has some intuitive appeal, it awaits scientific validation. Various other approaches to subcategorization abound, but they fall prey to a similar problem—a lack of empirical validation for their classification schemes. At this time, it is appropriate to assume that a syndrome of hyperactivity does not exist and that no reliable means of subclassifying the group has been found.

Another problem with the concept of a syndrome is that the symptoms noted for hyperactivity are also found in other groups of psychiatrically disturbed and developmentally disabled children. Mentally retarded children frequently display problems with activity level and attention span, although for many these problems are consistent with their mental age. Psychotic children also may display periods of highly active or manic behavior, while frequently also having problems with inattention. Finally, as many as 60% of children with language delay manifest behavior problems, especially noncompliance. If hyperactivity is to have any meaning as a diagnostic concept, it must be capable of discrimination from these other conditions.

The primary symptoms of hyperactivity appear to vary as a result of several factors. Recent research by Jan Loney at the University of Iowa (1978), as well as by other scientists, has shown—as indicated earlier—that both the prevalence of hyperactivity and the severity of its symptoms increase as SES decreases. Similarly, SES is also a significant predictor of prognosis or outcome. Current research suggests that hyperactive children of lower SES are more likely to experience problems across a wide array of social, academic, emotional, and occupational areas than children of higher SES who are also hyperactive. An identical situation has been observed in the effects of pregnancy and obstetrical complications on a child's later development. Children experiencing highly similar biologically compromising events during pregnancy or delivery were observed to differ substantially in their outcome, depending on their social class. As expected, those of lower SES showed more developmental problems as a result of the early complication than those of higher SES, whose developmental patterns were closer to normal. There is no reason to think that a similar continuum of caretaker casualty or stress is not also operating with respect to children at risk for developing hyperactivity.

One important yet relatively unaddressed issue regarding symptomatology is that of whether hyperactive girls are different in these respects from hyperactive boys. Clinical lore and experience suggest that there are some sex differences in presenting complaints, although research has yet to address their validity. Girls who are hyperactive seem more likely to present with problems in mood, affect, and emotional lability, in addition to their overactivity and inattention. They may also have fewer difficulties with physical aggression, although this may be more apparent than real, considering that fewer girls are referred for hyperactivity. The only study to date to compare hyperactive boys and girls suggests that learning and language disabilities are more prominent in the girls, though the study suffers from many methodological shortcomings. Certainly, the prognosis for these groups may differ, at least in terms of those adult disorders for which they are at risk. In any case, serious scientific attention is needed in this area.

As noted earlier, the primary problems with hyperactivity may differ in their expression, severity, and frequency across differing situations. Many clinicians mistakenly assume that unless the symptoms are present across *all* situations, hyperactivity is not a viable diagnosis. This, in fact, could not be further from the truth. My own research and that of others clearly indicates that hyperactive behaviors are common in some settings while not in others. This can be seen in Table 1.4, where parental ratings of occurrence and severity of symptoms across various situations are displayed for hyperactive and normal boys. These findings suggest that hyperactive boys are much more likely to display problems when they play with other children, when their parents are on the phone, when visitors are at the home or when they

TABLE 1.4. Percentage and Parent-Rated Severity of Problematic Situations for 60 Hyperactive Boys

Situation	Percentage having problems	Mean severity rating[a]
Play alone	57	2.4
Play with other children	88	4.9
During mealtimes	90	4.8
While dressing	72	4.2
While washing/bathing	53	2.8
When parent is on phone	93	6.1
Watching television	82	4.1
When visitors are in home	98	6.0
While visiting others	95	5.2
In public places	93	5.3
When father is home	73	3.4
Chore performance	88	5.0
At bedtime	83	4.5
While in the car	82	4.1

[a]Mothers were asked to note whether or not the child had behavior problems in each setting, and if so, to rate the problem on a scale from 1 (mild) to 9 (severe).

are visiting others, and when they are in public places (e.g., stores, restaurants). While these are the most problematic situations, a variety of other situations are more of a difficulty for hyperactive than for normal children. Nonetheless, hyperactive boys are much less likely to show problems when they are playing alone, when they are washing or bathing, when they are dressing, and when their fathers are at home. Similarly, I have noticed that hyperactive children are less likely to create problems in novel situations, especially if adult males are involved. Recently, Esther Sleator and Rina Ullman (1981) found that hyperactive children were much less likely to misbehave in the pediatrician's office.

These situational fluctuations in behavior problems are likely to lead to several difficulties for families seeking help for their hyperactive children. First, many clinicians use children's behavior in the office as a major source of information as to whether such children are hyperactive. Since clinic offices are highly novel situations for the children, and since the clinician involved is more likely to be a male, the children are much less likely to be problems. The clinician will fail to make the diagnosis and will often accuse mothers of being overly sensitive to their children and perhaps poor managers of the children's behavior at home. After all, if the children can behave for the doctor, they ought to be able to do so at home if their mothers handle them properly. Such an attitude frequently leads families to seek evaluations from multiple professionals; each evaluation generally has a similar result. Eventually, the families are accused of "shopping" for services and never being satisfied, whereas the real problem rests with the clinicians themselves. Second, because the children are more likely to behave when their fathers are at home, the fathers may feel (as the professionals do) that no problem exists for the children, or that it is less than their wives report it to be. Such differences in perceptions between parents often lead to conflicts in these families over child-rearing methods and the need for outside assistance with the children. Wives often find their husbands blaming them, as the professionals have done, for poor child disciplinary measures and oversensitivity to the children's behavior; neither accusation is necessarily true, as we will see in the next chapter.

Research by several investigators has shown that the primary symptoms of hyperactivity decrease with age, though it will be shown later that the problems hardly disappear by adolescence, as is still commonly believed. Similarly, the attention span, activity level, and impulse control of normal children have been shown to improve with age. An important point is that while the developmental curves for these two groups parallel each other for all measures, hyperactive children are still having more difficulties in these behaviors than normal children, even during their late teenage years. Thus there is no evidence as yet for the "normalization" of hyperactive symptoms, even by the teenage years.

Related to these developmental trends is the issue of the precise age at which hyperactive symptoms are likely to appear. Many investigators have failed to address this question in selecting hyperactive children for research, yet, clearly, a hyperactive 9-year-old whose symptoms first developed several months ago is probably quite different from one whose symptoms have existed from 2 years of age onward. Quite likely, the age of onset of symptoms is partly a function of the particular etiology involved with a given child. Nevertheless, some research suggests that as many as 60% to 70% of hyperactive children are identifiable as problems by 2 years of age or earlier. Some hyperactive children certainly show problems in temperament during their infancy. "Temperament" is here used to refer to regularity of habits (eating, sleeping, etc.), response to stimulation, emotionality, activity level, and sociability. But other hyperactive children may not show any problems, at least in their parents' opinion, until they begin grade school. Douglas and her colleagues have argued strongly that hyperactive behaviors that do not develop until a child is several years into grade school are quite probably different from those arising in the preschool years. The former are often seen as a response to classroom failure or other environmental stress events, while the latter may prove to be disturbances of temperament of a more biological origin. My own clinical research suggests that the vast majority of hyperactive children manifest their problems prior to 5 years of age, with the exception of those few children who develop hyperactivity secondary to head trauma or other neurologic insults.

Despite an onset of symptoms in early childhood, many hyperactive children may not come to the attention of professionals until later in their lives. In some cases, the family has recognized the child as problematic from an early age but has felt little compulsion to seek treatment until after entry into grade school, when the school staff begins to pressure the family to seek outside assistance. In other cases, families do seek help from their family physicians quite early, only to be rebuffed with statements that all young children are like that or that the child is merely passing through a phase. In a few cases, parental naivete as to normal child behavior creates a situation where the child is in fact a problem but is not recognized as such until he or she begins school. The facts that many parents of hyperactive children are below the average child-bearing years in age, and that hyperactive children are more often firstborn, suggest that this explanation may well be tenable for certain children. Regardless of the circumstances, it seems fair to assume that hyperactivity in most children develops in late infancy or early childhood.

RELATED PROBLEMS

Numerous problems seem to coexist with hyperactivity, though they do not necessarily occur in all hyperactive children. Some have viewed these problems as secondary to or caused by the primary symptoms noted above, while others view them simply as related problems of lesser frequency than those considered primary. Both explanations probably apply to some degree, depending on which of the following problem areas one is discussing.

Behavioral

Two related behavioral problems occurring with greater frequency in hyperactive than normal children are distractibility and aggression. While often confused with short attention span, "distractibility" does not refer to a child's length of persistence at responding to a given task, but to his or her likelihood of being drawn off task by extraneous stimuli. That is, "poor attention span" refers to a child's inability to persist with a task, especially beyond the point where it becomes boring, regardless of the presence or absence of distractions. "Distractibility," however, concerns the child's inability to inhibit orienting to task-irrelevant stimuli. Hyperactive children clearly have short attention spans, but whether they are actually more distractible remains controversial. One recent study has shown that the appeal value of the distractor may play a role in determining how distractible the child is. In contrast, a second study using more naturalistic high-appeal distractors found hyperactive *and* normal children alike to be more distractible than they were in low-distracting conditions. At this time, it is difficult to state that distractibility is in fact related to hyperactivity.

This is not the case with aggression, whether physical or verbal. Aggressiveness is observed frequently in many, though not all, hyperactive children, and it becomes more prevalent in hyperactive children of lower SES. Loney has shown that while aggression and hyperactivity are often seen together, they do not correlate to any significant degree. That is, it is not necessarily true that the more hyperactive a child is, the more aggressive that child will be, or vice versa. Similarly, early childhood hyperactivity does not predict later aggression, nor does early aggression predict later hyperactivity. In spite of this apparent dissociation, aggresion, not severity of hyperactivity, seems to be a better predictor of adolescent social adjustment. The severity of hyperactivity in childhood seems to best predict later academic difficulties in adolescence.

Another often-cited problem of hyperactive children is their general frequency and level of vocal noisiness. These are not necessarily verbal excesses, though hyperactive children are frequently noted to be quite talkative. Many, however, often engage simply in excessive vocal noises, thereby proving quite disruptive of others' ongoing activities both in class and at home. In a recent study of ours (see Barkley, Cunningham, & Karlsson, 1981, in "Suggested Reading"), it was demonstrated that not only do hyperactive children verbalize more than normal, but *mothers* of hyperactive children also verbalize more while with these children than mothers of normal boys. Although the direction of effect here is not completely clear, the results of a related drug study suggest that the mothers' excessive verbalizations were probably a reaction to those of their children.

Another frequently noted characteristic of hyperactive children is their high rate of risk-taking behavior. While undoubtedly related to their poor impulse control, this problem often leads them to experience more accidents, poisonings, bumps, scrapes, bruises, and broken bones than other children. The child seems unable to appreciate the short- or long-term consequences of such behavior, other than the possible "thrills" or satiation of curiosity that the activity might provide. Such behavior proves quite frustrating to parents, who must supervise the child almost constantly to prevent accidents from occurring. For this reason, idle time, especially during the summer months, is to be avoided for these children, as it seems only to increase the likelihood that problems will occur.

Some research efforts have also been made to determine if hyperactive children respond differently to behavioral consequences than normal children. The results are quite tentative, due to the small number of studies involved. Up to this time, they suggest that hyperactive children respond better to negative feedback during task accomplishment and may also respond better to mild punishment. This may be more characteristic of younger hyperactive children, according to one recent report. In addition, once reinforcement for target behaviors is discontinued during treatment, there appears to be a more rapid recovery of negative behaviors to baseline levels of responding. Finally, hyperactive children have shown a greater deterioration in on-task and appropriate behavior where schedules of reinforcement are changed from continuous to partial or intermittent. Paul Wender at the University of Utah Medical School has speculated that hyperactive children may have a diminished experience of pleasure and pain, which may account for their lesser responsivity to behavioral consequences. Wender (1971) has suggested that, in order for behavior therapy programs to be successful, they must utilize stronger than normal consequences over more learning trials and with greater consistency. At present, data are lacking on these conjectures. However, the results suggested by research so far obviously have some bearing on the ways in which treatment programs are designed—a point to be discussed more thoroughly in Chapter 7.

Cognitive

In addition to problems with attention span and impulsivity, hyperactive children are more likely to manifest a variety of other cognitive deficits. Not all hyperactive children will have all of these problems, and, among those who do, not all will show them to the same degree. One area that has received little scrutiny is the question of whether hyperactive children, on the average, are more or less intelligent than normal children. An early report suggested that hyperactive children were significantly less intelligent than other children from the same neighborhood. Since hyperactive children are typically more difficult to assess, differences indicated in the testing may be more the result of problems in the testing situation than a reflection of actual intellectual differences. More recently, some research has found that hyperactive children are not necessarily less intelligent than normal children, but that they show select deficits in those aspects of intellectual performance related to attention span, short-term memory, and freedom from distractibility. This area clearly remains in need of future research.

Another area of interest has been the question of whether hyperactive children show problems in the processing of information in any sense modalities. One recent paper has suggested that these children have more trouble processing auditory information than visual information. Many parents often believe that their hyperactive children have auditory memory problems because of the need to repeat instructions to them more than to normal children. In either case, inattention may well be the cause of these problems, rather than actual deficits in auditory processing or memory. The paucity of research to date prevents any conclusions from being made.

Some investigators have also speculated that hyperactive children are more likely than normal children to have problems in language development. One report found that as many as 54% of hyperactive children had poor speech development. Again, the studies examining the issue are quite scarce. In a paper previously mentioned, we compared the language of 14 hyperactive and 14 normal children during interactions with their mothers. The results are obviously tentative, considering the small sample sizes. They suggested, however, that while both hyperactive boys and their mothers talk more than normal mother–child dyads, there are no significant differences in any of several measures of language complexity. Thus, deficits in language skills remain a matter of clinical conjecture at this time.

One area of possible cognitive deficits that has received little or no attention from scientists but is frequently commented upon by parents is the hyperactive child's lack of conscience or perspective about his or her own behavior. That is, many hyperactive children are said to have little appreciation for the social, ethical, moral, or even legal consequences of their behavior. Basic notions of right and wrong do not seem to govern their actions, nor do they seem to show as much respect for the feelings, rights, or property of others as they should for their age. Whether this stems from an inability to consider the consequences of one's behavior toward another person from that person's point of view, or whether it reflects a deficiency in the chain of complex cognitive processes underlying the notion of a "conscience," is simply not known. Are these children merely so impulsive as not to take the time to reflect upon their behavior, and would it improve their display of a "conscience" if the basic defect in impulse control were improved? Or does the problem with "conscience" reflect a deficit at more complex, higher levels of cognition? Certainly, these are matters for scientists to address in future research.

Related, perhaps, to this lack of perspective regarding the consequences of one's behavior toward others may be the often-deplored lack of a current or future perspective in hyperactive children in general. Specifically, hyperactive children appear to show little awareness of their own behavior and its immediate consequences and implications, or even of the ways in which such behavior gets them into trouble. They often appear to accuse the world of being at fault when they are disciplined and to show little comprehension of the ways in which their behavior repeatedly leads to trouble. Perhaps they also show little awareness of their own talents and deficits—a major deficiency in basic self-awareness. We should not be surprised, then, to find that they have little concern for the future consequences of their behavior or for their future in general. All-consumed with the immediate situation and their desires, they at times seem as if they are at the mercy of some force beyond their control, as many parents seem to suggest. At this time, these problems in the child's perspective taking, whether with current or future situations or with other people, await future investigation as to their presence, frequency and intensity of occurrence in this group of children.

Academic

Obviously associated with the possible cognitive deficits of hyperactive children are the deficits believed to exist in the areas of academic behavior and learning. As noted earlier, hyperactive children frequently manifest disruptive and noncompliant behavior in the classroom. High rates of off-task and out-of-seat behavior are reported in studies of classroom performance with these children. It is no wonder, then, that few classwork or homework assignments are completed by these children. While these classroom behavior problems are quite likely related to the primary symptoms of hyperactivity noted above, such a relationship does not readily account for the sizeable percentage of hyperactive children with specific learning disabilities in one or more areas of scholastic ability. A learning disability is viewed as a significant deficit compared to expected grade level in one or more areas of academic achievement, despite normal intelligence and educational opportunity. Some authorities estimate that as many as 60% to 80% of hyperactive children are likely to have such learning problems. However, no single learning disability seems to be more prevalent than others in this group. Recent research by Dennis Cantwell and Jerome Satterfield at the University of California at Los Angeles (1978) has shown that as many as 76% of the hyperactive children examined were underachieving in at least two academic subjects. While these deficits in academic functioning would at first appear to be related to possible lower levels of intellectual functioning in hyperactive children, several studies have partialled out the influence of such children's IQ on their academic measures and yet still find these children to be underachieving in all major academic subjects. The risk of school failure has been estimated to be two to three times higher in hyperactive than normal children, with many being retained at least one grade before entry into the middle or junior high school years.

Deficits in handwriting skills have also been reported to be more common in these children. Whether this is related to their generally greater motor incoordination, possible visual–motor problems, deficits in higher cortical–cognitive planning, or simple impulsivity is not known.

Social

Some of the behavioral deficiencies (and excesses) of hyperactive children have already been mentioned, while others, particularly those involving interactions with family members, will be discussed in some detail in the next chapter. In general, hyperactive children are frequently noted to be socially immature. Parents often report that the few friends these children have are likely to be younger than they are. In addition, their selection of toy preferences may also be immature for their age. Aggression, described earlier, is commonly observed in their interactions with peers, as are selfishness, lying and dishonesty.

Direct behavioral observations of the interactions of hyperactive children with their peers and teachers have only recently been conducted. The most extensive work on peer interactions has been conducted by Carol Whalen at the University of California at Irvine (see Whalen & Henker, 1980, in "Suggested Reading"). These studies have typically observed hyperactive children in classroom or task-oriented settings and seem to suggest that they are more vocal, noisy, off-task, and disruptive than other children. Hyperactive boys tend to initiate more social interactions with other children and to engage in more inappropriate behavior than normal boys. Since no studies have yet used a behavior coding system that captures reciprocal influence in interactions, there is no way of knowing precisely how other children react to these high-rate, intense, and inappropriate behaviors.

Research on the interactions of hyperactive children with their teachers have generally paralleled the findings from research on mother–child interactions to be reviewed later. In one recent study, hyperactive children were observed during a teaching lecture situation with their regular teachers to be more interactive, more questioning, less attentive, and more negative and inappropriate in their general behavior than normal classroom children. In turn, their teachers were more interactive, commanding, and negative toward hyperactive than toward normal children. Surprisingly, however, the teachers proved to be more responsive to the hyperactive children's interactions and questions than to those of normal children. This may reflect the fact that hyperactive children are more intrusive in their interactions, making them less likely to be ignored than normal children. During an independent study period, the hyperactive children were again more interactive, less compliant, and more off-task and negative than normal children. Again, their teachers were also more interactive and directive toward the hyperactive than normal children. When the teachers were not attending to or responding to the children, the hyperactive children were more likely to engage in off-task and negative behavior. Similar results were reported by Whalen and her associates. Taken together, the results indicate that hyperactive boys are clearly more noncompliant, more negative, and more interactive generally than normal boys when interacting with their teachers. Their teachers are clearly more negative, more directive, and more generally controlling in interactions with hyperactive than with normal children. At first glance, it seems difficult to determine the direction of effects here. Do more directive, commanding teaching styles make hyperactive children less compliant and more negative?

Or is the teacher's behavior simply a response to the child's hyperactive interaction pattern? The results of stimulant drug studies on these interactions suggest that, like the behavior of mothers of hyperactive children, their teachers' behavior is a reaction to such children's problems, since it becomes indistinguishable from teacher interactions with normal children when hyperactive children are receiving stimulant therapy.

To summarize, hyperactive children display a wide array of difficulties in social behavior toward others, appearing to be more disruptive, intense, negative, and noncompliant than normal children. In addition, their lack of concern for others and deficient awareness of the short- and long-term consequences of their own behavior cause great consternation in those who must live with, care for, teach, or simply interact with these children. These adults often have to respond to these children with greater supervision, control, and discipline than is necessary for same-age normal children. The effects of these interaction patterns on both the child and others over time remain to be sufficiently examined. Speculations as to what may happen in the long run are offered in Chapter 2.

Emotional

The emotional characteristics and development of hyperactive children have not been well studied. Parents often complain that their hyperactive children are immature in the control of their emotions; they are more likely to become angered and frustrated over events and are perhaps more labile and capricious in their moods. Follow-up studies, to be reviewed later, indicate these children to be at greater risk for depression and (especially for hyperactive girls) hysteria or a tendency to become easily emotionally upset or excitable.

In a recent study, I had the mothers of 60 hyperactive boys complete the Achenbach Child Behavior Checklist with respect to their sons' home behavior. Significantly abnormal scores were obtained on the scales of hyperactivity, aggression, delinquency, and, surprisingly, obsessive–compulsive symptoms. The latter finding is misleading, since many items on this factor of the scale pertain to daydreaming, sleeping problems, excessive talking, and so on—items likely to be endorsed by parents of hyperactive children who are not actually obsessive–compulsive. This profile is set forth in Figure 1.2.

One commonly noted, though little studied, emotional problem of these children is their low self-esteem. This typically does not emerge as a problem until later childhood and is probably a reaction to the years of chronic failure in familial, social, and academic areas. Often the children complain vaguely of having few friends and of getting punished so often. Veiled threats of suicide may occur, though there is no evidence that the actual occurrence of suicide attempts is higher than in normal children. In spite of these

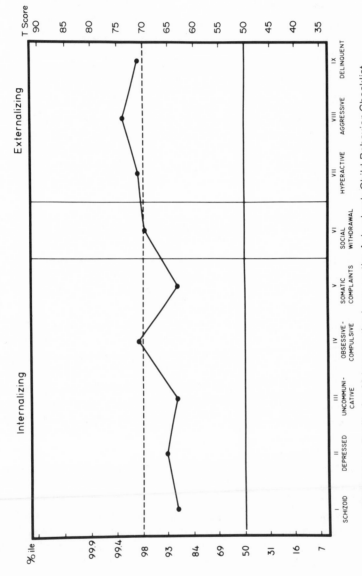

FIGURE1.2. Profile for 60 hyperactive boys on the Achenbach Child Behavior Checklist.

depressed feelings, the children rarely capitalize on them as a source of motivation to change themselves. Instead, they continue to see other people as their problem, as well as the rules these other people expect them to follow. Clearly, hyperactive children have a wide array of emotional problems, although which are primary disorders and which are secondary or reactive may be hard to distinguish.

Another aspect of the hyperactive child's emotional behavior upon which many parents comment is its variability and unpredictability from one moment to the next. At times, the child may seem content, calm, and generally well-behaved, yet may switch to temper outbursts, destructiveness, negative behavior, and in some cases rage attacks on others with minimal provocation or frustration. This is often hard for parents and many professionals to comprehend, and they may tend to believe that such children's behavior problems are purely "emotional" or volitional in nature. That is, they come to believe that if such children can be calm and unexcitable some of the time, they must be able to do it all the time if they so desire; some even come to think that these children may not be hyperactive at all. Yet this variability of mood and behavior is so common among hyperactive children as to be a virtual hallmark of the disorder itself. As will be shown later, such variability in responding is also seen on various measures of psychophysiologic functions.

Physical

A substantial amount of research has been done on the physical correlates of hyperactivity, probably because of the widespread belief that it results from physiological or neurological problems. Much of this research has proven equivocal, partly because the criteria for selecting hyperactive children vary across the studies. Those findings listed below should therefore be viewed as tentative and in need of more definitive investigation.

Much of the research findings suggest physical immaturity in some, though not all, hyperactive children. Clinicians have long noted that many of these children are smaller and thinner than other children their age. Recent research seems to bear this out in suggesting that 7- to 8-year-old hyperactive children have bone ages from 5 to 12 months younger than their chronological ages. Similarly, studies of psychophysiological functions find some hyperactive children to show more "slow-wave activity" or signs of cortical underarousal than normal children do. These results are interpreted as suggestions of cortical immaturity. In addition, several reports have found hyperactive children to have more neurologic "soft signs" than normal; these again are interpreted by some as indications of neurologic immaturity. These signs usually consist of motor incoordination, mildly abnormal reflexes, and marginally abnormal sensory findings. It should be remembered, however, that just as many studies have not found such differences from normal. Again, as has been shown before and will continue to be mentioned throughout this text, hyperactivity is a heterogeneous diagnostic entity for which one is unlikely to find a common set of symptoms or etiology. Some hyperactive children are undoubtedly physically immature, but these studies do not permit any sweeping generalizations to be made for the group as a whole.

Findings from other studies intimate that some hyperactive children have physical problems not easily explained on the basis of simple immaturity or a developmental lag. First, psychophysiologic studies suggest that a fair percentage of these children are underreactive to stimulation (see Hastings & Barkley, 1978, in "Suggested Reading"). That is, they are not necessarily underaroused in their basal or resting levels of heart rate, respiration, skin conductance, or cortical activity. However, when stimulated, their responses appear to be smaller in amplitude, slower to occur, and generally faster to habituate on a variety of psychophysiological measures. Furthermore, their responses on these measures seem to be more variable from moment to moment than is typical of normal children. While intriguing, such observations do not permit widespread "neurologizing"—speculation often seen in this area of research as to the neurologic mechanisms underlying these results. It is tempting to conclude that hyperactive children's inattention is the result of underarousability to stimuli that do not capture their attention as readily or for as long as such stimuli do with normal children. However, the findings in this area are purely correlational and do not permit such causal inferences. It could just as easily be that both the inattention and the underreactivity are the result of some as yet unknown central neural mechanism.

Second, and possibly related to this underarousal, is the frequently reported negative reaction of hyperactive children to sedatives, especially phenobarbital. These drugs apparently make some children even more hyperactive than they were prior to drug treatment—an observation reported as long as 40 years ago. Perhaps what is happening is that the subgroup of children already neurologically underreactive is made further so by the sedatives, which thus further decrease central inhibitory controls over behavior. More recently, however, it has been shown that as many as 35% to 40% of normal children display a worsening of behavior as a reaction to certain anticonvulsant drugs having sedative properties, chief among them phenobarbital (see Wolf & Forsythe, 1978, in "Suggested Reading"). It may be, then, that hyperactive children are actually no different from normal children in showing a negative reaction to these drugs.

A third set of observations inconsistent with an immaturity hypothesis is that of the frequent sleeping problems often reported for hyperactive children. Many clinicians believe that it is virtually diagnostic for hyperactive children to show shorter than normal sleeping periods and greater night waking than normal children. Recent research has failed to confirm this, however. Nonetheless, clinical anecdotes abound of hyperactive children requiring nets over their cribs or toddlers needing locks on their bedroom doors to prevent their nighttime wanderings. Some young hyperactive children have left their houses and have been found wandering the neighborhood or playing in the driveway at early hours of the morning. Others, though remaining within the house, have been found at night mixing foods in the kitchen or playing in the bathroom with substances from the medicine cabinet. A few hyperactive children create such problems in this respect that they require a sleeping medication at bedtime to insure a longer night's sleep. This is not always successful and may, as noted above, actually exacerbate the children's behavior and sleeping problems.

A fourth observation, seemingly unrelated to immaturity, is the hyperactive child's apparently high tolerance for pain. Interestingly, no scientific studies have examined this commonly noted clinical anecdote. Perhaps it is related to the neurologic underreactivity of some of these children, although this relationship in individual hyperactive children has not been examined.

Finally, hyperactive children show a higher number of physical ailments and anomalies than normal children—ailments that do not appear related to the concept of developmental lag. Parents often report a proneness to more colds, upper respiratory infections, ear infections, and allergies than are typical of normal children. With respect to allergies in particular, research suggests that as many as 50% of hyperactive children have allergies, the most frequent being reactions to grain substances, milk, and pollen. In addition, hyperactive children (boys especially) display more minor physical anomalies or dysmorphic features than normal children—findings that have held up over a number of replications. "Minor physical anomalies" refers to slight deviations in the physical appearance of the child, and these can be assessed during the newborn period with modest but acceptable degrees of reliability. Most prominent in this area has been the work of Patricia Quinn and her colleagues at Georgetown University Hospital and the National Institute of Mental Health. A list of some of the anomalies examined in her research are provided in Table 1.5. This research has found that higher anomaly scores are related to more pregnancy complications in the mother, more hyperactivity in the father's history, and increased symptom severity and an earlier onset of hyperactivity in the child. While the exact cause of such anomalies is uncertain, the belief has been that they are associated with problems during the first trimester of pregnancy. Whether such minor anomalies in appearance intimate similar anomalies in neurologic structures or development is only speculative at this time. Furthermore, other groups of psychiatrically disturbed children seem to show as much proneness to these ailments and anomalies as hyperactive children, making them nonspecific to hyperactivity.

Hyperactive children are frequently clumsy, awkward, and incoordinated in their fine and gross motor skills; this frequently puts them at a social disadvantage because of poor athletic prowess. A recent study found that as

TABLE 1.5.   Anomalies and Scoring Weights for Obtaining "Stigmata" Scores

Anomaly	Scoring weights
Head	
Head circumference	
1.5 *SD*	2
1 to 1.5 *SD*	1
"Electric" hair	
Very fine hair that won't comb down	2
Fine hair that is soon awry after combing	1
Two or more whorls	0
Eyes	
Epicanthus	
Where upper and lower lids join at the nose, point of union is:	
deeply covered	2
partly covered	1
Hypertelorism	
Approximate distance between tear ducts:	
1.5 *SD*	2
1.25 to 1.5 *SD*	1
Ears	
Low-set	
Bottom of ears in line with:	
mouth (or lower)	2
area between mouth and nose	1
Adherent lobes	
Lower edges of ears extend:	
upward and back toward crown of head	2
straight back toward rear of neck	1
Malformed	1
Asymmetrical	1
Soft and pliable	0
Mouth	
High palate	
Roof of mouth steepled	2
Roof of mouth moderately high	1
Furrowed tongue	1
Smooth–rough spots on tongue	0

TABLE 1.5. (Continued)

Anomaly	Scoring weights
Hands	
Fifth finger	
Markedly curved inward toward other fingers	2
Slightly curved inward toward other fingers	1
Single transverse palmar crease	1
Index finger longer than middle finger	0
Feet	
Third toe	
Definitely longer than second toe	2
Appears equal in length to second toe	1
Partial syndactyly of two middle toes	1
Gap between first and second toe (approximately ¼ inch)	1

Note. From "Minor Physical Anomalies and Neurologic Status in Hyperactive Boys" by P. Quinn and J. Rapoport, *Pediatrics,* 1974, *53,* 742–747. Copyright 1974 by the American Academy of Pediatrics. Reprinted by permission.

many as 62% of the hyperactive children examined experienced poor motor coordination. This incoordination, combined with their poor impulse control, seems to make them more accident-prone than other children. Early research by Mark Stewart at the University of Iowa (1970) discovered that hyperactive children experienced more accidental poisonings than normal children. Clinical reports also find them to have more bumps, scrapes, bruises, broken bones, and lacerations requiring sutures than same-age normal children. Again, this seems to necessitate closer parental supervision for hyperactive than for normal children, which is likely to enhance the frustration of the parents and contribute to poorer family interaction patterns—a point to be taken up in the next chapter.

Related to these physical problems are those difficulties hyperactive children seem to have in developing normal toileting skills. Several research reports have found that as many as 50% of these children were bedwetting and that up to 25% had problems with encopresis or soiling. It is not known whether these problems are related to immaturity in neurologic development or to problems in toilet training that result from their generally noncompliant and inattentive behavior. In either case, interventions with hyperactive children frequently must address more than the hyperactive symptoms; they necessitate multiple intervention strategies, if not multiple professional disciplines.

In summary, hyperactive children appear more likely to experience a wide array of physical difficulties, some of which support the notion of general physical immaturity or a developmental lag. The basis for these difficulties remains to be satisfactorily explained, and it is far from certain that such problems are specific to hyperactive children rather than characteristic of psychiatrically disturbed children in general.

EARLY PREDICTORS OF HYPERACTIVITY

Within the past five years, scientific attention has been directed toward discovering possible early signs or risk factors for children likely to become hyperactive. Since hyperactive children seem to manifest their problems by at least early childhood, it seems reasonable to assume that some earlier signs in the child's developmental or family history might be useful in predicting later hyperactivity. One well-studied predictor is that of minor physical anomalies in the newborn. As noted earlier, high physical anomaly scores seem to be related to more severe hyperactive behaviors having an earlier onset than in babies with lower anomaly scores. Although these relationships are statistically significant, the size of the correlation is sufficiently small to be without much utility in a clinical setting.

One of the more useful predictors to be studied is infant temperament. Infants with difficult temperament are often seen to have problems with feeding (such as colic or finicky eating preferences), sleeping, and irritability of mood. They are likely to be less cuddly or interactive and may show greater reactivity to environmental stimuli, especially in a negative way. Some research has found that infants with difficult temperament were likely to experience behavior problems in general and hyperactivity in particular by the time they were 2 to 3 years of age.

High activity level by itself has also been shown to be related to lower intelligence estimates, poorer cognitive skills, and poorer interactions with others by age 7. While not predictive of hyperactivity in particular, early peer judgments of other children have been shown to be quite reliable predictors of later conduct problems in adolescence and adulthood.

Paul Nichols of the National Institutes of Health (1980) recently examined a number of variables collected during the Collaborative Perinatal Project, which followed a large group of children from their pregnancies until 7 years of age. Variables found to have some statistical association with later hyperactivity were maternal smoking during pregnancy, obstetrical and birth complications, presence of hyperactivity in a sibling, and father absence from the home. Again, while intriguing, the degree of relationships involved were not of much clinical utility. In addition, prospective studies on the relationship of perinatal complications to later behavioral and academic problems have shown them to be of only a low order and to "wash out" over time. That is, the older the group of children one was predicting to, the less of a relationship there was between these variables and later outcome.

Retrospective studies of hyperactive children have found a greater occurrence of parental psychiatric problems, such as conduct problems, alcoholism, and hysteria, in parents of hyperactive children than in those of normal children. This might suggest that a parental history of hyperactivity in childhood or of conduct, alcohol, and emotional problems in adulthood would be useful predictors of which families are more likely to have hyperactive children. However, the necessary prospective studies using families with these risk factors remain to be done. Thus, the utility of parental psychiatric history remains purely conjectural at this time.

While research on possible predictors of hyperactivity holds some promise, present findings are of little help to the clinician in dealing with individual cases. If valid and useful predictors can be identified, then the next task will be to evaluate early intervention strategies for their effectiveness in altering the likelihood of hyperactivity in children tagged as at risk.

DEVELOPMENTAL COURSE

Although some aspects of the developmental course of hyperactive children have been intimated above, it is worth examining hyperactivity at various developmental stages in more detail. An excellent description of these stages has been provided in the scholarly review of research on hyperactivity by Dorothea Ross and Sheila Ross at Stanford University (1976). Some of the earliest research on hyperactive children optimistically held that they tended to outgrow their problems by adolescence. More recent research has shown that many of the problems of hyperactive children, though lessening with age, are still present in late adolescence and young adulthood.

Not all hyperactive children show difficulties during their infancy, though a large percentage do. Those problems which do occur are more likely to be difficulties with temperament—with eating, sleeping, and activity level. Often colicky and irritable, they are fussy eaters, showing irregularity in their feeding patterns. Some show allergies to milk, thereby requiring special formulas for feeding. Many will show disturbances in sleeping patterns, often having shorter periods of sleep than other babies. Active and restless, they may be difficult to hold, preferring not to be cuddled, and may require extraordinary measures to restrain them in their cribs or to prevent them from inadvertently destroying their cribs or mattresses.

By 2 to 3 years of age, those who were not difficult as infants are now likely to begin manifesting problems with their behavior, as those who have been temperamental since birth will continue to do. Parents are more likely to date the onset of problem behaviors to this period. The children are often described as noncompliant, requiring repeated instances of commands before even partial, though temporary, compliance occurs. Always restless and "on the go," these children will begin to show their clumsiness and proneness to accidents during this age. "Childproofing" the house becomes mandatory if serious accidents or destruction are to be even partially avoided. Many parents tend to dismiss the problems at this age as being simply the "terrible 2's" or just a phase their children are going through, especially if such a child is the first child. The parents may also complain that the children have difficulty taking naps or playing alone without frequently demanding attention from the parents. Because of the children's noncompliance, toilet training may prove more time-consuming, frustrating, and less successful than with normal children.

In early childhood, when these children are between 3 and 5 years of age, the parents may begin to seek professional help if they have not done so already. This is especially likely if the children enter day care, preschool, or kindergarten programs, where school staff may begin to describe these children as problems and in need of psychological help. Still, a few may not be identified by the school staff as problematic, even though such children's behavior at home is becoming progressively more difficult to manage. This discrepancy in behavior may stem in part from the limited amount of time spent in school at this age (usually a half day or less) or to the relatively unstructured nature of these programs. Upon entry into first grade, the picture may change dramatically as the children are asked to limit their behavior within structured routines for longer periods of time. In our opinion, the child who does not develop hyperactivity until after school-entry age is relatively rare and perhaps unique, with a different etiology and prognosis. I am in agreement with Douglas that, where problems with hyperactivity emerge only in later childhood, they are probably a reaction to the school failure common to children with emerging learning disabilities, to environmental stress events, to head trauma, or to toxic drug reactions often seen with anticonvulsants.

Between the ages of 3 and 5, noncompliance, especially in public, and poor peer interactions are likely to come to the forefront as major problems, as are school behavior problems in some children. With increasing exposure to broader social situations, problems with social conduct become progressively more obvious and of primary concern to the parents. Sleeping and toileting problems may continue in a smaller percentage of children. The parents may now begin to complain that their children have less of a conscience, or concern with the consequences of their behavior, than other children. In addition, the parents may become bewildered at the children's lack of responsiveness to typical disciplinary methods. And, when disciplined, such children may become quite angry, may be prone to temper tantrums, and may show rage outbursts in some cases. Acceptance of responsibility for their behavior is often deficient, as seen by the children's frequent blaming of others for all of their difficulties. Aggression toward other children is also likely to be seen with many hyperactive children during this age; selfish with their own possessions and demanding of those possessions of other children, they may cause frequent fights. Destructiveness is also common by this age, though frequently nonmalicious in nature. These children often seem incapable of not touching everything in view at this age. They may inadvertently break or destroy objects, more out of curiosity, clumsiness, and impulsivity than anger; when they are angered, however, destruction of articles is more commonly seen than in normal children. Parents may now begin to have trouble with finding babysitters for such a child, and family shopping trips may have to be rearranged so that one parent remains at home with the child while the other gets the shopping done. The reduction in parental socializing that may occur secondary to the problem only adds to the tension in these families and between the parents and hyperactive children in particular. Parental depression may emerge as a significant problem, if it has not already done so.

Once hyperactive children reach school age (5 years or older), the problems with school behavior and performance will have emerged, if they have not during the preschool period. Parents will now have to contend with the complaints of school staff and their often overly negative, judgmental attitude toward the parents' role in causing these children's problems. Decisions about retaining such children in kindergarten or first grade may have to be made, because of obvious immaturity or poor academic readiness. By second grade, the appearance of learning disabilities becomes highly probable, although some school staff will erroneously attribute the academic failure to the children's behavior problems rather than to a cognitive deficit. Because of such children's already growing reputation for immature, aggressive, selfish and hyperkinetic behavior, as well as poor athletic ability, they may be shunned by most children, finding themselves "loners," though hardly by choice. Over the years, their academic performance remains quite variable and their grades are more likely to decline. The question of retention or transfer to a special class for behavior disorders may appear necessary. These children are likely to continue to blame others for their problems, and lying as well as petty thievery may arise. Parents now begin to complain that they cannot trust such children to do what they say they will when left alone.

In the later childhood years, hyperactive children are increasingly likely to show signs of depression and low self-esteem. Success at school, at home, and in social relations has been rare. Acting-out behavior may increase as a result of the frustration that must accompany their chronic failure. Bragging of fictitious accomplishments, lying, and cheating in school are often seen as these children begin to try any means possible to gain success or acceptance with peers. By now, truancy may begin, and such children may have their first contact with juvenile authorities for status offenses (e.g., violating curfew, truancy, incorrigibility), although these are more likely to emerge during the teenage years. Increasingly, family arguments and home tensions erupt into confrontations with these children.

With adolescence is likely to come the most tumultuous period in the lives of hyperactive children and their families, despite declines in the children's activity level. Peer problems continue unabated, contacts with juvenile authorities become more likely, and truancy is more common. The best information available on this phase of development has come from Gabrielle Weiss and her colleagues at Montreal Children's Hospital (1978). This research suggests that many children have been retained in school at least one grade, and actual school performance may in fact be several grades below current placement. Families are often fed up with these children and with the likelihood that any intervention may actually help. More so than many adolescents, hyperactive teenagers are likely to be argumentative, rebellious, and unwilling to listen to authority. Depression is very common with this age group, with as many as 40% to 60% reporting low self-esteem. Sadness, low expectations of future success, and poor self-confidence have been found to be more likely in hyperactive than in normal teenagers. In later adolescence, alcohol abuse becomes more common than in normal or learning-disabled children, while abuse of other substances has not as yet been observed to be more frequent. Car accidents have also been noted to occur more often with hyperactive teens and young adults.

In adulthood, the problems for these children may be less than in adolescence, partly as a result of the greater freedom afforded adults. Thus hyperactive children are able to seek jobs and life styles which are more likely to allow them their behavioral excesses. They are still more impulsive, inattentive, and restless than others, however, and geographic moves appear more common. Contacts with the law may be less than those seen during the teenage years. Hyperactive children as adults are often less educated than, and less likely to attain the economic status of, their parents or nonhyperactive siblings. Whether they are more likely to have marital problems, divorces, job changes, or contacts with mental health workers has not been well researched. The few studies of this age group find that their job status and their employers' satisfaction with them are not different from those of normal adults. It is not known whether hyperactive children as adults are more likely to have hyperactive children once they marry than are adults with normal childhood and adolescent backgrounds.

PREDICTING OUTCOME

Given that hyperactive children seem to have problems in many areas throughout their childhood and adolescence, there would seem to be some value in determining which factors predict better or worse outcomes within the hyperactive population. Much of the work in this area has come from Loney and Weiss. One of the best predictors of social and occupational outcome in many childhood disorders, including hyperactivity, is the SES of the family. As noted earlier, SES is associated with both the prevalence and severity of hyperactivity, so its association with outcome for these children should not be surprising. The lower the SES level of the family, the worse the outcome for the child in terms of academic, social, and occupational adjustment. A second predictor of later adjustment, especially in terms of academic success, is the child's intellectual level, which is partially related to the parents' own educational and SES level. Intellectually brighter children obviously tend to do better in school than children of lesser intelligence. The extent to which the child is accepted by his or her peers, even at an early age, has been consistently found to predict adult social adjustment; obviously, children who are more sociable with and acceptable to their peers have a better social outcome. Loney's work in particular has shown that the level of aggression in childhood predicts adolescent social outcome. The more aggressive hyperactive children are, the worse their adjustment in adolescence. On the other hand, the level of hyperactivity in childhood seems to be predictive of only academic outcome in adolescence, rather than social adjustment. Loney believes that this may be why stimulant drugs do not alter the eventual outcome of hyperactive children. Since these drugs appear to influence hyperactive, not necessarily aggressive, behaviors, then they would have less influence over later social adjustment. In any case, this necessarily brief review suggests that highly hyperactive children of low intellectual and socioeconomic levels who are highly aggressive and not well accepted by their peers are likely to show an extremely poor outcome as adolescents or adults.

ETIOLOGY

At the present time, the knowledge available regarding etiology is of no help in selecting treatment approaches for hyperactive children. Research on this aspect of hyperactive children has been slow, producing conflicting results. Few specific etiologies have been identified, although a few have recently begun to show promise. Certainly, hyperactivity is not the result of one etiology. Most scientists view it as a final common pathway for a variety of etiologies. Five main areas have been studied for etiologic factors, and these are briefly reviewed below.

Before considering this literature, the reader should be cautioned about a mistake all too often made by scientist and layman alike. This is the problem of construing correlation as causation. As any student of elementary statistics is taught, the simple covariance of two events does not mean that one necessarily causes the other. Yet it seems that this simple fact is grossly ignored in interpreting findings in the area of etiology. For instance, it has been shown that hyperactive children have more allergies than normal children and that their mothers smoke more during their pregnancies than those of normal children. Many clinicians have leaped to the conclusion that allergies or maternal smoking cause hyperactivity, though neither conclusion is warranted from the relationships so described. These covariations among events are simply covariations and provide no indication of causality. An extreme example will illustrate the point. It is not well known that there is a sizeable correlation between the number of heart attacks in a given period and the extent to which road pavement has melted. No one would propose that heart attacks cause roads to melt, or vice versa, yet the conclusions noted above about hyperactivity are tantamount to doing precisely that. In this illustration, it is obvious that a third variable, temperature, causes these two events. Similarly, some third as yet unknown variable may well cause the relationships shown above between allergies and hyperactivity, or maternal smoking and hyperactivity. Clinicians must therefore be extremely cautious in rushing to create causal conclusions from purely correlational data, as many scientists have unwittingly done.

Neurological Factors

The earliest and probably most frequently proposed etiology of hyperactivity was brain damage or injury, usually postulated to have occurred around the time of birth. Although the first descriptions of hyperactive children were of those recovering from encephalitis, the term "brain-damaged" was later applied to children with no obvious signs of damage or injury. It was assumed that because these latter children manifested behavioral problems similar to those of the children with encephalitis, they, too, must be brain-injured. The use of the term "brain damage" requires that one be able to establish, through autopsy, neurologic evaluation, or "hard" neurologic signs, that the brain has suffered structural injury or alteration. As previously noted, Rutter has pointed out that probably less than 5% of hyperactive children show any evidence of neurologic damage. Similarly, of those children with actual brain injuries, only a small percentage will develop hyperactivity, though others may be at greater risk for general psychiatric problems. In any case, the actual relationship of neurologic injury to hyperactivity is quite weak.

  Despite the lack of support for a brain damage hypothesis, the notion that hyperactive children may be suffering a neurologic dysfunction continues to receive widespread endorsement. Obviously, the evidence for dysfunction is quite inferential and often inconsistent, primarily based on greater neurologic "soft" signs and psychophysiologic findings suggestive of arousal problems in the CNS. As noted earlier, research on CNS arousal has shown that some, but not all, hyperactive children show an underresponsive reaction to stimulation. It remains to be demonstrated that such arousal problems actually create the hyperactive behaviors. Some investigators have proposed that hyperactivity stems from neurotransmitter deficiencies within given brain structures, while others limit their speculations to inefficient or dysfunctional brain structures without necessarily proposing neurochemical abnormalities. At this time, such notions are purely conjectural, as the evidence available does not support a specific dysfunction in any circumscribed neurologic area for all hyperactive children.

While this may be the case, the similarities between hyperactive behaviors in children and the results of prefrontal injuries in adults and primates are quite striking and may yet prove to be more than coincidental. The prefrontal cortex in humans lies at the very anterior portion of both cerebral hemispheres, occupying the cranial area just behind the forehead. It is the most recently evolved area of the human brain, an area which humans possess more of than any other animal. This region is known to have abundant interconnections with the brain stem arousal mechanisms, the midbrain emotional centers, and the sensory–motor cortex and posterior association areas. While still not well understood, some of its functions have been elucidated. The prefrontal cortex appears to play a substantial role in inhibiting, modulating, planning, and regulating complex human behavior. Its place in permiting humans to anticipate and prepare for future events is generally accepted. It also seems to underlie human ability to generate motor behaviors from linguistic statements or rules. Such rule-governed behavior appears essential to the socialization of humans. Finally, there is little doubt that this structure is responsible for human ability to sustain attention for prolonged periods of time and to work toward goals some distance into the future.

Adults (and some children) with injuries specific to the prefrontal cortex are often noted to be inattentive, distractible, impulsive, restless, and unable to follow rules. Inappropriate social and sexual behavior may be seen, together with a general failure to be concerned with the present and future consequences of one's behavior. Anticipation of future events is often disturbed, as is the planning of complex voluntary acts (apraxia), despite the preservation of normal sensory–motor functions. Such behaviors are quite similar to those noted above for hyperactive children, offering the possibility that future neurophysiologic studies may reveal select cortical inefficiencies, immaturities, or dysfunctions in the prefrontal cortex of hyperactive children. For the moment, the similarities remain coincidental.

For years, clinicians believed that the positive response of hyperactive children to stimulant drugs suggested norepinephrine or dopamine deficiencies. Recent studies with normal children by Judith Rapoport and her colleagues (1978) showed that they responded similarly to stimulant medication, thus weakening the major support for the idea of neurotransmitter deficits. The best one can conclude from this area is that neurologic dysfunction may some day prove to be causal in some hyperactive children, although the nature of that dysfunction remains ambiguous.

An alternative to the damage or dysfunction models has been the concept of neurologic immaturity. Here the mechanism appears to be a delay in the maturation of CNS structures underlying attention and response inhibition, rather than a deficit in these structures. There is much inferential support for this concept, as noted above in the section on physical correlates of hyperactivity. Briefly, as many as 50% of hyperactive children show underaroused electroencephalogram patterns suggestive of cortical immaturity. Difficulties with physical, emotional, and cognitive immaturity have also been observed in many of these children. As with the dysfunction hypothesis, however, this concept requires greater specification and research support before its merits can be fully evaluated.

Presently, then, as appealing as neurologic hypotheses may be, evidence for their existence remains quite circumstantial. However, recent breakthroughs in neurologic methodologies, metabolic assay procedures, and psychophysiologic techniques provide promising means for elucidating the mechanisms involved in hyperactivity.

Genetic Factors

This area of research has begun to receive increasing attention and seems to hold great promise for specifying at least one of the several etiologies involved in hyperactivity. Studies conducted to date suggest that families of hyperactive children have higher rates of alcoholism, psychopathy, hysteria, and depression than those of normal children. Such disorders are quite similar to those for which hyperactive children are at risk during their adolescence and adulthood. These problems are not seen in the adopted parents of adopted hyperactive children. Some recent research has also found the parents of hyperactive children to be more inattentive and impulsive than other adults of similar age, intelligence, and SES. Further, there is evidence to suggest that up to 30% of the siblings of hyperactive children are also likely to be having psychiatric problems, chief among them hyperactivity. In addition to the familial nature of the disorder, the few studies of identical and fraternal twins that have been done are supportive of an hereditary basis to the disorder, although these studies can be faulted on numerous methodological grounds.

Related to this issue has been the research conducted on the heritability of activity level and temperament. One study of 93 pairs of same-sex twins revealed higher concordance rates for activity level between monozygotic twins than between dyzygotic twins. Similar studies of infant temperament have found it to have not only a high degree of stability over time, but to show higher heritability among monozygotic than among dyzygotic twin pairs. Nonetheless, the research in this area remains sparse, although promising, and more definitive studies will have to be done. One such study might be to examine the prevalence of hyperactivity among offspring of hyperactive children followed into adulthood.

Environmental Toxins

Recently, a variety of toxins and allergy-producing substances have been the subject of debate as to their contribution to the causes of hyperactivity. Chief among these have been the food additives and refined sugars, as proposed by Benjamin Feingold (1976) and Lendon Smith (1975). Their theories will be discussed in greater detail in Chapter 9. A number of scientific papers have addressed the Feingold hypothesis regarding the toxic behavioral effects of various food dyes and additives. To date, empirical support for this hypothesis is quite weak. The research has been reviewed by Eric Taylor (1980) and again by Conners (1980), with both reaching independently the conclusion that the effects of additives on behavior are quite weak, are limited to a very small percentage of children, and are apparently more likely to be seen in those 6 years of age and younger. Thus, food additives are probably not a major cause of hyperactivity, although they may yet be shown to exacerbate the symptoms of a relatively small group of hyperactive children.

The role of refined sugars and other foodstuffs such as milk, chocolate, and "junk" foods in causing hyperactivity has not received much scientific scrutiny. While Smith has pontificated widely on the issue, his opinions are based more on his clinical cases than on any sound scientific research. Like Feingold, Smith believes that a variety of childhood psychological disorders can result from these substances, yet no acceptable scientific evidence is provided to support such claims. At this time, the manner in which sugar and other foodstuffs affect hyperactivity is simply not known, with the burden of scientific proof falling to those who advocate these views so strongly.

Various degrees of lead poisoning have been examined for their contribution to hyperactivity. The findings, while provocative, remain equivocal because of serious methodological flaws in the few studies to date. The current studies suggest that as many as 30% to 35% of children with elevated blood lead levels are hyperactive. This research has also found that some hyperactive children with signs of elevated lead levels will show behavioral improvement following chelation therapy. This is a relatively intrusive and painful treatment that attempts to purge the lead from body tissues. While it seems plausible that elevated blood lead levels may cause some children to become hyperactive, it is unlikely to account for the vast majority of hyperactives who show no such elevations. In addition, it is possible that the hyperactivity precedes the lead exposure and may in fact account for it. That is, it is known that hyperactive children are more likely to suffer accidental poisonings than normal children because of their impulsive behavior. Perhaps such behavior leads them also to ingest leaded paint chips or other leaded materials more than normal children do. SES may be a factor that contributes further to this explanation, since both hyperactivity and elevated blood lead levels are more frequently found in lower-SES groups. It is possible that low-income families are more likely to have hyperactive children as the result of a variety of factors unrelated to lead poisoning. Since more of these families are likely to reside in older, substandard housing, their hyperactive children are more likely to ingest leaded materials. The relationship of lead poisoning to hyperactivity, then, is far from clear.

In the mid- to late 1970s, there was a brief flurry of attention to the possibility that the soft X rays emitted from fluorescent lighting in schools might contribute to hyperactive behavior in the classroom. A former photographer with Walt Disney Studios produced films of classrooms with and without shielded fluorescent lighting. Children in the unshielded room were more restless and off-task than those in the shielded classroom. However, a highly controlled effort to replicate these results failed to find any effects of such lighting on classroom behavior. It would appear that no sound scientific evidence presently exists to support the claim that certain types of fluorescent lighting create hyperactivity.

Toxic reactions to sedatives, wherein children placed on anticonvulsant or sedative drugs become unmanageable, have been reported. One recent paper suggested that over 30% of children placed on these drugs became hyperactive, with the symptoms diminishing in most of them once the drugs were discontinued. While more objective studies of this phenomenon are clearly called for, many who work in pediatric neurology clinics often see children manifesting hyperkinetic reactions to anticonvulsant compounds. It is intriguing to juxtapose these findings with those from psychophysiological studies of hyperactive children, in which underarousability of the nervous system is found in some of these children. Perhaps sedating the immature neurologic inhibitory mechanisms of some children results in hyperactive behavior. In any event, while sedatives may well create "hyperkinetic reactions," most hyperactive children are not receiving such compounds. Hence, these substances are unlikely to account for any sizeable portion of the hyperactive population.

As noted earlier, maternal smoking during pregnancy has shown a weak but significant relationship to hyperactive behavior at age 5 in children born to such women. In addition, retrospective studies of hyperactive children have found that their mothers reported consuming significantly more cigarettes during their pregnancies with these children than mothers of normal children do. It is tempting to conclude that the noxious effects of smoking affect fetal development in such a way as to create or contribute to hyperactivity in the early childhood of that fetus. However, it is equally as plausible that women who are more likely to give birth to hyperactive children are, as has been reported above, more likely to have anxiety-related and other emotional disorders themselves. Such women may be more likely to smoke cigarettes during the stress of a pregnancy, and yet the smoking itself may not be contributory to the likelihood of hyperactivity in the child.

A similar relationship exists with respect to maternal alcohol consumption during pregnancy. A recent research report noted that 15 of 87 mothers of hyperactive children reported drinking alcohol during their pregnancies with these children. An examination of these children found them manifesting several physical anomalies consistent with fetal alcohol syndrome. Again, while it is tempting to conclude that alcohol abuse during pregnancy causes hyperactivity in the offspring, these data do not necessarily prove a causal connection. Mothers likely to have hyperactive children may have an increased occurrence of emotional disorders likely to cause them to turn to alcohol while under the stress of pregnancy. As with maternal smoking, it is the mothers' psychiatric history that contributes to the risk of hyperactivity and not the effects of alcohol (or smoking) consumption during their pregnancies. The problem of inferring causation from correlational data, as discussed earlier, clearly applies in this area of research.

Biological Variation

One cause of hyperactivity discussed by Marcel Kinsbourne (1977) is the possibility that hyperactive children merely represent the extreme ends of the normal distribution for characteristics related to temperament. Assuming normal distributions along each of these dimensions of normal personality, some children as a matter of biologic variation are bound to wind up at the extremes of these dimensions. A child who is only at the extreme of activity may simply be viewed as an energetic, exuberant, bright, inquisitive child. But a child at the extremes of two or more dimensions at once may have a socially "explosive" combination of temperamental features, predisposing him or her to problems in a society geared to those within the more normal ranges of these dimensions. An extremely active, impulsive, and emotional child may prove to be much more at risk for social maladjustment than one who is further from the extremes of these dimensions. This notion is intriguing but awaits clearer elaboration and empirical support.

Psychosocial Factors

Very little research has been conducted on the possible psychological or social conditions that may create hyperactive behavior. Some investigators have suggested that hyperactivity is nothing more than poor stimulus control of behavior by parental commands. The not-so-subtle implication of this proposal is that the poor child management methods used by parents leads to hyperactive behavior. Whether for this reason or as a consequence of other, more psychodynamic explanations, child clinicians have, in our experience, been very quick to place the blame for hyperactive children's problems on their parents' child-rearing skills. The greater incidence of psychiatric problems among families of hyperactive children has probably given these clinicians ample clinical evidence upon which to build their case. That clinicians are likely to find parents using more commands, fewer rewards, and more punishment with these children than are seen in normal parent–child dyads may only further serve to cement the verdict against the parents. Granted, hyperactive behavior clearly varies with its consequences, can be diminished by behavior modification approaches, and can be influenced by the behavior modeled by others interacting with the children.

Upon closer inspection, an environmental theory is fraught with problems and inconsistencies. First, if parents are to blame for these behavior problems, how are we to explain the very early onset and cross-situational nature of the problems? Why would so many teachers, relatives, and babysitters also have problems with these children? While the notion that the parents could have trained the children in the hyperactive behaviors so that the behaviors generalize to other people who must deal with the child may sound plausible, it would argue that the parents are better able to get child behaviors to generalize to other people and settings than any skilled behavior therapist has been. Second, such a proposal must also account for the wealth of physical findings and specific learning disabilities associated with the disorder. Third, one would expect that if hyperactive behaviors were reduced by some intervention (say, stimulant drugs), then little if any change in the directive, negative parental behaviors would occur. This, however, has not been the case. Drug studies in mine and several other laboratories suggest that parental management styles shift dramatically to more normal ones when the hyperactive child is on medication. Finally, how does one explain the presence of normally behaved siblings in the family, or the fact that hyperactivity develops in children adopted into homes with quite capable adoptive parents? Support for a completely psychological or social cause of hyperactivity must be viewed as extremely weak at this time.

Conclusion

It therefore seems that no single etiology can adequately account for the symptoms and correlates of hyperactivity. A reasonable approach is to assume that, like mental retardation, psychosis, or other developmental disabilities, it is multietiolotic in nature. In my opinion, familial–hereditary factors seem to play a large role in this disorder, with obstetrical–pregnancy complications contributing another portion of the population. Much smaller percentages of children may be related to obvious neurologic damage or insult, or to toxic reactions. Biological variation might well fit into the familial–hereditary hypothesis. Nonetheless, our knowledge of etiology is as yet of no help in early intervention or prevention programs or in designing treatments having any long-term impact on the outcome of these children.

A BEHAVIORAL ANALYSIS OF HYPERACTIVITY

Although hyperactivity may one day prove to have a clearly neurophysiologic basis, this does not imply that a functional analysis of hyperactive symptoms cannot be of value in further clarifying the nature of hyperactivity or in designing interventions. As with any other neurologic disorder having behavioral deficiencies associated with it, behavioral analyses may still offer the most promising approach to the management of hyperactivity. It is naive, however, to assume that, simply because behavioral symptoms can be manipulated by altering environmental consequences, they are not of neurophysiologic origins.

Inattention, Distractibility, and Impulsivity

In his classic book *Science and Human Behavior* (1953), B. F. Skinner presented an analysis of the terms "attention" and "self-control" from a behavioristic approach. His discussion of these long-debated concepts may help to shed some light on the nature of the behavioral symptoms of hyperactivity. Skinner proposes that attention is not itself a behavior or activity of the individual, but a relationship between a given discriminative or conditioned stimulus and a desired response to that stimulus. That is, attention simply describes the functional aspects surrounding a stimulus and a response. The length of time that a child responds to a stimulus is typically called the child's "attention span." The time that elapses between the presentation of a conditioned stimulus and the child's eventual response is generally referred to as "impulsivity," especially if the response given is not the desired one. The degree to which other stimuli, presented at the same time as the conditioned stimulus, are responded to by the child can be thought of as "distractibility." That is, how likely is the child to orient and respond to a stimulus competing with the one considered to be the more important by those involved with the child at the time? Finally, the aspects or characteristics of a given complex stimulus to which the child responds, such as size, color, shape, and so on, can be considered the child's "focus of attention."

To reiterate, the common problems of hyperactive children are not necessarily deficiencies in behavior *per se,* but in the functional relationship between a conditioned stimulus (usually deemed important by the social community) and a response (usually the one desired by the community). As noted earlier, hyperactive children seem to have their greatest deficits in impulsivity and attention span—that is, in the duration between stimulus presentation and response onset and in the duration of responding to that stimulus respectively. Interventions that can affect these two aspects of duration or timing are likely to be seen as successful treatments for hyperactive behavior. Irrespective of the initial causes of these relational or durational deficits, they can be affected by altering the characteristics of the conditioned stimulus; by altering the consequences provided for the response; and by altering the neurological substrate that mediates the relational properties between a stimulus and a response. One therefore does not actually directly treat poor attention span or impulse control, but instead manipulates the properties of the stimulus and response of which these deficiencies are a function.

Noncompliance, Poor Self-Control, and Poor Problem Solving

In addition to deficits in attention and impulse control, hyperactive children are often described as noncompliant and as having poor self-control. Both of these deficits, as well as that of poor social problem-solving skills, appear to be related to deficits in rule-governed behavior. Skinner discusses the notion that the presence or absence of self-control is actually related to rule-governed versus contingency-shaped behavior. "Contingency-shaped behavior" is that behavior that is produced or maintained by the immediately occurring natural consequences in a given situation. For instance, a child who touches a hot stove and quickly withdraws a burned finger learns to avoid the hot stove. The actual avoidance of the hot stove in subsequent situations is said to be contingency-shaped behavior. This is contrasted with "rule-governed behavior," in which the response is emitted to a verbal stimulus or rule directing the child to do something, and the response is consequated by socially, rather than naturally, arranged contingencies. Using the above example, when the child is told by the mother not to touch the hot stove and avoids the stove, the mother may reward the child's compliance to the command. The future avoidance of the stove at the request of the mother is rule-governed behavior. Eventually, when the child avoids the stove in the absence of the mother or her commands, the child is said to show self-control or to have "internalized" the rule. In fact, the child is probably responding to memory of the rule or to subvocalizing of the rule. In each case, the child avoids the stove, but the stimuli controlling the behavior, as well as the learning histories are quite different. In the first case, the stove itself serves as the controlling stimulus, while, in the second case, it is the rule or command that is the conditioned stimulus.

Rule-governed behavior, or the control of behavior by linguistic stimuli, appears to be essential to the socialization of children. First, it prevents children from being exposed to harmful or life-threatening events. Second, it prevents children's behavior from being shaped by the possibly spurious or inconsistent natural consequences in the immediate situation. And, third, it permits the community to bring children's behavior under the influence of future, rather than immediate, consequences. Children may thereby profit from the accumulated wisdom of the community through following its rules, instead of having to learn firsthand what prior community members have already learned. Rule-governed behavior permits the community to bring children's behavior under the control of its own rules and eventually to teach children to generate and follow self-generated rules—that is, to show self-control. Once children begin to ask questions of themselves when confronted with a problem, and to develop a solution or rule to follow, problem solving is said to occur. The questions in this case are considered to be second-order rules that make the occurrence of first-order rules or solutions more likely. Deficiencies in compliance, self-control, and problem solving in hyperactive children might therefore be the result of deficiencies in some aspect of rule-governed behavior. It is possible that the problems with rule-governed behavior are in part related to the child's deficits in attention span noted above.

The major processes leading to rule-governed behavior in children seem to be as follows:

1. The possession of a language by the community.

2. The presence of the neurologic substrate in the child necessary for acquiring and generating language.

3. The training of the child in the language of the community.

4. The presence of the neurologic substrate in the child necessary for converting linguistic stimuli into motor hehavior.

5. The training of the child to comply with the commands or rules of the community (compliance).

6. The training of the child to respond to memory or subvocalizing of those rules (self-control).

7. The training of the child to engage in self-questioning, or problem solving.

Problems that arise early in this sequence will probably affect later steps in the sequence. The earlier in the sequence the problem is, the more serious the later deficits in compliance, self-control, or problem solving will be. Obviously, some problems in self-control can have environmental causes (e.g., poor training) while others may have neurological bases (e.g., impairment in critical neurologic substrates, such as the left cerebral hemisphere for language and the left anterior frontal lobe in particular for rule-governed behavior). In either case, interventions based upon this developmental

sequence might show some promise in improving the misbehavior of hyperactive children. The parent training program outlined in Chapter 7 is in part
based upon this sequence.

SUMMARY AND CONCLUSIONS

Although much remains to be studied about the nature and etiology of
hyperactivity, some general conclusions can be made at this time. It seems
that "hyperactivity" is used to refer to the behavior of a relatively heterogeneous group of children who do not necessarily share a common set of
characteristics. However, most of these children appear to have primary
deficiencies in attention span, impulse control, and rule-governed behavior.
The disorder seems to have a variety of physical, academic, cognitive, and
social difficulties related to it; it has an early onset in the child's development
and lasts well into the adolescent or young adulthood years. Probably 3% to
4% of the school-age population could be identified as hyperactive, with the
disorder being more common in males and in lower socioeconomic groups.
It is associated with multiple etiologies, the most significant among them
being familial–hereditary factors and obstetrical–pregnancy complications.
Toxic agents, brain damage, and biologic variation may also contribute to a
lesser extent to this population. Environmental etiologies, most often related
to poor parental child-rearing practices, have not been well articulated or
supported in the literature. Certainly, however, such factors can serve to
modulate or exacerbate the child's hyperactive symptoms as well as the
eventual prognosis. Family socioeconomic status, and the child's own level
of intelligence, aggression, peer acceptance, and hyperactivity, all to some
extent predict adolescent or adult adjustment. Obviously, then, treatment
programs will have to be complex and long-term in nature, addressing the
wide range of problems these children are likely to experience throughout
their development. Simplistic, narrow, and short-term interventions, which
have been typical so far with this group, have not altered the prognosis of
these children to any appreciable degree.

IMPLICATIONS FOR ASSESSMENT

There are several broad implications of the previous review and discussion
for the assessment of hyperactive children.

   1. The primary behavior problems of hyperactive children appear to
have an early onset and to be chronic, making several demands on assessment procedures. First, the methods used should be reliable over time and

valid across age levels, permitting comparability of findings obtained from repeated assessments. Second, the changing nature of the disorder over time, especially with respect to increasing social and academic problems, necessitates the use of measures that assess social interactions and social skills, as well as cognitive and academic deficits. And, third, the use of measures that have developmental norms is imperative if one is to assess and reassess the age-appropriateness of the hyperactive child's behavior and to draw conclusions as to whether it is or remains problematic or statistically abnormal.

2. Hyperactivity is often cross-situational in nature, which suggests that more than one informant should be used in assessing the child's problems. Most often, parents, teachers, social workers, relatives, or other clinicians serve in this capacity, representing the different major situations in which most children participate—that is, home, school, clinic, and so on. We have found that mothers and fathers frequently disagree on the existence, nature, and severity of their children's problems. Such disagreement should not be construed as inaccuracy on either parent's part; it means only that a hyperactive child may behave differently for one parent than for the other. The opinion of each parent should be recorded and judged as credible *for that parent's interactions* with the child until proven otherwise.

3. The behavioral perspective on hyperactivity taken here—namely, that hyperactivity involves a deficiency in attention, rule-governed behavior, and self-control—leads to the inescapable conclusion that the assessment of the hyperactive child cannot simply focus on a single characteristic, such as motor activity levels. Instead, one must assess the child's ability to sustain attention to activities, as well as to follow commands, directives, and rules across a variety of situations at home, at school, or in public. Pertinent questions requiring attention during assessment include whether or not the child has trouble following rules (noncompliance), and if so, under what situations, with what types of commands, and with what individuals. As noted earlier, where problems in compliance and rule-governed behavior exist, so might difficulties with self-control and problem solving that require assessment. Since social conduct with others draws heavily upon one's knowledge of and ability to follow rules of conduct or etiquette, hyperactive children are also quite likely to manifest deficits in social skills. These, too, require some assessment.

4. Because the hyperactive child is also more likely to experience problems in various aspects of physical, self-help, academic, emotional, and social development, the evaluation must include, where needed, methods capable of evaluating these diverse areas of functioning. In some cases, the child may need to be referred to other professionals to accomplish this goal. Nonetheless, assessment of the hyperactive child cannot narrowly focus upon only one or two symptoms if a comprehensive picture of the child's problems is to be obtained and adequate treatment initiated.

SUGGESTED READING

Achenbach, T. The child behavior profile: Boys aged 6–11. *Journal of Consulting and Clinical Psychology,* 1978, *46,* 478–488.

Barkley, R. A. Recent developments in research on hyperactive children. *Journal of Pediatric Psychology,* 1979, *3,* 158–163.

Barkley, R. A. Specific guidelines for defining hyperactivity in children. In B. Lahey & A. Kazdin (Eds.), *Advances in clinical child psychology* (Vol. 4). New York: Plenum, 1981.

Barkley, R. A., & Cunningham, C. The effects of Ritalin on the mother–child interactions of hyperactive children. *Archives of General Psychiatry,* 1979, *36,* 201–208.

Barkley, R. A., Cunningham, C., & Karlsson, K. The language of hyperactive children and their mothers: Comparisons with normal and stimulant drug effects. *Journal of Learning Disabilities,* 1981, in press.

Campbell, S. Mother–child interaction: a comparison of hyperactive, learning disabled, and normal boys. *Developmental Psychology,* 1975, *45,* 51–57.

Cantwell, D. P. (Ed.). *The hyperactive child.* New York: Spectrum, 1975.

Cantwell, D. P. Hyperactivity and antisocial behavior. *Journal of the American Academy of Child Psychiatry,* 1978, *1,* 252–262.

Cantwell, D. P., & Satterfield, J. H. The prevalence of academic underachievement in hyperactive children. *Journal of Pediatric Psychology,* 1978, *3,* 168–171.

Carey, W. B., & McDevitt, S. C. Stability and change in individual temperament diagnoses from infancy to early childhood. *Journal of the American Academy of Child Psychiatry,* 1978, *17,* 331–337.

Chamberlin, R. W. Can we identify a group of children at age two who are at risk for the development of behavioral or emotional problems in kindergarten or first grade? *Pediatrics* (Supplement), 1977, *59.*

Conners, C. K. *Food additives and hyperactive children.* New York: Plenum, 1980.

Cunningham, C., & Barkley, R. A. The effects of Ritalin on the mother–child interactions of hyperkinetic twin boys. *Developmental Medicine and Child Neurology,* 1978, *20,* 634–642.

Cunningham, C., & Barkley, R. A. A comparison of the interactions of hyperactive and normal children with their mothers in free play and structured task. *Child Development,* 1979, *50,* 217–224.

Douglas, V. I. Stop, look and listen: The problem of sustained attention and impulse control in hyperactive and normal children. *Canadian Journal of Behavioural Science,* 1972, *4,* 159–182.

Douglas, V. I. Sustained attention and impulse control: Implications for the handicapped child. In J. A. Swets & L. L. Elliott (Eds.), *Psychology and the handicapped child.* Washington, D.C.: U.S. Office of Education, 1974.

Douglas, V. I. Perceptual and cognitive factors as determinants of learning disabilities: A review chapter with special emphasis on attentional factors. In R. Knights & D. Bakker (Eds.), *The neuropsychology of learning disorders: Theoretical considerations.* Baltimore: University Park Press, 1976.

Douglas, V. I., & Peters, K. G. Toward a clearer definition of the attentional deficit of hyperactive children. In G. A. Hale & M. Lewis (Eds.), *Attention and the development of cognitive skills.* New York: Plenum, 1980.

Feingold, B. *Why your child is hyperactive.* New York: Random House, 1975.

Halverson, C. F., Jr., & Victor, J. B. Minor physical anomalies and problem behavior in elementary school children. *Child Development,* 1976, *47,* 281–285.

Hastings, J. E., & Barkley, R. A. A review of psychophysiological research with hyperactive children. *Journal of Abnormal Child Psychology,* 1978, *7,* 413–447.

Kinsbourne, M. The mechanism of hyperactivity. In M. Blaw, I. Rapin, & M. Kinsbourne (Eds.), *Topics in child neurology*. New York: Spectrum, 1977.

Lambert, N. M., Sandoval, J., & Sassone, D. Prevalence of hyperactivity in elementary school children as a function of social system definers. *American Journal of Orthopsychiatry*, 1978, *48*, 446–463.

Lapouse, R., & Monk, M. An epidemiological study of behavior characteristics in children. *American Journal of Public Health*, 1958, *48*, 1134–1144.

Loney, J. Childhood hyperactivity. In R. H. Woody (Ed.), *Encyclopedia of clinical assessment*. San Francisco: Jossey-Bass, 1978.

Millichap, J. G. *Learning disabilities and related disorders*. New York: Year Book Medical Publishers, 1977.

Nichols, P. Early antecedents of hyperactivity. *Neurology*, 1980, *30*, 439.

Rapoport, J. L., Buchsbaum, M. S., Zahn, T. P., Weingartner, H., Ludlow, C., & Mikkelsen, E. J. Dextroamphetamine: Cognitive and behavioral effects in normal prepubertal boys. *Science*, 1978, *199*, 560–563.

Ross, D. M., & Ross, S. A. *Hyperactivity*. New York: Wiley, 1976.

Routh, D. K. Hyperactivity. In P. Magrab (Ed.), *Psychological management of pediatric problems* (Vol. II). Baltimore: University Park Press, 1978.

Rutter, M. Brain damage syndromes in childhood: Concepts and findings. *Journal of Child Psychology and Psychiatry*, 1977, *18*, 1–21.

Safer, R., & Allen, D. *Hyperactive children: Diagnosis and management*. Baltimore: University Park Press, 1976.

Skinner, B. F. *Science and human behavior*. New York: Macmillan, 1953.

Skinner, B. F. *Cumulative record: A selection of papers*. New York: Appleton-Century-Crofts, 1967.

Sleator, E. K., & Ullman, R. K. Can the physician diagnose hyperactivity in the office? *Pediatrics*, 1981, *67*, 13–17.

Smith, L. *Your child's behavior chemistry*. New York: Random House, 1975.

Stewart, M. A., Thach, B. T., & Freidin, M. R. Accidental poisoning and the hyperactive child syndrome. *Diseases of the Nervous System*, 1970, *31*, 403–407.

Taylor, E. Food additives, allergy, and hyperactivity. *Journal of Child Psychology and Psychiatry*, 1979, *20*, 357–363.

Trites, R. L. (Ed.). *Hyperactivity in children*. Baltimore: University Park Press, 1979.

Weiss, G., Hechtman, L., & Perlman, T. Hyperactives as young adults: School, employer, and self-rating scales obtained during ten-year follow-up evaluation. *American Journal of Orthopsychiatry*, 1978, *48*, 438–445.

Wender, P. H. *Minimal brain dysfunction in children*. New York: Wiley, 1971.

Werry, J. Developmental hyperactivity. *Pediatric Clinics of North America*, 1968, *15*, 581–599.

Werry, J., & Quay, H. The prevalence of behavior symptoms in younger elementary school children. *American Journal of Orthopsychiatry*, 1971, *41*, 136–143.

Whalen, C. K., & Henker, B. (Eds.). *Hyperactive children: The social ecology of identification and treatment*. New York: Academic Press, 1980.

Wolf, S. M., & Forsythe, A. Behavior disturbance, phenobarbital, and febrile seizures. *Pediatrics*, 1978, *61*, 728–731.

CHAPTER TWO

THE FAMILIES OF
HYPERACTIVE CHILDREN

As are families, so is society.—If well-ordered, well-instructed, and well-governed, they are the springs from which go forth the streams of national greatness and prosperity—of civil order and public happiness.—*William Thayer*

It seems to be a statement of the obvious that children's behavior does not occur in a vacuum, but in some setting or social context. In fact, the very diagnosis of hyperactivity implies that certain children have come into conflict with their social environment and that others have found their behavior to be intolerable. Hence, the referral for treatment. In spite of the obvious, however, most literature dealing with hyperactive children has virtually ignored this social context and the implications it has for assessment and therapy.

A greater understanding of the family context within which hyperactive children interact is imperative to the clinician for several reasons. First, as will be shown later, there appears to be an increased likelihood of psychopathology in parents and siblings of hyperactive children. Such problems must have some modulating influence over such children's symptoms. Second, many clinicians tend to assume that because hyperactivity may have an hereditary, neurophysiologic, or "organic" basis, the social context in which the hyperactive symptoms are emitted is of lesser importance and hence not worth much time during the assessment or treatment process. Not even the most ardent advocate of the neurophysiologic basis for hyperactivity, however, would deny the role of environmental consequences in the expression of children's behavior. Third, many clinicians either have become so discouraged at the enormous complexity of social interactions in families that they choose to ignore these interactions, or have blindly endorsed unempirical theories of "family systems" based more upon armchair hypothesizing than upon scientific analysis. Such an endorsement often leads to treatment programs for which there is little scientific support. Simply to state, as many clinicians do, that one has a "family system" orientation to treatment does not mean that the clinician has any awareness of the proliferation of scientific observations now accruing on parent–child interactions or of interventions that seem useful for altering those interactions. Furthermore, despite the seemingly wide endorsement of this "systems" approach, most clinicians seem in practice to have forgotten about the issue of reciprocity—that is, the fact that both the parent *and the child* may contribute equally to the status of interactions. Many child clinicians continue to scrutinize parental behavior for even the slightest flaw upon which to base their clinical judgments and conclusions. As we will see later, the issue of reciprocity makes finding fault with parents a clinical endeavor of little redeeming value.

FAMILY PSYCHIATRIC PROBLEMS

Within the past five years, studies of hyperactive children and their families have revealed a variety of psychiatric problems in the siblings and parents of hyperactive children—problems not typically seen in comparison groups of relatives of normal children. Research has shown that parents of hyperactive children are more likely to manifest symptoms of hysteria, depression, and psychopathy than parents of normal children. While this might suggest that hyperactivity develops because of the modeling and environmental effects these parental psychiatric problems may have on children, other studies do not support this notion. Studies of adoptive parents of hyperactive children do not find any greater prevalence of these psychiatric disorders in these parents than in the parents of normal children. As noted in Chapter 1, these findings strongly intimate an influence that is more hereditary than environmental. These and other investigations have also revealed a greater occurrence of alcoholism and smoking in the parents and relatives of hyperactive children than in either the families of normal children or the adoptive families of hyperactive children.

Recently, Phillip Firestone at the University of Ottawa not only replicated the above findings, but also found the parents of hyperactive children to have more difficulties with attention span and impulse control than adoptive parents of hyperactive children or parents of normal children. These groups were matched on the basis of education, age, and socioeconomic status; these factors were thus ruled out as possible explanations for the results. Parents of hyperactive children therefore seem to be having problems similar to those seen in the children themselves, especially as the children grow older. Finally, Firestone's research has revealed significantly greater marital dissatisfaction among the parents of hyperactive children than among parents in the other control groups noted above. Certainly, hyperactive children born into families where the parents may already be having psychiatric problems are likely to appear very different in their own symptom pictures from children born into families where no such problems exist.

Previous research has also noted that mothers of hyperactive children are likely to be having more difficulties managing such children than their fathers seem to have. While objective observations of these interactional differences remain to be done, rating scales and interview data collected in my own studies seem to bear this out. The reason for this apparent sex difference in parent management of child behavior problems is not known. Perhaps it relates to the fact that most mothers spend more time with their children than fathers do. Or it may be that mothers tend to use an approach based on reasoning with their children, an approach likely to be ineffective with children whose major deficits are in rule-governed behavior. Because fathers may discipline their children more intensely and more quickly for noncompliance than mothers do, they may obtain greater compliance from the children. Finally, it may be that the fathers' relatively greater physical size and strength prompts greater child compliance.

In any event, problems in the marital relationship and in the emotional well-being of the mother are likely to ensue from this discrepancy in child compliance to each parent. I have often encountered fathers who either do not believe that the children have any problems or refuse to admit that the problems are as serious as the mothers may make them out to be. In some cases, the fathers may believe that their wives are overly sensitive to what they themselves see as normal childhood exuberance. This can then lead to insistence by the fathers that their wives, not their children, seek psychiatric help. Since they are able to handle the children, why then can't their wives? At other times, the fathers may feel that their wives are too permissive and that firmer disciplining would make the children "normal." Similar scenes may also be re-enacted with the male pediatricians to whom the mothers go for help, especially since the hyperactive children are much less likely to act up in their offices. The result is that marital difficulties are quite likely to develop around child management issues, unless the fathers and pediatricians can be gotten to accept the idea that the children are probably behaving differently for different adults and really are presenting problems for their mothers.

This discrepancy in child compliance, at times coupled with marital discord, is likely to lead to ever-increasing feelings of frustration, incompetency, and low self-esteem in mothers. In any case, mothers of hyperactive children may see themselves as having more problems than other mothers in handling their children, and thus may believe that they are less capable in their role as parents. The result is frequently maternal depression and low self-image by the time a referral for professional help is elicited. While this may in part explain why mothers of hyperactive children are found to be more depressed than mothers of normal childen, it does not explain why adoptive mothers of hyperactive children are *not* more depressed than mothers of normal children.

Research on the siblings of hyperactive children has only recently begun. One study revealed that as many as 26% of the male siblings of hyperactive boys were also likely to be hyperactive, while only 9% of the male siblings of control children were found to be so. Both hyperactive children and their siblings were observed to be more depressed than control children. Other studies have found aggression and learning problems to be more common in the siblings of hyperactive children than in those of normal children. While these findings may support an hereditary basis for general conduct and learning problems in hyperactive children, they could just as easily suggest that these problems in siblings are the result of having to live with a hyperactive child. In either case, these sibling problems are likely only to add further to the confusion and negativism in the household, especially if the parents are also experiencing psychiatric and/or marital difficulties.

The typical picture of the household in which the hyperactive child resides is one of turmoil. Either as a direct effect of such children's difficult behavior, especially as it may be exacerbated by parental and sibling psychiatric problems, or through the indirect effect of such behavior on the emotional well-being of the parents (particularly the mothers) who must confront these difficulties day in and day out, hyperactive children can create disruptive and aversive family situations. A point to be raised repeatedly throughout this book is that both assessment and treatment tactics for hyperactive children must take this social context into consideration.

A BEHAVIORAL APPROACH TO DEVIANT FAMILY INTERACTIONS

Several promising developments in the objective analysis of parent–child interactions, when taken together, form a useful means of understanding and treating deviant family interactions.

Unidirectionality versus Reciprocity

One of the most influential developments of the past 15 years in research on the socialization of children has been the concept that the effects in parent–child interactions are bidirectional or reciprocal. Set forth most eloquently by Richard Bell of the University of Virginia, the idea was actually proposed as long ago as 1897 by J. M. Baldwin, who stated that a child was both a factor in as well as a product of his socialization experiences. Perhaps because of the complexity of studying the direction of effects in interactions, as well as a lack of proper methodology for doing so, investigators neglected this concept for over 60 years; instead, they focused on the role played by parental variables in determining the socialization and outcome of children.

In 1968, however, Bell forcefully demonstrated that the findings of much of the research on socialization in children that had previously been argued as evidence for the effects of parents on their children could be better understood as the effects of children on their parents. The point was not lost on investigators in the area of normal child development, but it has only been acknowledged within the past few years by many scientists studying abnormal child psychology. The exception to this has been Barclay Martin at the University of North Carolina at Chapel Hill, who for years has stressed the concept of reciprocity in studying deviant family systems. Simply stated, Bell's 1968 paper pointed out that children, including young infants, are not passive recipients of social interactions, as was once believed. The child is not a *tabula rasa* on which the parent shapes and molds an image, but an active participant in social exchanges—one, in fact, whose behavior has substantial stimulus control over parental reactions. As in many areas of the social and biological sciences, this point was accorded great respect by those studying animals before it was accepted by those who study man. Many clinicians still fail to appreciate the role of reciprocity in deviant family systems; abnormal parent–child interactions can as easily be attributed to certain child characteristics as to parental ones. How often have we been wrongfully quick to judge certain negative attributes of parents as causal? In the future, clinicians must heed the findings of their brethren in the basic social sciences and pay attention to the bidirectional effects involved in parent–child relations.

UNDERSTANDING CHILD EFFECTS ON ADULTS

In his 1968 paper, and later in his book with Lawrence Harper in 1977, Bell outlined a model for classifying and understanding the effects which children may have on adults around them. Bell primarily stressed the role of the child in accounting for parental interactions toward the child, not because the influence of the parent was not substantial, but because 60 years of research had overemphasized this influence and virtually ignored child effects on parents. While similar stress on child effects is given here, it should be made clear at the outset that both the parent and the child make substantial contributions to their social exchanges.

These disclaimers aside, the model proposed by Bell indicates that adults, parents in particular, have expectations or thresholds for a child's behavior in a given situation. If a child's behavior is inappropriately excessive in terms of frequency, duration, intensity, or age-appropriateness for a given situation, it is said to exceed that parent's "upper limit threshold." In contrast, when a child's behavior is deemed by a parent to be inappropriately deficient along the same parameters, it is said to exceed the parent's "lower limit threshold." Such thresholds or expectations may obviously differ across settings, parents, and time. According to Bell, the reactions of a parent to a child will differ quite radically, depending on which, if any, of these thresholds is violated by the child's behavior.

In the case where the child's behavior exceeds the upper limit threshold of the parent because it is excessive, high-rate, or aversive, the parent is likely to respond with "upper limit controls." Such controls frequently consist initially of ignoring the child's behavior, but they almost always progress to restrictive commands, negative affect, and even physical disciplining of the child. Bell is quick to point out that he is not yet specifying *why* parents respond in this manner to excessive child behavior. His system at this point is meant merely to be descriptive, not to address the functions of parent or child behavior. From a behavioral perspective, parental control behaviors may be emitted in response to excessive child behaviors because of their history of affecting such child behaviors. While Bell avoids this sort of functional analysis, the work of Gerald Patterson and others has not, and these notions are discussed later in this chapter. For the moment, Bell's model would predict that hyperactive behavior from a child would elicit parental upper limit controls.

Where the child's behavior remains within the parental expectations or limits, parental reactions are likely to consist of positive interactions, questioning, occasional praise, and perhaps mild physical affection. Bell has termed such behaviors "equilibrium controls" by the parent. Again, they are perhaps manifested by parents because of a prior learning history of success at maintaining ongoing appropriate child behaviors, though Bell himself does not offer any explanation for the parental reactions.

In the instance where the child's behavior falls below the parent's lower limit threshold, the parent will emit "lower limit controls." Such reactions seem to consist of drawing the child's attention to activities, coaxing, questioning, prompting, and encouraging, as well as providing provocative commands and physical guidance to the child. These behaviors seem designed to increase the behavior that appears infrequent or unresponsive in the child, and they are often seen in parents of retarded or language-delayed children.

Bell has also noted that parental reactions are probably hierarchically and sequentially organized such that when initial reactions prove unsuccessful, other reactions next in the hierarchy of that set of control behaviors will be emitted. Should no behaviors within the parental repertoire serve to affect a child's behavior, it is likely that disengagement from and future avoidance of the child will be the result.

The model set forth above stresses the child's behavior as the antecedent to parental reactions and places the child in a central position as controller over subsequent interaction sequences. It should be recalled, however, that such social exchanges have reciprocal influences. Thus, child behaviors may elicit particular parental responses, but these in turn will affect subsequent child behaviors to some degree. The selection of one person in the dyad as having the greater influence in the interaction sequence is not necessarily arbitrary, as it may at first seem. Studies in child development have attempted to isolate the effects of certain characteristics of children on adults, and vice versa, to determine the direction of effects. This research suggests that, while both parent and child influence each other, certain behaviors and charac-teristics of one person may have a disproportionate causal influence on the reactions of the other in certain exchanges. This research, however, is a long way from cataloging a common set of characteristics and their degree of influence.

Recent research in mine and other laboratories provides substantial support for Bell's descriptive model, especially with respect to hyperactive children. In some of the first studies of the parent–child interactions of hyperactive children, Susan Campbell (1975) compared the mother–child interactions of hyperactive, learning-disabled, and control children during accomplishment of a series of tasks. The results suggested that hyperactive children were more likely to request help from their mothers and to be more noncompliant than the other groups of children. The mothers of hyperactive children were more likely to engage in commands and directives and to give more help and encouragement than mothers of the other children. More recently, Charles Cunningham and I compared the mother–child interac-tions of hyperactive and normal children during both a task situation and in free play. These results are set forth in Table 2.1 and indicate that hyperactive boys were more negative and less compliant in both situations than normal boys. The mothers of hyperactive boys gave more commands and negatives and were less responsive to their sons' interactions than mothers of normal boys. While it is possible, as Bell would suggest, that the noncompliance of the hyperactive child leads the mother to be more directive and negative, it is equally possible that the mother's directiveness provokes the child's non-compliance. The results of these studies cannot address this issue of causality or direction of effects in the interactions.

However, a series of studies in my own laboratory, as well as subsequent studies by Thomas Humphries, Marcel Kinsbourne, and James Swanson (1978) at the Hospital for Sick Children in Toronto, have addressed this issue. These studies examined the effects of stimulant drugs on the mother–child interactions of hyperactive children. If the child's behavior is the result of parental directiveness, then reducing the child's hyperactivity with stimu-lant medication should result in little change in parental behaviors. But, if the mother's directiveness is in fact a response to her child's excessive behavior, as Bell's model suggests, then decreasing the child's excessive

TABLE 2.1. Results for the Comparison of the Mother–Child Interactions of Hyperactive and Normal Children during Free Play and Task

Behavioral measure	Normal[a]	Hyperactive[a]	p
Free-play setting			
Mother initiates interaction	54.3	37.4	.01
Child responds	83.9	93.9	.01
Child initiates interaction	67.7	60.9	NS[b]
Mother responds	91.8	67.3	.01
Child plays independently	29.9	35.2	NS
Mother encourages play	53.2	22.5	.01
Mother controls play	6.1	27.9	.01
Task setting			
Mother commands	21.3	40.8	.01
Child complies	95.4	70.5	.01
Compliance duration	8.9	4.9	.01
Mother rewards compliance	9.1	4.3	.01

Note. From "The Parent–Child Interactions of Hyperactive Children and Their Modification by Stimulant Drugs" by R. Barkley and C. Cunningham. In R. Knights and D. Bakker (Eds.), *Treatment of Hyperactive and Learning Disordered Children.* Baltimore: University Park Press, 1980. Copyright 1980 by University Park Press. Reprinted by permission.

[a]All measures are presented as percentages of total number of interactions or as conditional percentages within a given type of interaction: for example, the child complies 95.4% of the time to the mother's commands for the normal mother–child dyads. Mean compliance duration represents the number of intervals of child compliance divided by the number of intervals of mother commands.

[b]NS indicates that the means are statistically not significantly different.

behavior should reduce maternal directiveness. The findings from this area of research are best illustrated in a study we conducted with two hyperactive identical twin boys and their mother. Each boy was observed individually with his mother in both free-play and task periods on four different occasions. Using a double-blind drug–placebo reversal design, the boys were placed on and off Ritalin, a stimulant drug, across the four observation sessions. The results appear in Figure 2.1. These findings clearly indicate that, in this case, the mother's directiveness was a reaction to her boys' excessive behavior. When medication reduced the hyperactive behavior and increased compliance, the mother dramatically reduced her level of commands. These results have been replicated several times, using larger groups of hyperactive children and studying both mother–child and teacher–child interactions.

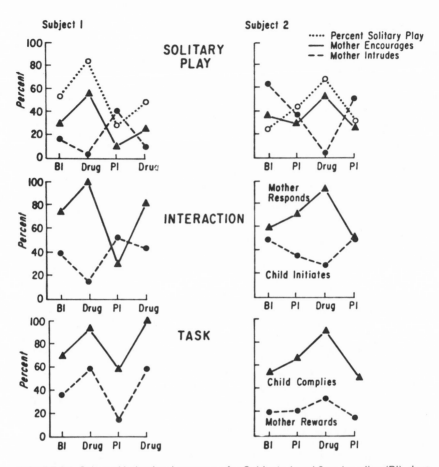

FIGURE 2.1. Selected behavioral measures for Subjects 1 and 2 on baseline (BI), drug, and placebo (PI) sessions. Solitary play and interaction measures were derived from the free-play periods. Task measures were calculated from the structured task situations. (From "The Effects of Ritalin on the Mother–Child Interactions of Hyperkinetic Twin Boys" by C. E. Cunningham and R. A. Barkley, *Developmental Medicine and Child Neurology*, 1978, *20*, 634–642. Copyright 1978 by Spastics International Medical Publications. Reprinted by permission.)

As this study suggests, parent and child behaviors are best viewed as a reciprocal feedback system in which the behavior of one person serves as both a controlling stimulus and a consequating event for the responses of the other. It further serves to underscore the notion that the child's behavior exerts a great deal of control over parental responses, in addition to the traditional view that parental behaviors influence child responses.

My own clinical and research work with hyperactive children has helped to clarify the hierarchy of responses through which parents are likely to progress, should earlier behaviors prove unsuccessful in controlling the child's excessive behavior. Initially, parents seem to try to ignore, or withhold attention from, hyperactive behavior. As the child's behavior intensifies, parents are likely to give frequent restrictive commands, often repeating them five or more times before becoming more upset. Such commands may then be coupled with threats of disciplining, which may be repeated several times. Parents may then progress to disciplining the child physically or to acquiescing with the behavior insofar as their commands and threats go unenforced. The parents may even comply with their own commands—they may wind up picking up the child's toys themselves, for example. Over time, parents do not continue to start at the beginning of this hierarchy with each new instance of hyperkinetic or inappropriate behavior. Instead, they are likely to dispense with those controlling behaviors that were unsuccessful and to begin at that level of the hierarchy at which they last succeeded to any small degree. Some parents may show intense anger or physical disciplining of a child when hyperactive behaviors occur—responses that, on the face of it, seem too intense for the child's inappropriate behavior. Yet, if one considers the parents' learning history with respect to this child, it may be that other, less intense types of reacting to misbehavior have met with little success. Intense initial reactions may therefore be the only even partially successful management tactic the parents have. Or the parents may simply acquiesce or fail to confront the child for noncompliance. Such an approach may be successful for the parent only in that it reduces the likelihood of intense confrontations with the child, keeping the level of tension within the family lower than if disciplining were used.

While we do not have sufficient scientific data to support the point, it is our contention that some parents of hyperactive children eventually wind up in a response pattern known as "learned helplessness" with respect to managing the child's behavior. In this condition, parents make no, or very few, efforts to give or enforce commands to the children, leaving them in essence to do as they please. This seems to be the final state for parents, culminating a long history of difficult interactions with the children, in which few if any tactics for managing the children have proved at all effective. Along the way, such parents become progressively more disengaged from the children, monitoring behavior and confronting transgressions less and less, until little if any supervision is exerted over the children's hyperactive behaviors. "Learned helplessness," as the term is applied here to severe child management cases, is seen as the result of failure to effect change in children's behavior in spite of all previous efforts by the parents to cope. At this point the parents, especially mothers, are clinically depressed, showing very low self-esteem and displaying few reactions toward the children, either positive or negative.

That such a condition may develop for some mothers was supported by data I collected on 68 hyperactive boys and their mothers during free-play and task situations. These data showed that mothers of older hyperactive children (ages 8–12 years) spent less time interacting with or supervising their children's play and compliance than mothers of younger hyperactive boys (ages 4–7 years). In addition, the mothers of the older boys were much less responsive to those positive interactions and questions initiated by their boys than were mothers of the younger boys. This pattern suggests a progressive disengagement of mothers from their hyperactive children over time.

On many occasions, I have witnessed clinicians who, after observing mothers in this pattern of acquiescence or disengagement, leap to blame such mothers for the children's behavior problems because of their apparent incompetence or unwillingness to manage the children. Such clinicians ignore the years of learning history the mothers have acquired in social exchanges with the child and assume that they are ignorant of or deficient in appropriate child management methods. The mothers' deficits are quickly pointed out to them, and training in child behavior modification (using positive reinforcement and parental ignoring) is quickly begun, with the therapists secure in the knowledge that they are on the right track with these families. In such cases, therapy may fail outright or show only temporary and superficial progress. Specific reasons for such failure and better approaches to therapy are given later in this chapter. For now, suffice it to say that such a clinical approach has (1) ignored the parents' learning history with the children; (2) assumed a deficiency in child management skills where none may actually have existed; (3) ignored the mothers' own depression, low self-esteem, and general emotional status; (4) possibly contributed further to maternal depression by implicitly criticizing the mothers' prior efforts at management; (5) assumed that the children's misbehavior is motivated by a desire to gain attention; and (6) ignored the contributions made to the situation by other intra- and extrafamilial factors.

How might such negative interactions develop, and what maintains them? Despite the fact that child or family therapists would have a wide range of opinion on this point, there is very little objective data to address the question. Probably the most large-scale studies of the matter have been conducted by Gerald Patterson and his colleagues at the Oregon Research Institute, who have proposed a coercion theory of aggressive–aversive child behaviors.

Coercion Theory

Patterson's work on aggressive child behavior has spanned 15 years or more, making it the most enduring and prolific series of investigations in this literature. Although referred to as "aggressive," the children and adolescents studied by Patterson show a variety of behaviors that could be called

TABLE 2.2. Parent-Rated Aversive Behaviors

Negative response to command	Noncompliance
Crying	Negativism
Disapproval	Physical negative response to command
Dependency	Teasing
Destructiveness	Whining
High-rate behavior	Yelling
Humiliation of others	Social aggression
Ignoring others	Hostility

Note. Adapted from "The Aggressive Child: Victim and Architect of a Coercive System" by G. R. Patterson. In E. J. Mash, L. A. Hamerlynck, and L. C. Handy (Eds.), *Behavior Modification and Families.* New York: Brunner/Mazel, 1976.

hyperactive. In fact, it is quite likely that the majority of these children would be diagnosed as hyperactive by other clinicians.

In the early studies, Patterson set out to define the nature of aggressive-aversive child behaviors and to understand their development and maintenance within the context of family interaction patterns. An objective, reliable, and highly specific observation coding system was developed for recording interactions among family members. It was unique for its coding of sequential interactions, giving the ability to study reciprocity between family members in their interactions. A list of 16 negative child behaviors was developed as part of the coding system; the basis for selecting these behaviors was the belief that parents and siblings would generally view such behaviors as aversive. These behaviors are listed in Table 2.2.

In order to determine whether others in fact believed these child behaviors to be aversive, Patterson had mothers of both normal and clinic-referred children rate these behaviors as to their perceived aversiveness. All of the behaviors classified as negative by the coding system were in fact judged by the parents of both groups to be quite aversive. Patterson, however, also required that aversive events be defined as events that people would attempt to escape from or avoid, and, that furthermore, as events that would reduce the probability of a subsequent occurrence of some behavior when they occurred following that behavior. Studies by the Patterson group showed that in normal families these aversive behaviors did indeed tend to suppress the behaviors of other family members that they followed.

With this highly rigorous and specific observation system, Patterson went about recording numerous hours of family interactions, primarily within the homes of many families referred to the clinic for children with negative and aggressive behaviors. Patterson's initial hypothesis, like that of many clinicians, was that these negative child behaviors were motivated by "positive reinforcement." That is, they occurred because of the increased social attention and positive consequences they brought the child. It was logically assumed that if one ignored the occurrence of these aversive child behaviors, they would extinguish or diminish because they no longer brought positive reinforcement to the child. This initial working hypothesis was later radically altered because of the failure of the data on family interactions to support it. Whereas parental punishment of negative child behaviors in normal children tends to suppress the behaviors or at least to reduce their likelihood of recurring, Patterson found that the opposite seemed to occur with the clinic-referred children. Parental punishment appeared to accelerate or increase aversive child behaviors. Such aversive behaviors, when they occurred, had a "bursting" quality in that they were highly likely to continue once emitted. Patterson also noted that parental commands were likely to produce negative or aversive child behaviors, and that their rate of occurrence was likely to be even higher if the command was accompanied by disapproval. Finally, both Patterson and others began to find that training families of children with severe behavior problems to ignore negative behaviors in the children actually resulted in *increased* negative behavior. Clearly the notion that negative child behaviors are motivated by positive reinforcement required some modification. This is not to say that some aversive child behaviors are not positively motivated—only that such motivation does not account for many such child behaviors in the families of aggressive children.

Patterson and his colleagues then proposed that aversive child behaviors may be under the control of negative reinforcement. In learning theory, "negative reinforcement" occurs when an ongoing aversive event (say, electric shock) is terminated by the occurrence of a particular behavior (say, pressing a lever). In this case, the probability of a recurrence of behavior that terminated the aversive event will increase in future such situations and is said to be negatively reinforced. The concept seems to apply to the data on aversive child interactions. Patterson hypothesized that parental *and sibling* aversive behaviors, such as commands, disapproval, negative behavior, and aggression, are emitted toward aggressive children. Such children may respond toward other family members by emitting aversive, aggressive, or negative behavior of their own. If this reaction is successful in terminating the aversive behaviors of others toward these children, then the children's aggression has been negatively reinforced. Hence, in subsequent similar situations, aversive child behaviors would increase in probability. The children's aversive/aggressive behavior becomes a successful means of coping within such families. Their negative behavior is said to "coerce" other family members into discontinuing their aversive behavior toward them.

The wealth of data on family interactions produced by Patterson and others appears to support the idea that, in some families, certain aversive child behaviors are developed and maintained by the operation of negative reinforcement. For one thing, Patterson has shown that parental commands, disapproval, and punishment within those interactions only serves to accelerate aggressive child behaviors further rather than to diminish them. On many occasions, the aversive child behaviors, such as whining, are quite successful at terminating parental commands and disciplining. Furthermore, efforts to teach parents to ignore such child behaviors, as noted above, have resulted in increased negative behaviors in some children. Patterson has also shown that, even in normal children, manipulating parental behaviors so that commands or disapproval are terminated by negative child behaviors can result in a dramatic increase in the negative behaviors in as few as four learning trials. Finally, when the rates of each type of negative child behavior in clinic families were examined, those followed by the least amount of parental punishment occurred most frequently, as would be expected. That is, the negative behaviors that were more successful occurred more often.

THE DEVELOPMENT OF COERCIVE CHILD BEHAVIORS

Patterson suggests that by 3 to 4 years of age, most normal children have acquired a wide range of coercive behaviors, although they do not display them in most situations because of parental sanctions against them. Such behaviors are probably acquired through direct experience with other children, watching such displays of coercive exchanges on television, or observing them firsthand with siblings or other people. Patterson reports that normal children seem to increase their use of coercive behaviors until they are approximately 4 years of age, when such behaviors begin to decline. Perhaps this decrease is the result of increased efforts by parents to suppress such behaviors because of their recognized inappropriateness for the children's age. For whatever reason, this decrease is contrary to what has been observed in clinic-referred children, in whom coercive behaviors occur at high rates well into the later childhood years.

Patterson has argued that children develop aggressive–coercive behaviors because of their effectiveness within a family system in which most members are displaying high rates of commands, disapproval, and generally aversive behaviors. As evidence of this, Patterson points to the data that show that other family members of aggressive children do indeed show higher than normal levels of aversive behaviors. The family system is therefore viewed as the primary etiology in developing aggressive child behavior. Whether children display such coercive behaviors initially at school, in the neighborhood, or at home toward siblings is not important, as the behaviors may eventually be used within the home toward parents. Presumably, after being exposed to the aversive or aggressive behavior of others, such children emit aversive responses of their own as a counteroffensive. The other individuals then terminate their aversive behavior, and the children have now been negatively reinforced for reacting with coercive behaviors. As shown earlier, after a few such learning trials, such children will develop a high probability for displaying aggression or coercion in response to others.

While this hypothesis for developing coercive behaviors probably applies to some children, it is certainly not the only possible manner of generating such behaviors. Other avenues for developing coercive behaviors must be invoked to account for what is known about hyperactive children. First, not all parents or siblings of hyperactive children seem to show high rates of coercive behaviors toward each other in addition to those displayed toward the coercive hyperactive child. My own studies comparing the interactions of mothers with their hyperactive children to those of the same mothers with normal siblings reveal that these mothers resemble normal mothers when interacting with the normal siblings. This contrasts with the high rates of commands and negative behaviors shown by the mothers toward the hyperactive child. Second, the management styles of mothers of hyperactive boys more closely resemble those of mothers of normal boys when the hyperactive children are placed on medication. And, third, hyperactivity would not show as much, if any, heritability if the environment were the sole contributor to the child's coercive behaviors.

In our view, it is certainly plausible that some hyperactive children develop their aversive behaviors in the manner outlined by Patterson, especially given the higher level of conduct and psychiatric problems in their parents. Such parents may in fact show high levels of aversive behavior toward all members of the family system. Hyperactive children may also be more likely to develop coercive behavioral repertoires because of their high rates of activity, poor attention, high impulsivity, poor compliance, and poor rule-governed behavior. Irrespective of the etiology of the hyperactivity, the hyperactive behaviors themselves predispose these children to emit behaviors that could potentially develop into a coercive interaction pattern with others. This, of course, would hinge on the reaction of others to these potentially coercive behaviors. In families who capitulate to the initial aversive child behaviors, coercive patterns of interaction could easily develop.

It should be noted that this explanation distinguishes between "hyperactive" and "coercive" behaviors. Each can occur without the other, or, as just discussed, they can occur together. "Hyperactive" behaviors are those noted earlier to consist of higher than normal rates of inattention, impulsivity, and noncompliance that have an early onset in development and are cross-situational in nature. Whether these behaviors result in the termination of aversive behavior by others is not relevant to the diagnosis. "Coercive" behaviors, on the other hand, are those aversive or high-rate behaviors that are developed and maintained by their negatively reinforced effects. That hyperactive children may be more likely to utilize coercion is quite possible, but coercive children need not be hyperactive, at least as hyperactivity is defined in Chapter 1. The overlap between these two populations of children may, however, be considerable. In any case, regardless of the initial factors that lead children to emit their first potentially coercive responses, the eventual development and maintenance of these responses can be accounted for on the basis of negative reinforcement as explained by Patterson.

THE REINFORCEMENT TRAP

Patterson points out that, in some family systems, coercive child behaviors may prove effective not only in terminating parental aversive behaviors, but also in obtaining positive parental attention and other reinforcers. For instance, a mother may begin to give a child a series of restrictive commands and disapproval for a given misbehavior. The child reacts by whining, berating the mother, and yelling, and perhaps by stomping his or her feet and throwing things. The mother responds by ceasing her commands and threats and leaving the situation. This is a typical coercive interaction. But if, rather than leaving, the mother responds by saying she is sorry, offering to play with the child, and displaying physical affection, a "reinforcement trap" has developed. The child's coercion will be both negatively reinforced by the cessation of maternal disapproval and positively reinforced by the simultaneous provision of attention to the child. The mother is more likely to display her acquiescent–apologetic behavior in future situations, as it has also been negatively reinforced by the discontinuation of the child's temper tantrum. Patterson indicates that such behavior by the mother may in fact shorten the *duration* of coercive interactions when they occur, but will actually increase the likelihood of their occurring in future situations in which the mother gives commands or disapproval to the child. Hence, the mother's acquiescence, while apparently an effective response in the immediate context, is counterproductive in the long run. Like her child, she is both victim and architect of the coercive family interaction pattern in which she finds herself.

FURTHER ASPECTS OF COERCION THEORY

As stated above, both child and parental behaviors in coercive exchanges can be developed and maintained by the operation of negative reinforcement. This fact leads to the all-too-likely possibility that parents themselves may develop coercive behavior strategies in dealing with aversive child behaviors. Instead of capitulating to their children's aversive behavior, parents may respond with more intense aversive behaviors of their own. Such a reaction by the parents need only be successful part of the time to insure its recurrence. In cases in which both parent and child aversive responses are developed from a history of partial success in causing the other to terminate aggression, rapid bursts in coercive exchanges may occur between parent and child, for the aversive behavior by one only serves to *increase* the likelihood of an aversive response by the other. That these bursts of mutually coercive exchanges can lead to inordinately long negative exchanges between parent and child has been effectively supported by Patterson's data. These research findings have shown that an aversive behavior by one member of the dyad may double the likelihood of an aversive response by the other, which itself increases the probability of further aversive reactions by the first person. The results have also revealed that, once an aversive behavior is emitted by one person, the best prediction of the way in which the person will behave in subsequent time intervals is that the aversive behavior will be continued. This phenomenon, known as "bursting" or "chunking" of coercive behaviors, is an important revelation in the Patterson data and requires understanding by those who would attempt to treat coercive children and their families.

Besides increasing in frequency, these mutually coercive, negatively reinforced exchanges increase in intensity over time as well. Studying this possibility has been difficult because of the problems inherent in measuring "intensity" of responding. Nonetheless, it is generally accepted that such interactions may well escalate in "intensity" as each member becomes more aversive, louder, and more intense in his or her reactions to antecedent aversive behaviors by the other. Such escalation may lead quite plausibly to physical injury to the parent or physical abuse of the child.

The principles of mutual coercion and escalation of intensity raise the question of the ways in which such exchanges eventually terminate. Patterson offers the observation that each person must be at least occasionally successful at coercion, or termination of the other's aversiveness, if these exchanges are to continue. At some point, therefore, each must play victim to the other's coercion. Patterson believes that who the victim will be may be determined in part by the rapidity with which each person escalates to intensely aversive behaviors and by the ultimate level of that intensity. In short, the person who escalates most rapidly in intensity of negative behavior will cause the other to concede. These concepts overlap with the idea of hierarchically organized parental upper limit controls, as discussed by Bell and reviewed earlier in this chapter. It may also explain why, in this hierarchy many parents vacillate between aggression and acquiescence toward negative child behaviors.

Like almost all parents, those of coercive children are likely to show inconsistency in using punishment for coercive child behavior. Patterson believes that in such cases where inconsistency is high, the eventual use of consistent punishment for coercion will prove less effective with the child than it might if it had been used consistently from the beginning. This relates to the well-known observation that partial or intermittent schedules of consequences result in behaviors less likely to diminish than those developed by consistent or continuous schedules. In other words, if the child is even partly successful at coercing parental reactions, then the child will continue the coercive behavior in the face of intermittent punishment.

Another important aspect of coercive child interaction patterns is that they do not necessarily show generalization to other settings. Patterson reports that almost all coercive behaviors show little correlation between home and school settings. Children more likely to use coercion at home are not necessarily as likely to employ it at school, and vice versa. This is hardly unexpected, since coercion depends on the reactions of others, and the people with whom the child interacts in one setting are likely to react differently from those in the other setting. Coercion, then, like hyperactivity, varies across situations, depending on the persons with whom the child interacts. There appears to be one exception to this observation, and that is for child noncompliance. Patterson has found a significant positive relationship between noncompliance at home and at school. This agrees with our previous published data and that of Rex Forehand and his associates at the University of Georgia (1979), which revealed that parental ratings and direct observations of noncompliance at home were significantly predictive of noncompliance in clinic playroom situations used to observe parent–child interactions.

Besides differences in settings and personalities that affect the appearance of coercive–aversive child behaviors, other factors may influence the occurrence of such behavior. A review of the situations in which hyperactive children are more likely to present problems, described in Chapter 1, suggests that aversive child behaviors are more likely to occur (1) when a child is with the mother rather than the father; (2) when the situation is familiar rather than novel for the child; (3) when there is less likelihood of adult supervision; (4) when there is less likelihood of punishment for these behaviors; (5) when the setting places great demands for self-control on the child; and (6) when there is a high rate of positive social exchanges between other people while the child is present.

LONG-TERM EFFECTS OF COERCIVE FAMILY INTERACTIONS

A number of consequences seem to develop over long periods of time in which high-rate, coercive interaction patterns occur. Obviously, reduced levels of positive consequences are being exchanged among family members. As a result, feelings of frustration and of lack of appreciation are likely to develop in both the parents and the children. In addition, high rates of negative behavior that can only add to the tension within the home are being maintained. Family members begin to disengage from one another, often decreasing the amount of recreational time they spend together. Eventually, low self-esteem and depression develop in those members, especially the mothers, who spend a disproportionate share of their time as victims of the coercion. This may in turn reflect itself in greater marital dissatisfaction and divorce in these families. Furthermore, Patterson has shown that the children increasingly devalue their parents' positive attention when it does occur. That is, the effect of such attention on the child may be minimal in comparison to similar attention given by individuals outside the family. All of these factors need to be considered when designing interventions for hyperactive, coercive children.

OTHER FACTORS INFLUENCING PARENT-CHILD INTERACTIONS

In addition to the reactions of parent and child to each other, factors outside their specific interactions may have some influence upon these interactions. Some of these factors have been better studied than others, especially those that seem to affect a parent's ability to care for and interact with a child. This probably results from the considerably greater interest over the last 60 years in parental effects on children than in child effects on parents. The pendulum of research focus has swung the other way now, and we are likely to see an increasing amount of literature in the near future on child variables and their effects on family interactions.

Parent Variables

Many factors affecting the parent seem to have some modulating effect, even if indirect, on a parent's interactions with a child. Chief among these factors seem to be socioeconomic status, intelligence, and educational attainment. Research has repeatedly demonstrated that socioeconomic factors are strong predictors of a child's eventual academic, social, and occupational outcome. More specifically, lower-class parents show different interaction patterns from those of middle-class parents; lower-class parents are generally less rewarding and nurturant and more quick to discipline. Although this point is not well studied, parents of lesser intelligence and educational level may reflect less upon the best ways to respond to child behaviors, especially deviant ones.

Physical characteristics of parents, such as age, sex, physical constitution, and health, must certainly have some direct or indirect influences on the ways in which parents respond to child behavior. Very young or very old parents are likely to show unique patterns of interacting with children in comparison to parents in the typical child-bearing years. The direction these differential effects may take is not known, though clinical lore suggests that parents in late middle age or retirement years may be less likely to discipline a child for misbehavior. In Chapter 1 and earlier in this chapter, differences in interaction patterns related to the sex of parents were discussed. It seems that mothers are more likely to experience problems in managing deviant child behaviors than fathers. Recent research also suggests that parents of the same sex as the child are likely to show more direction and control over that child's behavior than over that of an opposite-sex child. A parent's general physical endowment or constitution may place broad limits on the types of activities in which the parent is able to engage with the child. Finally, health and general physical well-being influence the way in which one treats a child, as is well known to any parent who has had a cold or headache and yet still has had to deal with one or more children. While periodic illnesses of the typical sort may leave only transient effects on parental reactions to children, chronic, more widespread, or more serious illnesses may drastically alter parent–child interactions in a more enduring way. One parent in our clinic who suffered from lupus remarked that she was simply too tired to chase after her child to discipline him for transgressions. In other cases, parents with recurrent migraine headaches have remarked that they must frequently disengage completely from interactions with their children because of their temporary yet pervasive debilitation with the headache. The list of medical maladies and handicapping conditions that could potentially affect parental exchanges with children is virtually endless. The point to be made here is simply that such conditions require more consideration than is typically given by clinicians who strive to evaluate deviant child behaviors.

Related to medical and health concerns is the issue of those parents who use behavior-modifying drugs, whether for medical, social, or recreational ends. Given the reciprocity which exists in parent–child interactions, substances that alter parental behavior are obviously going to have some effect on the way in which the child is treated, and also on the way in which the child responds to the parent. Currently, we are not aware of any literature on behavior-modifying substances that has examined in any objective or rigorous way the manners in which such substances specifically alter parent–child interactions. In one unpublished clinical case, I studied the effects of diazepam (Valium), an antianxiety agent, on the interactions of a mother and her unmedicated hyperactive son. The results are tentative and should be viewed cautiously because of the lack of a completely experimental design to evaluate the drug's effects. Double-blind drug–placebo procedures were utilized, however, and the results, displayed in Table 2.3, are quite intriguing. It can be seen that Valium appeared to reduce this mother's high level of commands and negative behavior toward the child, while also decreasing her positive interactions. In turn, her child's noncompliance and negative behavior improved somewhat, suggesting that they were, in part, a reaction to the mother's directive style. The child's attention span and activity level were not visibly improved, however, which suggests that the drug had only reduced

TABLE 2.3. Effects of Valium on Mother-Child Interactions

Measure	Baseline[a]	Drug[a]	Placebo[a]
Mother interacts	37	40	27
Child responds	86	100	88
Mother directs	27	13	32
Child complies[b]	44	75	32
Mother behaves negatively	12	2	12
Child behaves negatively	12	2	23
Child total compliance[c]	35	77	32
Mother responds positively	14	7	26
Mother responds negatively	48	22	42

[a]All measures are presented as percentages of total number of interactions or as conditional percentages within a given type of interaction.
[b]This measure refers to the percentage of mother commands to which the child complies.
[c]This measure refers to the total percentage of possible interactions in which the child is scored as complying.

the mother's likelihood of confronting the child's transgressions or supervising his compliance. Nevertheless, any substance, such as alcohol, caffeine, tranquilizers, or stimulants, may have some effect on parental exchanges with children. What these effects and their long-range implications are can only be conjectured. Still, they must be given some consideration by clinicians who find that such drugs are being used in families with deviant children.

Affective, emotional, or psychiatric disorders in parents must surely make the manner in which those parents react to their children different from that of parents without such disorders. Such variables are important to consider, since they are more likely to occur in parents of hyperactive children. Mothers of hyperactive children are often more depressed than those of normal children. Whether this is a reaction to a chronic history of inability to manage the child or an endogenous disorder in the mother, it will have some effect on the way in which she responds to the child. Hysteria, or a tendency to overreact emotionally to events, is also more common in these mothers, perhaps leading them to discipline misbehavior too frequently or to overindulge the child with affection and permissiveness. That the greater impulsivity and inattention in some parents of hyperactive children might alter their interactions toward their children is certainly plausible. Whatever the psychiatric problem, it must be weighed if present in the drawing of clinical judgments about the deviant family interactions. Research is sorely needed on the manner in which such characteristics of parents specifically influence parent-child relations.

There is no question that marital problems and dissatisfaction alter the patterns of interactions within families. Again the exact nature of these effects has been the object of much debate but little study among child clinicians. As noted earlier, parents of hyperactive children are likely to report more marital dissatisfaction than parents of normal children report. While this may well stem from the disagreements in child management that might arise with a hyperactive child, similar marital problems in adoptive parents of hyperactive children are not seen to any significant degree. In either case, marital problems deserve some attention in assessing families of hyperactive children. This is made all the more important by studies (corroborated by my own clinical experiences) that find marital problems one of the most important predictors of failure in coping with developmental problems and in responding to parent training programs. It is my practice not to undertake child management training with parents with whom serious marital problems are occurring—at least not until they have been resolved.

According to clinical lore, a number of other factors seem to play a role in the ways in which parents manage their children. This may occur through the way in which these factors change parental attitudes and expectations toward or knowledge of child behavior and its management. In any event, they deserve attention from investigators who study parent–child relations. Among these factors are relatives and friends and the problems or stresses that may result from their interaction with the parents. Other factors are the religion of the parents and the stresses presented by various types of parental occupations, as well as the previous experience of the parents with children and the fact whether this child's pregnancy was planned or accidental.

One possible factor, related to those above, that has received some attention is the "insularity" of the mother in terms of her extrafamilial interactions and activities. Robert Wahler at the University of Tennessee (1975) classified mothers of deviant children as "insular" or "noninsular." "Insular" mothers were those who had few social contacts outside of the family and few nonfamily activities. "Noninsular" mothers were those having higher levels of extrafamilial social exchanges. Wahler found that insular mothers were likely to have more serious behavior problems with their children and to have less success in child management training than noninsular mothers. While these results may suggest that the decreased community contacts result in the greater problems with children and poorer response to parent training in these mothers, the data are correlational and may indicate just the opposite. That is, they could mean that parents of more seriously deviant children are unable to socialize outside their families as much as those with less seriously deviant children because their children present greater difficulties for baby-sitters or in public situations. It might therefore be the child's deviant behavior that interferes with the family's socializing and hence restricts it. Similarly, more deviant children would be expected to have a poorer response to treatment programs. Again, as Bell has shown us, the direction of effects in such correlational findings is not at all clear. Studies that directly manipulate parental social contacts outside the family and measure subsequent changes in deviant family interactions would seem highly desirable in answering this question.

Finally, certain variables associated with the conditions of the setting in which the parent–child interactions take place must have some influence on how parents respond to their children, and vice versa. Such things as temperature, ambient noise level, number of other people in the room (degree of crowding, visitors versus family members, etc.), and type of activity in which a parent was engaged immediately before or during an interaction with a child could conceivably have some effect on the interactions. For instance, some research suggests that parents are likely to interact more positively with children when they know they are being observed than when they are unaware of such observations. Similar effects might occur within the home when visitors are there or when a parent is in a public place, such as a store. The direction of effects that these factors would have on family interactions is not known but seems deserving of attention.

Child Variables

Equally important to a complete understanding of parent–child interactions are those variables which influence, either directly or indirectly, the interactions of children with their parents. In some cases, these factors remarkably resemble those already discussed as parent variables. For instance, children's general health and the occurrence of illnesses can affect their interactions with others as much as these factors in others can alter their interactions with the children. Again, chronic illness probably creates more widespread and enduring changes in children's interactions than do transient illnesses. Related to this, of course, are the children's physical characteristics and general constitution. Smaller, weaker children or those with physical handicaps may interact differently with parents than do those children without such characteristics. A critical aspect of these factors and those discussed below is the general effect of physical development or maturation on children's ability to interact with others. The changing status of the children across their development may, apart from these other factors, exert unique effects on parent–child relations. This was seen in the preliminary results of an unpublished study in which I compared the mother–child interactions of hyperactive and normal children across five age levels (years 5 to 9). It was observed that hyperactive and normal children differed in their social interactions, as noted earlier, but in no instance were the groups different in the ways in which they changed with age. All children showed greater on-task behavior and compliance with age, while their mothers showed less commanding and less negative reactions to poor-quality compliance.

Related to these health and development factors are those effects associated with drug treatment of children, especially the use of psychotropic medications. It was shown earlier in this chapter that using Ritalin with hyperactive children resulted not only in changes in their behavior but also in the manner in which they are treated by their mothers. Other drugs used to alter behavior would also seem to influence parent–child interactions, though the specific effects await investigation.

Children's intellectual ability has been shown to influence their social interactions with parents, just as this factor in parents influences interactions with children. Retarded children interact less with and ask fewer questions of their parents than do normal children. They are also more likely to be noncompliant with parental requests. Similarly, levels of specific mental abilities such as language ability, also affect the children's interaction patterns with others. Perhaps because social interactions rely quite heavily on language, children delayed in this ability show social interactions that are similar in some respects to those of retarded children. It is often believed that school achievement might affect a child's relations with his parents. Those who do poorly in school may reflect their frustration, depression, and low self-image in their manner of interacting with their parents.

Research has shown that the temperament of children may influence their reactions toward their parents. This has been more widely studied with infants. Temperament, as described in Chapter 1, is comprised of a child's regularity of eating and sleeping habits, emotionality (response to stimulation), sociability, and activity level. Children who are colicky, show night waking, or have short sleep patterns are likely to be treated by their parents differently from those who do not have these problems. This is especially true in those interactions surrounding feeding and sleeping periods. Similarly, children who are irritable, less likely to initiate social exchanges, or more active are likely to respond to and be treated by others differently from those without these characteristics. That these infant temperament variables may irreparably alter early mother–infant attachment (now viewed as crucial to later childhood adjustment) suggests that even early differences in temperament among children may have far-reaching developmental effects.

It has already been shown that children's attention span and degree of impulse control affect the ways in which they interact with others and hence the ways in which they are treated by them. Children with problems in these areas seem to show greater problems with compliance and play and are more likely to elicit commands, supervision, and discipline from parents than are normal children.

Although not well studied, children's prior experience with adults, as well as their level of acceptance from peers, could conceivably influence the manner in which they react or interact with their parents. The effects of insularity on parents, noted earlier, may be similar in children. Finally, as noted for adults, setting factors also play some role in influencing parent–child interactions from the children's side. Number of observers and their relationship to the child in the setting, temperature, time since last sleeping or eating period, attractiveness of stimuli in the setting, and so on, all probably have some effect on social interactions; the nature of this effect requires further study.

This necessarily cursory review of variables outside specific parent–child interactions shows that they may directly affect the parent or child, or they may indirectly influence their social exchanges and perhaps their success in treatment. As a result, these factors deserve careful attention during the assessment process. While this may seem gratuitous to the sophisticated clinician, it has become apparent in my observations of and discussions with other clinicians that obvious aspects of deviant parent–child interactions have been overlooked or given slight import in understanding these interactions.

SUMMARY

Dramatic increases in scientific research on normal and deviant family interactions over the past decade have revealed much that is relevant to clinical work with the families of hyperactive children. These families are more likely to have psychiatric problems, particularly depression, psychopathy, hysteria, and alcoholism. There is also an increased probability of hyperactivity, as well as conduct and learning problems, in the siblings of hyperactive children. Both findings have led to speculation about the role of genetic factors in hyperactivity. Irrespective of genetic theories, the increased incidence of psychopathology in these families broadens the scope of assessment and treatment from the children themselves to the family context in which they interact.

Research by many investigators clearly stresses the reciprocity or bidirectional effects involved in parent–child interactions. The importance of understanding the effects of children on their parents is demonstrated in the research of Bell and others—a point that should not go unheeded by child clinicians. Parental reactions to child behaviors appear to be sequentially and hierarchically organized, depending in part on their effectiveness at influencing those child behaviors. Thus, the history of parent–child exchanges requires attention in the clinical setting. The work of Patterson and his associates has illuminated the mechanisms of deviant, coercive parent–child interactions and the role of negative reinforcement in generating and maintaining these aversive exchanges. Both parent and child coercive behaviors are explicable in the light of these theories. In addition, some parent–child exchanges do seem to be developed and maintained by their positive consequences—a notion long advanced by many behaviorists in their studies of deviant child behavior.

Beyond the specific actions and reactions of each member of the dyad, variables outside parent–child interactions have some indirect effects on their outcome. Both parents and children are affected by variables that spill over into their treatment of each other—for example, the health of a parent or a child may drastically alter the person's actions and hence the reactions of the other. Substantial research is needed to clarify the role of these variables and interaction processes. That they exist at all is sufficient justification for their consideration by child clinicians working with deviant family interactions.

IMPLICATIONS FOR ASSESSMENT

The theories and research findings in this chapter have numerous implications for evaluating hyperactive children; only the more general of these will be reviewed here.

1. Assessment methods must focus not only on the specific problem behaviors of the children and the history of such behaviors, but also on the context in which they occur and their effects on others, especially parents and siblings. Approaches that stress this reciprocity are the subject of the next two chapters.

2. Since the problems of hyperactive children permeate many interactions with others, there is a need to assess more than one or two response classes if the evaluation is to be at all thorough. Methods that stress only activity level, attention span, and impulse control are outdated if they do not take into account the social interactions that these factors influence and the consequences that result.

3. Because parent–child interactions are complex and often have years of learning history behind them, the evaluation of deviant interactions requires reference to this historical context. What is often seen in the clinic is the culmination of years of social exchanges, which should not be judged in isolation from that context. It requires great clinical skill and empathy and much inquiry in the assessment process to tease out the direction of effects in these interactions and the ways in which their evolution may have occurred. In doing so, the clinician must acknowledge to some extent the impact which a hyperactive child may have on any family, especially if the child has been difficult to raise since infancy. Parental fatigue, depression, low self-esteem, marital difficulties, and social insularity may evolve from these parent–child interaction problems. Increased parental guilt, shame, anger, resentment, jealousy of other parents, and negativism toward the child must certainly arise out of the years of confrontation with the child, and these deserve some recognition by the clinician during the evaluation. That these parental reactions may spawn abuse or neglect of the child seems probable in cases where other factors place the family under greater stress than usual. Because of the increased time these children demand of their parents, some parents may elect to forego the chance to have other children, fearing that they will not have the nurturance or stamina to raise both children properly. How hyperactive children might affect their siblings remains to be studied, yet some influence must occur, considering the effects these children have on their more resilient parents.

4. The evaluation must also broaden in scope to the extent that it must consider other intra- and extrafamilial factors. Characteristics of parents and children impinge upon the outcome of their social interactions. Parental health-related, marital, financial, cognitive, social, and affective characteristics, as well as other factors, deserve investigation. Similarly, developmental, physical, cognitive, temperamental, social, and health-related characteristics of children also demand attention again to the degree that they may affect exchanges between the children and other family members.

5. Finally, greater empathy and compassion is needed by most clinicians evaluating families with hyperactive children. All too often the blame for such children's difficulties is placed on the parents, with no more than the flimsiest piece of clinical evidence to support such blame. Since family interactions are reciprocal, fault-finding is groundless.

IMPLICATIONS FOR TREATMENT

Again, the specific implications of this chapter for therapy are left to subsequent chapters. General considerations for therapy include the following:

1. Initially, intervention is likely to be at the level of social interactions between parents (or teachers) and children in present contexts. As with assessment, treatment methods focusing solely on activity level or attention seem to be without efficacy. Those that focus on child compliance and responsiveness to adult commands, and that alter parental actions toward children, seem more useful. This is especially true, given the data on generality of child noncompliance across various settings.

2. Beyond intervention at this level, additional therapies may have to contend with the myriad of other social problems in settings outside the home involving others, such as peers or teachers. Multisetting interventions will probably have to be devised and implemented if generalization of treatment across settings is to occur.

3. The possibility that other individuals in a family may also have social or psychiatric problems means that they must at least be considered in the

types of treatment to be used for the child, if not in the types to be selected for the parent. Referral to others more expert in the parental problems may coincide with or precede interventions with the child, depending on their severity.

4. Before launching into the therapies that are to be offered, the clinician must take care to avoid undue blaming of the parents. This is particularly true where poor maternal self-esteem and depression are evident in regard to child management issues. Fault-finding is likely to undercut parental motivation for treatment and may only contribute further to parental affective disorders.

5. Patterson has shown that, over time, the reinforcement value of parental attention decreases in its effects on child behaviors. Initial steps in parent training must be designed to reverse this decline before parental social praise can be used as an effective reinforcer of appropriate child behaviors. Methods for doing so are outlined in Chapter 7.

6. When disciplinary methods are to be taught, parents should be advised that these methods may *increase* child coercive behaviors temporarily and that they are not to capitulate if this proves true. Such methods may take longer to suppress coercive–aversive child behaviors when consistently applied, simply because of their intermittent and unsuccessful use in prior interactions.

SUGGESTED READING

Baldwin, J. M. *Social and ethical interpretations in mental development: A study in social psychology* (3rd ed.). New York: Macmillan, 1902. (Originally published, 1897.)

Barkley, R. A., & Cunningham, C. E. The parent–child interactions of hyperactive children and their modification by stimulant drugs. In R. Knights & D. Bakker (Eds.), *Treatment of hyperactive and learning disordered children.* Baltimore: University Park Press, 1980.

Barkley, R. A., & Cunningham, C. E. The effects of Ritalin on the mother–child interactions of hyperactive children. *Archives of General Psychiatry*, 1979, *36*, 201–208.

Battle, E. S., & Lacey, B. A context for hyperactivity in children, over time. *Child Development*, 1972, *43*, 757–773.

Bell, R. Q. A reinterpretation of the direction of effects in studies of socialization. *Psychological Review*, 1968, *75*, 81–95.

Bell, R. Q. Stimulus control of parent or caretaker behavior by offspring. *Developmental Psychology*, 1971, *4*, 63–72.

Bell, R. Q. Socialization findings reexamined. In R. Q. Bell & L. Harper (Eds.), *Child effects on adults.* New York: Wiley, 1977.

Bell, R. Q., & Harper, L. (Eds.). *Child effects on adults.* New York: Wiley, 1977.

Campbell, S. Mother–child interaction in reflective, impulsive, and hyperactive children. *Developmental Psychology*, 1973, *8*, 341–347.

Campbell, S. Mother–child interaction: A comparison of hyperactive, learning-disabled, and normal boys. *American Journal of Orthopsychiatry*, 1975, *45*, 51–57.

Cantwell, D. P. Psychiatric illness in the families of hyperactive children. *Archives of General Psychiatry*, 1972, *27*, 414–427.

Cunningham, C. E., & Barkley, R. A. The effects of Ritalin on the mother–child interactions of hyperkinetic twin boys. *Developmental Medicine and Child Neurology*, 1978, *20*, 634–642.

Cunningham, C. E., & Barkley, R. A. A comparison of the interactions of hyperactive and normal children with their mothers in free play and structured task. *Child Development*, 1979, *50*, 217–224.

Forehand, R., Sturgis, W., McMahon, R., Aguar, D., Green, K., Wells, K., Breiner, J. Parent behavioral training to modify child noncompliance: Treatment generalization across time and from home to school. *Behavior Modification*, 1979, *3*, 3–25.

Harper, L. V. The young as a source of stimuli controlling caretaker behavior. *Developmental Psychology*, 1971, *4*, 73–88.

Humphries, T., Kinsbourne, M., & Swanson, J. Stimulant effects on cooperation and social interaction between hyperactive children and their mothers. *Journal of Child Psychology and Psychiatry*, 1978, *19*, 13–22.

Lamb, M. E. Influence of the child on marital quality and family interaction during the pre-natal, perinatal, and infancy periods. In R. M. Lerner & G. B. Spanier (Eds.), *Child influences on marital and family interaction: A life-span perspective*. New York: Academic 1978.

Morrison, J. R., & Stewart, M. A. A family study of the hyperactive child syndrome. *Biological Psychiatry*, 1971, *3*, 189–195.

Morrison, J. R., & Stewart, M. A. The psychiatric status of the legal families of adopted hyperactive children. *Archives of General Psychiatry*, 1973, *28*, 888–891.

Patterson, G. R. The aggressive child: Victim and architect of a coercive system. In E. J. Mash, L. A. Hamerlynck, & L. C. Handy (Eds.), *Behavior modification and families*. New York: Brunner/Mazel, 1976.

Wahler, R. G. Some structural aspects of deviant child behavior. *Journal of Applied Behavior Analysis*, 1975, *8*, 27–42.

Wahler, R. G. Deviant child behavior within the family: Developmental speculations and behavior change strategies. In H. Leitenberg (Ed.), *Handbook of behavior modification and behavior therapy*. Englewood Cliffs, N.J.: Prentice-Hall, 1976.

THE EVALUATION OF HYPERACTIVE CHILDREN: CLINICAL INTERVIEW AND RATING SCALES

Education is the knowledge of how to use the whole of oneself. Many men use but one or two faculties out of the score with which they are endowed. A man is educated who knows how to make a tool of every faculty—how to open it, how to keep it sharp, and how to apply it to all practical purposes.—Henry Ward Beecher

The previous chapters suggest a number of issues that must be considered in the evaluation of hyperactive children. These are reiterated in specific sections of this chapter. Several, however, require emphasis here to set the tone of the evaluation. Foremost among these is the need to focus on the social behavior and interactions of such children with other significant individuals. Despite the particular physical, cognitive, or behavioral deficits of the children, it is most likely to be their social behavior, and particularly their noncompliance, which is the basis for their referral for treatment. A second consideration is that, because of the reciprocity involved in social interactions, the evaluation process must be nonjudgmental. The goal of clinical assessment should not be to blame, to find fault, to accuse, or to deprecate. It should be to establish problem areas and to design effective interventions. While constructive criticism may be necessary in this process, it should not degenerate into a "witch hunt" intended to crucify or exact punishment from parents. Third, the assessment approach itself will need to be of a broad spectrum, for hyperactive children will present with a variety of secondary and associated problems other than hyperactivity that are likely to require treatment. The point is illustrated in Table 3.1, which lists the myriad of problems often seen in hyperactive children. Hence, a narrow approach addressing only one or two symptoms will be both simplistic and ineffective. Finally, there is an obvious need for considering the cross-situational nature of the child's problems and the opinions of those individuals who must deal with the child in each setting. It is imperative that the evaluation extend beyond the confines of the clinic office to encompass those individuals who frequently interact with the hyperactive child.

TABLE 3.1. Problems Associated with Hyperactivity in Children

General area	Specific problems
Behavioral	Short attention span
	Distractibility
	Restlessness
	Poor impulse control
	Destructiveness/noisiness
Social	Poor peer relations
	Noncompliance to commands
	Aggression/lying/stealing
	Belligerent and disrespectful language
	Poor self-control/high risk-taking
	Poor social problem solving skills
Cognitive	Immature self-speech (internal language)
	Inattention/distractibility
	Low average intelligence
	Lack of conscience
	Poor perspective on future consequences of behavior
Academic	Underachievement for intelligence
	Specific learning disabilities
Emotional	Depression
	Low self-esteem
	Excitability
	Immature emotional control
	Excessive frustration
	Unpredictable/variable moods
Physical	Immature physical size
	Immature bone growth
	Enuresis/encopresis
	Increased upper respiratory infections
	Increased frequency of otitis media
	Increased frequency of allergies
	Greater number of minor physical anomalies
	Underreactive central nervous system
	Short sleep cycles
	High pain tolerance
	Poor motor coordination

APPROACHES TO DEVIANT SOCIAL BEHAVIOR

Before addressing the specific procedures involved in evaluating hyperactive children, it is worthwhile to review the various approaches by which a child's behavior may be diagnosed as pathological or deviant (see Furman, 1980, in "Suggested Reading"). The approach probably followed by most clinicians, whether consciously or not, is that related to adult discomfort with the child's behavior. This approach merely labels as abnormal any child behaviors which the parents or other adults view as distressing, atypical, or discomforting. Since evaluation of child behaviors rests heavily on parental or teacher reports, these adults are given inordinate weight in establishing deviancy. Such a view, while necessary as an adjunct to other approaches discussed below, is fraught with many problems. Primary among these is that adults often base their complaints about child behavior problems on their own subjective norms and expectations for appropriate child behavior. How representative such reference points are of actual normal child behavior and development may be questionable. All clinicians at one time or another have encountered parents whose expectations of children's behavior are too high or demanding, or who are naive about normal child development. In these cases, the children's behavior is not necessarily deviant in comparison with that of their peers, and thus the focus of treatment should be on altering parental expectations or knowledge. A second problem is that adults are not as accurate, objective, or reliable in their observations as clinicians would like. Often, other events or stressors in families may interfere with parents' judgment of the children's problems. For instance, research has shown that, when under stress, parents may increase their punishment of children's behavior, even though the behavior is no different from periods where less stress is occurring with the parent. Thus, parents' view of a problem hinges partly on their level of tolerance for certain child behaviors. Parents may also tend to overestimate the frequency of a problem behavior, and such an overestimation contributes to their view of its severity or need for treatment. Finally, as many courts are beginning to realize, there may exist a conflict of interest between the parents and the children that precludes nonpartisan opinions about the children. Obvious examples of this come from cases involving litigation over children's problems, as in accident-related cases, or from cases in which parents no longer want children in the home. The courts have partly resolved the problem by appointing guardians *ad litem* for the children to look after the children's interests independently of the attorneys representing the parents. Clinicians do not have this advantage and so must be careful to consider points at which conflicts of interest may taint parental opinion and to ensure that other sources of information about the child's behavior are obtained. For these and other reasons, parents' opinions are necessary but not sufficient to establish deviant social behavior in a child. Other approaches to establishing deviancy must be followed.

One approach often used in conjunction with parental discomfort is the normative approach. In this case, the quantity or quality of a particular child's behavior is compared against information already available on normal children of a similar age. Those child behaviors that deviate from the average for normal children are viewed as pathological. This statistical criterion incorporates developmental changes in rates of child behaviors, since children are compared against only their own age groups. It also allows one to determine how effective interventions are at returning children's behavior to within normal rates. Although better than parental judgments alone, this approach is not without its problems. Normative data on many child behaviors are either not available or not readily accessible to the clinician, and this makes many comparisons impossible. In other instances, norms for child behaviors vary with social class, race, or cultural background, and this may make it difficult to know what reference to use for a particular child. The setting (time and place) or the way in which the norms were collected may make them invalid for behaviors observed under different circumstances. Finally, some clinicians may argue that average rates of behavior may not always be the most desirable ones. This approach, then, while helpful in establishing statistical deviancy, may not be so useful in determining whether behavior is really a "problem."

Another approach to establishing problem behaviors is that of social validation. Here, either other children, the target child himself, or experts in the field judge whether or not certain child behaviors are appropriate. Clinicians often implicitly use the "expert in the field" approach; after all, to the parents at least, they are the "experts" on appropriate child behaviors. In many cases, however, clinicians' opinions hinge on their knowledge of the developmental literature; this approach is thus open to the same criticisms applied to the normative approach. Furthermore, other "experts" may not always concur with the opinion of the clinician, and it is then open to question whether or not the child has a problem. Nonetheless, this approach is more advantageous than parental opinion alone.

A different perspective on deviancy, and probably the most clinically desirable one, lies in the "current and future adjustment" approach. The relationship of the potential problem behavior to others known to facilitate or impair social adjustment is used to judge its need for treatment. For instance, as shown in Chapter 1, high levels of childhood aggression predict innumerable social problems in adolescence; this makes aggression worthy of treatment, regardless of statistical deviancy or peer/expert opinion. Like the other approaches, this one requires that clinicians remain familiar with a broad range of scientific literature on normal and abnormal behaviors *and their contribution to future adjustment.* Unfortunately, the weakest area of child development literature is often prospective follow-up research. Furthermore, problems arise in attempting to define the adequacy of present or future "adjustment." If this approach is used, clinicians need to consider both the current and future adjustment problems associated with the behavior in question, as some childhood behaviors may create immediate difficulties but show a high rate of spontaneous remission over a short time.

At present, the best way out of this quagmire of establishing the deviancy of child behaviors is to employ several approaches. Relying on parental opinion alone is inadequate but necessary and should always be used with one of the other approaches. Regardless of which of the others are used, it is imperative that clinicians remain reasonably abreast of child development literature (covering both normal and abnormal behavior) if their judgments are to have any credibility. The all-too-common situation of clinicians' dramatically decreasing their reading of current child development journals after graduation is both professionally self-destructive and irresponsible.

DIAGNOSTIC CRITERIA

As noted in Chapter 1, clinicians may agree on what symptoms occur in hyperactivity but may agree less often on which children should be called hyperactive. The problem arises both in different definitions of hyperactivity and in the ways in which these definitions are operationalized for clinical or research purposes. While there is no general consensus on the exact criteria to be used in diagnosing hyperactivity, I have found that the following definition and criteria meet with wide acceptance among those doing research in this field:

Hyperactivity is a developmental disorder of age-appropriate attention span, impulse control, restlessness, and rule-governed behavior that develops in late infancy or early childhood (before age 6), is pervasive in nature, and is not accounted for on the basis of gross sensory, motor, or neurologic impairment or severe emotional disturbance.

The goals of diagnosis are clear from this definition. Problems with attention span, impulse control, restlessness, and noncompliance must be demonstrated (usually through interviews, rating scales, and objective observations). These problems must be deviant for the child's age; that is, as noted in Chapter 1, they must be two standard deviations above the mean for normal children of the same age on some rating scale or method of observation for which there are norms. A better reference group is that of children of similar *mental* age, as some retarded children can also be hyperactive in relation to their level of intellectual development. The age of onset and duration of symptoms are established through the interviews; as noted, the child's problems should have begun before 6 years of age. Most hyperactive children are reported as problems by age 2–3 or earlier. If the child is under 6, the problems should have existed for at least one year. The pervasiveness of the problem is established through interviews with and completion of rating scales by parents *and* teachers, or by direct observation across several settings. In my clinical practice, I require that a child have problems across 50% of those 16 situations listed on the Home Situations Questionnaire to be discussed later, or that direct observations across several settings demonstrate pervasiveness. The absence of gross sensory (blindness, deafness, etc.), motor (cerebral palsy, etc.), or neurological disorders (epilepsy, tumors, strokes, etc.), or of psychosis, is established through a medical history, interviews, observation of the child, and a medical–neurologic exam, where necessary.

Children whose behavior problems fall short of these criteria may be diagnosed as having borderline hyperactivity, conduct disorder, or situational behavior problems. While some clinicians may take issue with one or another of the criteria in this diagnostic process, some starting point in objective diagnosis is required if confusion is to be reduced in both research and clinical practice. I have used these criteria for the past three years with several hundred hyperactive children and have been quite satisfied with its clinical utility, especially in justifying the diagnosis to parents, courts, insurance carriers, school staff, or others with a need to know how the diagnosis was established. Note that the diagnosis relies on more than simply the parents' or clinician's feelings that the child is a problem.

WHO SHOULD CONDUCT THE EVALUATION?

There is often debate among various professionals as to which of them is best qualified to evaluate and treat hyperactive children. This seems to arise from the variety of physical, psychiatric, and social problems often associated with hyperactivity, and from the diversity of treatment methods available. Physicians are likely to believe they are best equipped to care for the "total child" because of the many physical problems, temperament difficulties, allergies, upper respiratory infections, toileting problems, and neurologic "soft" signs seen with these children. That drug treatment is often used with these children frequently guarantees the physician some role in the care and management of the hyperactive child.

Social workers may also believe that they are necessary to the care of these children because of their many social problems, the need for counseling of their families, and the probable need for assistance from social service agencies in times of crisis with the child. Psychologists, too, may feel best qualified to provide primary care to hyperactive children because of their cognitive, behavioral, and familial problems. The need for child management training, individual and family therapy, and classroom management are viewed as justification for their involvement. Lastly, educators and school psychologists may believe that a role for their services is created by the numerous academic and social problems occurring at school for many of these children.

It therefore appears that no single profession can meet all the needs of hyperactive children and their families. Multidisciplinary cooperation in evaluation and treatment is imperative if even partially adequate services are to be given. The profession that plays the central role with the child will vary from one locale to another and one child to another, depending on the agency from which the family initially seeks assistance. The answer to the question "Who should conduct the evaluation?" the professional who can take the necessary time to provide effective assessment, treatment, and follow-up care for the hyperactive child and the family. Each profession needs to respect its individual competencies and limitations and not fail to involve other professions when the need should arise.

PREPARATION FOR THE EVALUATION

The assessment of hyperactive children should not be undertaken lightly or by the inexperienced. The complexity of their problems, their family context, and their interactions within that context demand adequate preparation, time, and execution of the procedures set forth in this chapter. A 20-minute assessment in an examining room in a pediatric outpatient clinic is not enough. Nor, however, is a 90-minute school psychological evaluation that uses only psychometric and projective measures. Although it is crucial, time is not the only factor controlling the adequacy of the assessment; the areas which are to be assessed are just as important if not more so. Since a satisfactory evaluation usually consists of parent and child interviews, completion of behavior rating scales, psychometric assessment, and observations of parent–child or teacher–child interactions (where possible), a minimum of 2 to 3 hours will be needed for the initial examination.

Examiners, of course, should have prior experience in child clinical assessment or should be supervised by persons who have. This book is not intended to replace more general texts on or training in the style and content of general clinical assessment, particularly with respect to interviewing. Several excellent books on interviewing and assessment are listed at the end of this chapter and deserve reviewing even by experienced clinicians. A few of the important aspects of the style of assessment, however, are worth briefly acknowledging here, as they may often be overlooked even by experienced examiners. Throughout an evaluation, it is imperative that the examiner periodically stop the procession of questions and evaluative instruments to reflect upon and summarize what has been gained so far. This is especially pertinent while conducting interviews and reviewing parent questionnaires;

it insures that what the examiner is hearing accurately represents what the parents, child, or even teacher are trying to say. While this sort of "checking it out" procedure should not be overdone, it can greatly enhance the parents' belief that the examiner in fact "understands" the problems when it is used properly. Equally important is the need for the examiner to pay attention not only to *what* is said, but to *how* it is said and how the parent or child *feels* about what is said. The focus on "body language" can be carried to ridiculous extremes, but manner, tone of voice, and particular facial expressions are key sources of information that may be overlooked in the rush to obtain hard data and begin treatments. Discussion of how the child or the parents feel about the answers they give or the reactions they have provides a direct way of "checking out" the more subjective impressions the examiner may be forming during the evaluation. This can be extended to inquiring of one parent his or her feelings about what the other parent or the child has said. These points on assessment intimate that the style in which the examination is conducted can be as important in the evaluation as the specific questions or methods themselves.

Where other professionals have previously been involved with a child, their records, when pertinent, should be sought for review prior to the evaluation. This is, of course, done with the consent of the child's parents or guardians. Since hyperactivity is chronic, has an early onset, and may have several problems associated with it, it is very likely that others have seen the child already and have provided certain treatments. Having these records and the impressions of other professionals can prove invaluable in avoiding previous mistakes, coordinating one's own efforts with others in treatment, and understanding the history and context of parental concerns more fully.

A number of questionnaires are discussed later in this chapter, and examiners should familiarize themselves with them and their norms before beginning evaluations. Some examiners choose to mail them out in advance of an appointment for the parent to bring in on the appointment date. Others provide them to parents while they themselves are interviewing or testing a child. In either instance, their utility and efficiency in assessing children's problems are widely recognized. When possible, the opinions of both parents should be obtained on these questionnaires or on the day of the evaluation in the parental interview.

PARENTAL INTERVIEW

Despite its possible unreliability, the parental interview is an indispensable part of the assessment of children. No adult is more likely to have the wealth of knowledge about, history of interactions with, or sheer time spent with a child than is a parent. In addition, the unreliability of parental reports can be dramatically reduced by the use of questions of a specific rather than a general nature.

The parental interview often serves several purposes. First, it establishes a necessary rapport among the parents, the child, and the examiner that will prove invaluable in enlisting parental cooperation with later aspects of assessment and treatment. Second, the interview is an obvious source of descriptive information about the child and the family; it also reveals the parents' view of the child's problems and helps to narrow the focus of later stages of assessment.

Furthermore, provided such an arrangement is feasible and acceptable to the parents, the child can remain within the room during part of the interview so as to permit an informal assessment of parent–child interactions. Since hyperactive children often present problems for their parents when visitors are at their home, similar problems may arise when the parents and the examiner attempt to talk. Where feasible, hyperactive children and their parents should be interviewed in a clinic playroom that will later be used for direct observations of parent–child interactions via a one-way mirror in the room. By doing so, this allows the child some time to habituate to the playroom before the observations occur. Because the behavior of hyperactive children has been shown to worsen over time and with familiarity to novel situations, conducting the interview in this way takes advantage of this phenomenon in the hope that the later playroom observations will be more representative of home behavior problems.

A fourth purpose of the initial interview with the parents is that it can help to focus the parent's perception of the child's problems on more important and more specific controlling events within the family. Parents often tend to emphasize developmental–historical causes of a global nature in discussing their children's problems. The behavioral–interactional interview discussed later can serve to shift the parents' attention to more immediate antecedent and consequating events surrounding child behaviors, thereby preparing them for the initial stages of treatment, which will involve training in observing child behaviors.

Perhaps a fifth and final purpose of the interview is that of formulating a diagnosis, though this is certainly not essential to treatment planning. The diagnosis of hyperactivity, however, may gain prognostic utility as more follow-up studies are done. Many child behavior problems are believed to remit in 75% of the cases over relatively short time periods. Hyperactivity, in contrast, rarely does so; thus, when diagnosed, it warrants more caution in drawing conclusions about prognosis and more preparation of families to cope with children's later problems.

The suggestions that follow for interviewing parents of hyperactive children are not intended as rigid guidelines, only as areas that clinicians should consider. Each interview will obviously differ according to individual child and family problems. Generally, those areas of importance to an evaluation include demographic information, child-related information, and details about the parents and other family members.

Demographic Information

Obviously, various details about a child's age, school, grade, and teacher, as well as about the family size, religion, and pediatrician, need to be obtained. Figure 3.1 shows a typical form to be completed by parents at the time of the evaluation on these details. It should be noted that knowing who referred a family for evaluation is important not only in knowing who should receive copies of the final reports, but also in determining what prompted the parents to seek help for the child and what other professionals will need to be advised or consulted on various treatment decisions.

Information about the Child

Once demographic data are obtained, interviews should progress to the current concerns of parents regarding their children. Parents are likely to state initially that the children won't listen to them, can't finish anything they start, can't sit still, and have to be supervised constantly. Such general descriptors, as well as those of restlessness, not thinking before acting (impulsivity), and stubbornness, require greater clarification from the parents. Often asking about recent examples of each concern can elucidate more helpful details. Separating home from school problems will prove useful in later discussions with the children's teachers, in cases where these are appropriate. In discussing parental concerns, examiners should focus on the more specific situations in which problem behaviors occur, the occurrences that seem to provoke them, the frequency with which they occur, and the parents' current methods of handling them. Be sure to clarify any differences in disciplinary methods between parents. Some time should be given to determining a brief history of the problems causing concern, the date of their onset, and prior attempts at management by the parents. If the parents are seeking help for problems of longstanding duration, why are they coming for help at this point in time? This question reveals much about parental motivation for treatment; it should be borne in mind that if parents are under pressure from some outside agency, such as a school or court, interest in therapy and compliance with it may be less than desirable. Examiners should also inquire about prior professional involvement with the children. Finally, parents should be asked what they believe may be causing their children's problems and how willing they are to change their own behavior, if need be, to cope with these problems.

Once these details are carefully obtained, examiners should review the children's current health and medical status. What chronic or recent acute illnesses have these children experienced? Are the children on any medication at this time? If so, what types and how much of each, and why are they being prescribed? Are they psychoactive or do they have behavioral side effects? When sedatives or anticonvulsants are being used, they should be discussed

FIGURE 3.1. A typical form for obtaining demographic information about hyperactive children and their families. (Adapted from *Hyperactive Children* by D. Safer and R. Allen. Baltimore: University Park Press, 1976. Copyright 1976 by University Park Press. Reprinted by permission.)

Child's name _____ Birth date _____ Age _____

Address _____

Town _____ Zip code _____

Place of birth _____Length of time at present address _____

Home phone _____ Other phone _____

School _____ Grade _____

Teacher's name _____

School address and phone _____

PRESENT FAMILY INFORMATION (Family currently responsible for child)

Father's name _____ Age ____ Education _____

Mother's name _____ Age ____ Education _____

Is father employed? _____ What type of work? _____

Where? _____ How long? _____

Is mother employed? _____ What type of work? _____

Where? _____ Full-time/Part-time? How long? _____

Is either parent a step- or adoptive parent? _____

Are the natural parents still married? _____ Separated? _____ Divorced? _____

Physician's name _____

       Address _____

            _____

       Phone _____

List all children in family (living or deceased)

Name	Age	School grade/vocation
_____	____	_____
_____	____	_____
_____	____	_____

Others in home (age and relationship)

_____	____	_____
_____	____	_____

in detail with the parents, as the medications may actually be causing or exacerbating the hyperactivity. Do the children have any known sensory, motor, or neurologic disorders? If so, what types, and how are they managed?

This leads logically to a consideration of the children's developmental and medical history. Is a particular child adopted? If so, how much is known about the pregnancy and delivery, as well as about the medical and psychiatric status of the natural parents? This is not a frivolous inquiry, since hyperactive children are at least four times more likely to have been adopted than normal children. If a child is a biological offspring, then parents should be questioned about any problems the mother had in carrying this child or previous children. Was the pregnancy desired? Did the mother consume drugs, tobacco, or alcohol while pregnant? Was she experiencing any type of chronic emotional stress during this time? Was the pregnancy full-term, premature, or postmature? Were delivery complications present (e.g., caesarean, forceps, breech)? Were immediate postnatal complications noted, such as respiratory distress or convulsions?

As infants, what sort of babies were these children to care for? Were feeding or sleeping problems present? What were the babies' temperaments like? Were there atypical medical problems in infancy? When did these babies sit up, crawl, and walk with and without support? When did the children begin to use single words, and later, phrases? Were any oddities of development noted? How were these children toilet-trained? Do they still have problems in bowel or bladder control? Were the children exposed to lead or toxic substances? Were neurologic disorders present (e.g., epilepsy, febrile convulsions)? Is sexual development normal? Have the children spent any significant periods of time under the care or supervision of persons outside the immediate family? It is also important to establish the date of the children's most recent physical examination by a pediatrician and to determine whether problems in physical growth were noted.

Interviews should then progress to the children's school history and current academic problems. Examiners should ascertain where and at what age the children began school and what problems in behavior and learning may have been noted. How have these children progressed through each grade to the present? Were any grades repeated or special classes required? Truancy, suspensions, expulsions, and tardiness are also frequent problems of hyperactive children, and the examiner should inquire about these. Have the children received any multidisciplinary school evaluation under Public Law 94-142, and, if so, can these records be obtained by the examiner? Are there impending plans or program changes by the school for these children in the future? Because of the frequency of specific learning diabilities in such children, the examiner should ask about specific subjects with which the children have particular trouble. Finally, the examiner should take note of the parents' attitude toward schooling and determine whether there have been problems in interactions between parents and schools, regardless of such problems' origins.

Next, examiners should focus on the children's social interactions with and acceptance by peers, both at school and in the neighborhood. How many close friends do these children have? What ages are they? What problems occur in these peer interactions? How are they managed? It is often found that such children prefer younger toys and friends and are likely to have problems keeping friends. How aggressive the children are appears important to establish, since it is of great prognostic value and will deserve intervention. Finally, how are the children perceived by other parents in the neighborhood?

Symptoms of other psychiatric disorders, such as neuroses or psychoses, deserve some attention in the interview. Do these children have any fears, and, if so, are they unusual? Are nervous habits or mannerisms present? Do the children show any obsessional behavior? Are signs of depression present? How do the children respond to new situations? Examiners should discuss with parents any signs of disturbances in thinking, hallucinations, or delusions in these children. Do the children show odd movements, postures, fascinations, or preoccupations? When nervous tics or psychotic symptoms are found, stimulant drug treatment is generally felt to be contraindicated.

In additon to the above, the examiner should ask the parents questions about the children in several other areas. Do these children show much awareness of their problems or the consequences of their behavior for themselves and others? Do the children have any responsibilities, such as chores, within the home, and how do they handle them? The parents can also be asked about the children's particular "strong points"—their positive characteristics and abilities. Finally, some time should be spent in discussing possible rewards that may be useful for later treatment of the children. A list of possible reinforcers about which examiners can inquire is provided in Table 3.2.

Information about the Parents and Family

As Chapter 2 reveals, information about the families of hyperactive children is as important to understanding such children's behavior as that already obtained about the children themselves. Parents' respective ages, levels of education, and current occupations are important in appreciating family backgrounds and expectations for the children. Parents of differing socioeconomic classes seem to differ in their expectations for their children and in approaches to their management. Information on the number of siblings, their sex, and their ages, as well as the presence of any psychological, educational, developmental, or medical problems in siblings, should be obtained. Next, examiners should inquire as to the general relationship of

TABLE 3.2. Possible Reinforcers for Hyperactive Children

Social reinforcers	Activities	Nonedibles	Edibles
Praise/attention	Shopping	Models	Candy
Affection (physical/verbal)	Movies	Records	Gum
Extra privileges	Gym/playground	Posters	Soda
Time on telephone	Hobbies	Clothes	Cookies
Time out of house	Camping	Toys	Cakes/pies
Awards/certificates	Travel	Sporting	Ice cream
Public display of work	Radio	goods	Hamburgers
Special playtime with parent	Television	Pets	Hot dogs
	Use of car	Bicycle	Fruit
	Baking/cooking	Go-cart	Juices
	Drawing/coloring		Nuts
			Vegetables

the children to each of their parents and siblings. For example, does the mother or the father have the closest relationship to a particular child? Which sibling(s) seem to compete most with this child? What activities on the part of other familiy members seem to provoke misbehavior from the child?

Interviews should then proceed to a consideration of historical details about the parents and their families. Is there a history of psychiatric, learning, or behavioral disorders in the parents, their own parents, or their siblings? Examiners should ask specific questions about alcoholism, conduct problems, and affective disorders, such as depression, in the parents or their relatives. Parents seem likely to answer "no" to global questions about psychiatric problems but will often answer "yes" to questions about specific types of problems. If parents are experiencing psychiatric problems, care should be taken to find out what help they have received or are now receiving. This is especially necessary if a parent is taking psychoactive drugs that can interfere with child management.

Some attention also needs to be given to parental health, especially to any history of chronic illnesses that might affect family interaction patterns. Some disorders, such as migraine headaches, may produce transient yet acute effects on child management, while disorders such as diabetes, lupus, or multiple sclerosis are likely to have subtle but lasting effects on family interaction patterns. In one instance, I treated a family in which the mother had diabetes. She seemed chronically anxious about the long-term complications of her disease, frequently raising her anxieties as an issue with other family members when they did not act in the way she expected. Both the father and hyperactive son in this family felt that the mother was too sensitive about her illness, and they were tired of hearing about it. Hence, they avoided much leisure interaction with her because of her complaining. This illustrates the way in which apparently irrelevant parental medical conditions may in fact alter family systems.

Of importance in understanding hyperactive children's problems may be information about marital problems, where these exist. How long have the parents been married? How would they describe their satisfaction in marraige? Have there been previous separations or divorces? If so, why did they occur? If current marital problems exist, what are the areas of dissatisfaction, and do the children seem to be aware of these problems? Has help been sought for resolving the areas of dissatisfaction? If not, would the parents be interested in seeking such help? When time permits, having the parents complete the Locke–Wallace Marital-Adjustment Test (shown in Figure 3.2) may reveal marital problems of which the parents are not cognizant or problems that they are reluctant to divulge in an interview. Recent research has shown that parents of hyperactive children are more likely to report marital problems on this scale than are parents of normal children. As shown in Chapter 2, marital stresses, whether they are the result of occupational, financial, sexual, social, or emotional problems, are likely to have a negative influence on interactions with hyperactive children, as well as on parents' response to child management training.

Finally, independent of possible marital problems, the parents need to be questioned as to their degree of extrafamilial social activities. This is particularly true for mothers, for research has shown that their degree of insularity from the community correlates highly with deviant child behavior. How much contact do the parents have with friends, relatives, and others in the community? How often do the parents get out of the home for recreational activities with other adults? What is the parents' perception of the quality of these interactions? Is one parent spending a disproportionate amount of time caring for a hyperactive child? Where insularity seems problematic, recommendations to the parents to increase extrafamilial activities may be necessary.

Information on Parent–Child Interactions

At this stage of the interview, examiners should return to a detailed assessment of the children's social interactions with their parents. This can, of course, occur in that part of the interview described above in which parents are asked to relate their concerns about their children. However, I have

1. Check the dot on the scale line below which best describes the degree of happiness, everything considered, of your present marriage. The middle point, "happy," represents the degree of happiness which most people get from marriage, and the scale gradually ranges on one side to those few who are very unhappy in marriage, and on the other, to those few who experience extreme joy or felicity in marriage.

0	2	7	15	20	25	35
.	.	.	.	.	.	.

Very unhappy   Happy   Perfectly happy

State the approximate extent of agreement between you and your mate on the following items. Please check each column.

	Always Agree	Almost Always Agree	Occasionally Disagree	Frequently Disagree	Almost Always Disagree	Always Disagree
2. Handling family finances	5	4	3	2	1	0
3. Matters of recreation	5	4	3	2	1	0
4. Demonstrations of affection	8	6	4	2	1	0
5. Friends	5	4	3	2	1	0
6. Sex relations	15	12	9	4	1	0

7. Conventionality (right, good, or proper conduct)	5	4	3	2	1	0
8. Philosophy of life	5	4	3	2	1	0
9. Ways of dealing with in-laws	5	4	3	2	1	0

10. When disagreements arise, they usually result in: husband giving in (0), wife giving in (2), agreement by mutual give and take (10).

11. Do you and your mate engage in outside interests together? All of them (10), some of them (8), very few of them (3), none of them (0).

12. In leisure time do you generally prefer: to be "on the go" ———, to stay at home ———? Does your mate generally prefer: to be "on the go" ———, to stay at home ———? (Stay at home for both, 10 points; "on the go" for both, 3 points; disagreement, 2 points.)

13. Do you ever wish you had not married? Frequently (0), occasionally (3), rarely (8), never (15).

14. If you had your life to live over, do you think you would: marry the same person (15), marry a different person (0), not marry at all (1)?

15. Do you confide in your mate: almost never (0), rarely (2), in most things (10), in everything (10)?

FIGURE 3.2. The Locke-Wallace Marital-Adjustment Test. A score of less then 100 is felt to signify maladjustment (places an adult in the bottom 4% of the normative sample). (From "Short Marital-Adjustment and Prediction Tests: Their Reliability and Validity" by H. Locke and K. Wallace, *Marriage and Family Living*, 1959, 251–255. Copyright 1959 by National Council on Family Relations. Reprinted by permission of the publishers.)

found it more useful to obtain all of the family and background information first, so that the parent–child interactions can be discussed in an established context and thus placed in perspective.

In determining the nature of parent–child interactions, the following interview format has proven most helpful. It is adapted from that used by Constance Hanf at the University of Oregon Health Sciences Center and appears in Table 3.3. Interactions in at least 16 situations are discussed with parents. Each set of interactions identified as a problem is followed up with a series of questions (listed on the right side of Table 3.3) designed to elicit information on the nature of the interactions, their course, their outcome, and the parents' feelings about them. Examiners should also ask about differences between parents in the ways in which these problem situations

TABLE 3.3.   Parental Interview Format on Parent-Child Interactions

Situations to be discussed with parents	Follow-up questions for each problematic situation
General interactions	1. Is this a problem area? If so, then proceed with questions 2 to 9.
When playing alone	
When playing with other children	2. What does the child do in this situation that bothers you?
When at meals	
When getting dressed in morning	3. What is your response?
When washing and bathing	4. What will the child do next?
When parent is on telephone	5. If the problem continues, what will you do next?
When watching television	
When visitors are at home	6. What is usually the outcome of this interaction?
When visiting others' homes	7. How often do these problems occur in this situation?
When in public places (supermarkets, shopping centers, etc.)	
When mother is occupied with chores or activities	8. How do you feel about these problems?
When father is at home	9. On a scale of 0 to 9 (0 = no problems; 9 = severe problem), how severe is this problem to you?
When child is asked to do a chore	
When going to bed	
When doing homework	
When in other situations (in car, in church, etc.)	

Note. Adapted from an interview format used by C. Hanf, University of Oregon Health Sciences Center, 1976. From "Hyperactivity" by R. Barkley. In E. J. Mash and L. G. Terdal (Eds.), *Behavioral assessment of childhood disorders.* New York: Guilford Press, 1981. Copyright 1981 by Guilford Press. Reprinted by permsssion.

are handled, as well as about the length of time for which particular management methods were tried before others were taken up. For examiners who lack the 30 to 40 minutes it may take to pursue this part of the interview, a parent rating scale based on this section—the Home Situations Questionnaire—is discussed later in this chapter; the questionnaire can be completed by the parents relatively quickly. Examiners can then follow this up by questioning the parents only about those situations rated as most problematic. Either approach to assessment is satisfactory, though I have found that parents tend to rate situations as more problematic when the more thorough interview procedures are followed. The most likely problem situations for hyperactive children, as revealed by the use of this method, have been displayed in Table 1.4. As noted in Chapter 1, more problems seem to occur in situations where a hyperactive child is playing with other children, when a parent is on the telephone, when visitors are in the home, when the family is in public places (e.g., stores, restaurants), and when the child is asked to do chores. Somewhat less problematic settings are dressing times, visits to other people's homes, and bedtime. Many parents also believe that riding in the car is a serious problem situation for some of the children.

By either procedure, examiners are likely to find a sequence of social exchanges between parents and children common to most of these settings. A flow chart of the hierarchically organized exchange is seen in Figure 3.3. Basically, it appears that when a mother gives a command to a child with which the child does not comply, the mother is likely to repeat this command quite frequently (say 4 to 10 times) until the child complies or until her own frustration leads her to begin threatening the child. The threats may be repeated several times until the mother, again quite frustrated and perhaps angry, either aggresses against the child or acquiesces. That is, the mother may overzealously discipline the child, in some instances losing control of herself, or she may give up trying to enforce the command and perhaps obey it herself. This is the coercive interaction pattern described in Chapter 2 and so often seen in families of hyperactive children. However the exchange ends, feelings between the two participants are not likely to be pleasant and will probably taint other interactions that subsequently occur. Many parents report feelings of guilt, anger, depression, and incompetency following these interactions. Treatment clearly must focus on altering these exchanges if anything positive is to be achieved with hyperactive children and their families.

An example of the type of description likely to occur in this part of the interview is set forth below:

EXAMINER: What is your child likely to do when you have visitors in your home?

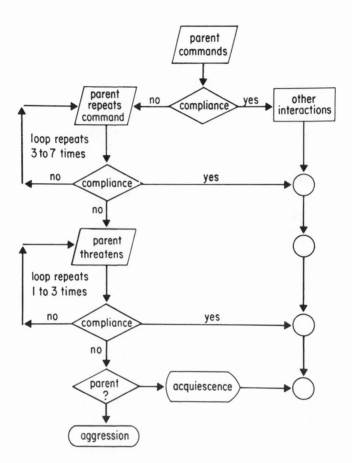

FIGURE 3.3 Flow chart of typical mother–child interactions occurring with noncompliant children.

MOTHER: He usually acts silly and disrupts whatever conversation we may be trying to have, or he starts hanging on the guests and trying to impress them with all sorts of stories.

EXAMINER: How will you respond to him at that point?

MOTHER: I'm likely to tell him to go play with his brother or sit quietly and watch television.

EXAMINER: What happens then?

MOTHER (*looking depressed and ashamed*): Well, he generally doesn't pay much attention to me. He might leave the room and get in mischief in the kitchen or bathroom. I frequently have to interrupt what I'm doing to get him to do as I asked or go see what he is getting into.

EXAMINER: How is this situation likely to end up?

MOTHER: After repeating myself to him many times, I may get frustrated and either hold him on my lap so he doesn't continue to dance around in front of us or send him to his room. None of this seems to work very well. If I send him to his room, he will likely leave his room without permission. If I hold him, he almost always continues to make noises and bother us.

EXAMINER: I can see that he is quite a handful for you at these times; how often does this type of problem occur?

MOTHER: Almost every time we have company over to the house. It gets very frustrating for my husband and me.

EXAMINER: How do you feel about these difficulties your child causes for you in front of others?

MOTHER (*beginning to cry now*): I'm extremely embarrassed that my friends see that I can't handle my child. Some of them don't come by to see us anymore because of our son's behavior and he is so bad for babysitters that we have a tough time getting them to stay with him anymore. I resent having to give up what little social life we have and this is likely to make me hate him for a long while. I know I shouldn't feel that way, but I need to have some time for my friends and activities and I can't seem to get it because of the problems we are constantly having with him.

This case illustrates the valuable information about parent–child interactions that can be gleaned from this interview format. It also provides ample evidence of the coercive exchanges described by Patterson, as well as suggestions of possible treatment for the hyperactive child and his parents.

If possible, it is often helpful (though not essential) to supplement the information obtained from interviews with that from diaries kept by parents on several of their children's behavior problems over a 1-week interval (or more). The parents can be asked to record this information the week prior to their evaluations for review by their examiner. Otherwise, examiners can select one or two of the most severe problem behaviors from those listed in Table 3.1 and ask the parents to record these behaviors for 1 to 2 weeks prior to the start of training the parents in effective child management methods. In either case, the parents should record the date and time at which a problem behavior occurs, what precipitates it, the parental response to it, and perhaps the number of times the commands given in that setting are repeated. This will often reveal more useful information for treatment planning than that derived simply from the interview.

CHILD INTERVIEW

Depending upon the children's age and intellectual level, some time in the assessment should be given to direct observation and interviewing of the children themselves. If the children have been present during the parental interview, then some impressions have already been obtained as to their language, behavior, and social skills. Examiners, however, need to obtain greater information on the children's perceptions of the need for evaluation and the specific problem interactions at home or school. If the children seem oblivious to any problems, as young hyperactive children often are, then more direct questioning on issues and problem settings described by the parents should occur. What is the children's relationship to their parents and siblings? What is their perception of their friendships with peers? Where school problems exist, the children need to be questioned on their awareness of these problems, the reactions of the teacher and classmates toward themselves, and which subjects are most difficult for them.

In conducting interviews, it is equally if not more important that examiners pay close attention to the style and quality of the children's responses and not simply to their content. Hyperactive children frequently are unaware of the difficulties they pose for others or are less concerned about them than others are. They often view the other people in their lives, not their own behavior, as the source of their problems. Since cognitive reflection is poor in these children, their responses to questions will be impulsive, sometimes distorted or fabricated, and based on spur-of-the-moment feelings or perhaps a desire to impress the examiner. For instance, I have often found that parents describe hyperactive children as having few, if any, friends, only to have the children tell me later that they have lots of friends and few problems with them. Thus, the child interview may not be especially useful in gaining further details or insights into the children's problems, but it is still a necessary component of the evaluation process.

With older hyperactive children, signs of depression, low self-esteem, and antiauthoritarian behavior may be present and should be noted. The interview may be of somewhat greater utility than with younger hyperactive children, since the children may now have some awareness of their problems. In either case, interviewing the children as to possible reinforcers for later use in therapy should be done.

Examiners should be extremely cautious about drawing conclusions about the children's behavior in other settings (home or school) on the basis of their behavior in the office and toward examiners themselves in particular. Hyperactive children are frequently well behaved while in a clinic office or examining room, yet they will probably be serious management problems for parents and teachers. Acknowledging this fact to the parents can often make them feel more comfortable during evaluations and help them to establish greater rapport with examiners. Parents often feel that they will be accused of contriving their children's problems or being overly sensitive to them if the children fail to misbehave for examiners. This can also lead the parents to question their own competence further as they see the children behaving well for someone else but not for them at home.

TEACHER INTERVIEW

Next to parents, teachers will have spent more time with the children than virtually any other adults. Their opinions of the children should be solicited and respected. If personal interviews are not possible, then examiners should initiate telephone contact with teachers. Obviously, the teachers should be questioned about the children's problem behaviors in the classroom. The teachers are likely to describe the children as restless, off-task, noncompliant, underachieving, and generally unable to complete assignments without supervision. Relations with classmates may be described as disruptive, immature, and perhaps aggressive. Noisiness; difficulties in handling themselves in special assemblies, on the bus, or on the playground; and lying or petty thievery are also likely to be problems for hyperactive children at school. As in parental interviews, examiners may have to question teachers further about specific parameters of the problems. How often do they occur? What seems to provoke them, in what context do they frequently appear, and how are they managed? The teachers should also be questioned about other learning and social problems. Do the children do much more poorly at one academic subject than at another? If so, have these children received an educational assessment recently? If not, examiners may include such an assessment as part of the evaluation or may refer the child to other professionals more skilled in the endeavor. Since many hyperactive children have learning disabilities, this may be a common procedure in the assessment process. In addition, are the children having difficulties with peer acceptance in the class or on the playground? Who seems to initiate the problem interactions? How often do they occur, and how are they resolved? Again, understanding the social context of the children's behavior is important to designing treatment strategies. As with parents, it may prove useful to have teachers keep diaries on the children's particularly severe or high-rate behavior problems in the classroom over a period of a week or so. Recording the same information suggested above for the parents diaries would be helpful; additional information on the reaction of the child's classmates to his behavior problems should also be kept for later analysis by the examiner. This, of course, assumes that such record-keeping chores are feasible within the teachers' daily routine. If not, direct classroom observations by examiners may be needed to gather more objective data on the children's problems.

BEHAVIOR RATING SCALES

One way of attempting to objectify adult opinions about children is to try to quantify their responses and to develop normative data on those responses. This is generally done through the use of questionnaires with multiple-choice or numerically scaled answers. No other area of child psychopathology has spawned more rating scales than that of conduct problem or hyperactive children. The most common and best standardized of these scales will be reviewed separately under those specific to parents and those meant for use by teachers.

Before reviewing these scales, it is worth remembering that a clinically and scientifically useful scale should meet certain standards other than the fact that some expert in the field has created it. First, it should have items that are worded so as to be easily understood by the vast majority of adults who must use it. Second, it should have a sufficient number of items to assess the construct(s) under study but not so many as to be inordinately time-consuming and hence discouraging to those who must complete it. Third, the answer format should allow for some indication of degree of the problem being endorsed, rather than merely for a "yes" or "no" answer. Fourth, it should have "face validity." That is, its items should appear to pertain to the construct under study. This does not necessarily mean that the scale actually does assess that construct; this is another requirement of rating scales known as "construct validity." This latter requirement is rarely met by most rating scales dealing with hyperactivity. Attempts to correlate these scales with more objective measures of hyperactive symptoms have not generally been successful. It is also helpful if the scale has some "predictive validity" in that it has been found to correlate with other useful measures at the same time that it is completed or at a future time. For instance, ratings of aggression in children predict poor social and academic adjustment during adolescence; such ratings are thus very useful in a clinical context. A seventh criterion of import to diagnosis is a scale's "discriminant validity," or the degree to which it distinguishes between children who score high on one construct, such as hyperactivity, and those who are "normal" on that construct. A scale should produce a satisfactory level of correctly classified children if it is to be helpful in diagnostic problems. Eighth, a rating scale, like any other measure, should have acceptable reliability not only between two points in time with the same rater, but between two raters using it at the same time with one child. Ninth, in the area of child psychopathology, the scale should have normative data available for children at differing age levels when age is likely to influence the construct being studied. Finally, virtually all of the rating scales for hyperactivity do not meet the requirement of "prescriptive utility." That is, they do not provide much information that is particularly useful in planning interventions, although they have frequently been used as one measure of the success of such treatment programs. The prescriptive utility of most scales is particularly limited because the social context in which the behaviors occur is of utmost importance to treatment planning. This aspect of the situation, however, is virtually ignored by the rating scales currently in use.

Since most rating scales of hyperactivity do not meet one or more of these standards, of what value are they to the scientist or clinician? In some cases for which adequate normative data are available, they can be of some diagnostic help to the clinician in determining whether the parental concerns are statistically different from those ratings provided for normal children. In addition, clinicians can use these same scales as a measure of treatment effectiveness by both determining change from the initial ratings and comparing the posttreatment scores with the normative data. Many rating scales of hyperactivity have been shown to reflect the effects of treatments, but only recently have they been used to show that most treatments do not change the child's behavior to "normal," depending on the way in which "normal" is defined. A third advantage of the rating scales is their ability to obtain information across a wide array of problem areas that would otherwise prove quite time-consuming if covered within an interview. Beyond these three advantages, however, the rating scales may prove disadvantageous in the false sense of security they may provide clinicians, who may think they have collected an additional, more "objective" source of data on the child than simple parental opinion. The errors encountered in using parental opinion are in many respects equally prevalent in the rating scales parents complete; in the scales, however, they are hidden under the guise of numerical scores. Rating scales are also limited by their inability to provide information on the antecedent and consequent events surrounding a particular problem behavior within a given situation. Yet this is the information of greatest value to planning behavior modification programs for a particular child.

Parent Rating Scales

While parents may have spent more time with their hyperactive children than teachers have, parents ratings have been found to be less reliable than those of teachers over time and between parents. This may result from the fact that teachers observe the children within a more restricted range of settings than the parents do. There is also data to suggest that teachers may be more likely to rate a child as hyperactive than parents may be; this may result from the same restriction of range noted above or from the teachers' typically broader experience with children and knowledge of what may be considered normal. Despite their lesser reliability and sensitivity, parent ratings are still considered indispensable to the assessment of hyperactive children because of the normative data they can provide. Where parents and teachers disagree sharply on their ratings, clinicians should pursue several possible clinical hypotheses for this. One is simply that sharp differences may exist between situational factors in the settings that parents and teachers are asked to evaluate. Clinicians should look closely at these factors, as knowledge of any differences may prove of some help in designing therapies. Another hypothesis is that one rater, a parent or a teacher, may be denying the actual presence or severity of a child's problems. When this occurs with one parent, talking to the other alone may give a more accurate indication of the child's problems. In the case of the teacher failing to rate the child as a problem, this can result from inexperience with children if a relatively young teacher is involved, or from a fear that the child may be medicated if the ratings are so severe. Some teachers may even feel that severe ratings reflect indirectly on their competence. Both problems may exist for some parents as well.

Probably the most commonly used rating scale of parental opinion of hyperkinetic behavior is the Parent Symptom Questionnaire (PSQ), developed by C. Keith Conners. The original scale consisted of 93 items grouped into 25 major headings, but the version in more frequent use is a 48-item scale recently factor-analyzed and found to yield the following major groupings: conduct problems; learning disability (inattention); psychosomatic problems; impulsivity–hyperactivity; and anxiety. Only four questions load on the hyperactivity factor, although 10 questions are used to comprise the hyperactivity index. The mean score of the index is often used in selecting children for research on hyperactivity. The 48-item version of the PSQ is set forth in Figure 3.4. Each item is answered "not at all," "just a little," "pretty much," or "very much," and the number of points assigned to each answer is 0, 1, 2, or 3, respectively. The questions that comprise each factor are listed in a footnote to Table 3.4; the norms for males and females aged 3 to 17 years are listed in the table itself. Scores for each factor are computed by summing the points across all items comprising that factor and dividing by the number of items in that factor. A mean score of 1.5 on the hyperactivity index is generally accepted as the lower limit for establishing hyperactivity. However, some researchers use a score of two standard deviations above the mean for age to make a diagnosis. The scores have been shown to be highly related to children's sex and age. Boys tend to be rated as more problematic than girls. (Parental ratings also differ by sex; mothers' ratings of children are more severe than fathers'.) Furthermore, the scores tend to decline as children grow older, a fact which should be given some respect in cases where very young (<5 years) or very old (>12 years) hyperactive children are being evaluated. Early studies of the longer PSQ found it to vary less with the age and social class of children than the shorter version did. These studies also found that the PSQ correctly identified 77% of neurotic children, 70% of clinic-referred children, 83% of normal children, and 74% of hyperactive children from its factor scores. My own research has found that the hyperactivity score and total score on the shortened PSQ do not correlate significantly with objective measures of activity or attention, but do correlate with measures of child noncompliance to parental commands. This suggests that child noncompliance may be the overriding concern of parents answering the hyperactivity items on the questionnaire. The scale and its factor scores are quite sensitive to drug treatment and parent training in child behavior management, and they also have satisfactory test–retest reliability over short time periods. Children scoring higher on the PSQ are more likely to have academic problems both as children and adolescents, and are also more likely to respond favorably to drug treatment, than those with lower scores. Furthermore, it is now believed that children with nervous tics or anxiety are likely to respond poorly to stimulants; this suggests that high anxiety factor scores may contraindicate drug therapy.

Another parent rating scale of some utility is the Werry–Weiss–Peters Activity Rating Scale (WWPARS). This questionnaire contains 31 items dealing with the child's behavior across seven settings: meals, television, homework, play, sleep, public places, and school. Each item can be answered "no," "some," "much," or "not applicable." Scores of 0, 1, or 2 are given to each answer and summed to yield a total score. The scale was shortened to 22 items (the school and homework items were deleted) and data were collected on 140 normal children aged 3 to 9 years by Donald Routh, now at the University of Iowa, and his colleagues. This modified scale appears in Figure 3.5, and the norms by age appear in Table 3.5. A score of two standard deviations above the mean for age is considered indicative of hyperactivity. While the scale has the advantage of assessing behavior in different settings, it does not take this into account in its scoring. Clinicians should inspect the items in each setting to enhance the clinical utility of the items. The ratings of fathers and mothers as a group did not differ from each other in the normative sample. However, the mean correlation between mothers' and fathers' ratings was only .33, suggesting that parents may not agree in their opinions of their children. Test–retest reliability has not been reported for this scale. Its scores do vary significantly with age; thus, the age norms should be employed for a child whose age falls within that of the normative sample. Otherwise, a score of 20 or higher may be taken as a sign of hyperactivity. The scale effectively discriminates between hyperactive and normal children and is sensitive to drug treatment or parent training programs. Children scoring high on this questionnaire tend to respond better to stimulant drugs than those with lower scores. The scale correlates highly with the PSQ hyperactivity factor. Like the PSQ, the WWPARS does not show acceptable correlations with objective measures of activity level or attention span, but does correlate with child noncompliance to parental commands. Factor analysis reveals these different item groupings: television

Parent's Questionnaire

Name of Child _____ **Date** _____

Please answer all questions. Beside *each* item below, indicate the degree
of the problem by a check mark (✓)

	Not at all	Just a little	Pretty much	Very much
1. Picks at things (nails, fingers, hair, clothing).				
2. Sassy to grown-ups.				
3. Problems with making or keeping friends.				
4. Excitable, impulsive.				
5. Wants to run things.				
6. Sucks or chews (thumb; clothing; blankets).				
7. Cries easily or often.				
8. Carries a chip on his shoulder.				
9. Daydreams.				
10. Difficulty in learning.				
11. Restless in the "squirmy" sense.				
12. Fearful (of new situations; new people or places; going to school).				
13. Restless, always up and on the go.				
14. Destructive.				
15. Tells lies or stories that aren't true.				
16. Shy.				
17. Gets into more trouble than others same age.				
18. Speaks differently from others same age (baby talk; stuttering; hard to understand).				
19. Denies mistakes or blames others.				
20. Quarrelsome.				
21. Pouts and sulks.				
22. Steals.				
23. Disobedient or obeys but resentfully.				
24. Worries more than others (about being alone; illness or death).				

25. Fails to finish things.			
26. Feelings easily hurt.			
27. Bullies others.			
28. Unable to stop a repetitive activity.			
29. Cruel.			
30. Childish or immature (wants help he shouldn't need; clings; needs constant reassurance).			
31. Distractibility or attention span a problem.			
32. Headaches.			
33. Mood changes quickly and drastically.			
34. Doesn't like or doesn't follow rules or restrictions.			
35. Fights constantly.			
36. Doesn't get along well with brothers or sisters.			
37. Easily frustrated in efforts.			
38. Disturbs other children.			
39. Basically an unhappy child.			
40. Problems with eating (poor appetite; up between bites).			
41. Stomach aches.			
42. Problems with sleep (can't fall asleep; up too early; up in the night).			
43. Other aches and pains.			
44. Vomiting or nausea.			
45. Feels cheated in family circle.			
46. Boasts and brags.			
47. Lets self be pushed around.			
48. Bowel problems (frequently loose; irregular habits; constipation).			

FIGURE 3.4. The 48-item version of the Conners Parent Symptom Questionnaire. (Reprinted by permission of C. K. Conners.)

109

TABLE 3.4. Category (Factor) Norms for the Conners Parent Symptom Questionnaire

Age (years)	n^a	(I) Conduct problems		(II) Learning problems		(III) Psychosomatic problems		(IV) Impulsivity– hyperactivity		(V) Anxiety		Hyperactivity index	
		$\bar{x}$	SD	$\bar{x}$	SD	$\bar{x}$	SD	$\bar{x}$	SD	$\bar{x}$	SD	$\bar{x}$	SD
						Males by age							
3–5	45	.53	.39	.50	.33	.07	.15	1.01	.65	.67	.61	.72	.40
6–8	76	.50	.40	.64	.45	.13	.23	.93	.60	.51	.51	.69	.46
9–11	73	.53	.38	.54	.52	.18	.26	.92	.60	.42	.47	.66	.44
12–14	59	.49	.41	.66	.57	.22	.44	.82	.54	.58	.59	.62	.45
15–17	38	.47	.44	.62	.55	.13	.26	.70	.51	.59	.58	.51	.41

Females by age

Age	n^a												
3–5	29	.49	.35	.62	.57	.10	.17	1.15	.77	.51	.59	.78	.56
6–8	57	.41	.28	.45	.38	.19	.27	.95	.59	.57	.66	.59	.35
9–11	55	.40	.36	.43	.38	.17	.28	.80	.59	.49	.57	.52	.34
12–14	63	.39	.40	.44	.45	.23	.28	.72	.55	.54	.53	.49	.34
15–17	34	.37	.33	.35	.38	.19	.25	.60	.55	.51	.53	.42	.34

Note. The norms are taken from "Normative Data on Revised Conners Parent and Teacher Rating Scales" by C. H. Goyette, C. K. Conners, and R. F. Ulrich, *Journal of Abnormal Child Psychology*, 1978, 6, 221–236. Copyright 1978 by Plenum Publishing Corp. Reprinted by permission. The scores are derived by assigning 0, 1, 2, and 3 points to the answers "not at all," "just a little," "pretty much," and "very much," respectively, for each item. The scores for those items assigned to each factor are then summed and divided by the number of questions assigned to or loading on that factor. The items assigned to each factor from the Conners Parent Questionnaire are as follows:

Conduct problems: questions 2, 8, 14, 19, 20, 21, 22, 23, 27, 33, 34, and 39.

Learning problems: questions 10, 25, 31, and 37.

Psychosomatic problems: questions 32, 41, 43, 44, and 48.

Impulsivity–hyperactivity: questions 4, 5, 11, and 13.

Anxiety: questions 12, 16, 24, and 47.

Hyperactivity index: questions 4, 7, 11, 13, 14, 25, 31, 33, 37, and 38.

$^a n$ = number of subjects per age group.

Child's name _____ Date _____

Parent's name _____

Instructions:
    Please answer each of the questions below by circling the word NO if the child does not do this behavior or almost never does it, SOME if he or she does it some of the time, MUCH if he or she does it quite a bit, and NA if the item does not apply to your child.

 1. During meals, is the child up and down at the table?
    NO   SOME   MUCH   NA

 2. During meals, does the child interrupt others without regard for what they are trying to say?
    NO   SOME   MUCH   NA

 3. During meals, does the child fiddle with things?
    NO   SOME   MUCH   NA

 4. During meals, does the child wriggle?
    NO   SOME   MUCH   NA

 5. During meals, does the child talk too much?
    NO   SOME   MUCH   NA

 6. When watching television, does the child get up and down during the program?
    NO   SOME   MUCH   NA

 7. When watching television, does the child wriggle?
    NO   SOME   MUCH   NA

 8. When watching television, does the child play with objects or his or her own body?
    NO   SOME   MUCH   NA

 9. When watching television, does the child talk too much?
    NO   SOME   MUCH   NA

10. When watching television, does the child do things which interrupt others' ability to watch the program?
    NO   SOME   MUCH   NA

11. Is the child unable to play quietly?
    NO   SOME   MUCH   NA

12. When at play, does the child keep going from one toy to another?
    NO   SOME   MUCH   NA

13. When at play, does the child seek the attention of an adult?
    NO   SOME   MUCH   NA

14. When at play, does the child talk too much?
    NO   SOME   MUCH   NA

15. When at play, does the child disrupt the play of other children?
    NO   SOME   MUCH   NA

FIGURE 3.5. (*Continued*)

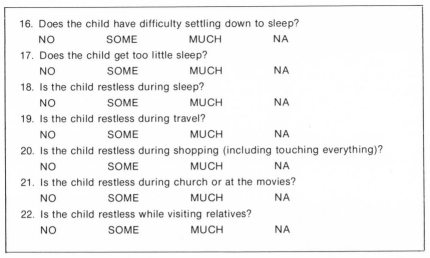

16. Does the child have difficulty settling down to sleep?
     NO   SOME   MUCH   NA
17. Does the child get too little sleep?
     NO   SOME   MUCH   NA
18. Is the child restless during sleep?
     NO   SOME   MUCH   NA
19. Is the child restless during travel?
     NO   SOME   MUCH   NA
20. Is the child restless during shopping (including touching everything)?
     NO   SOME   MUCH   NA
21. Is the child restless during church or at the movies?
     NO   SOME   MUCH   NA
22. Is the child restless while visiting relatives?
     NO   SOME   MUCH   NA

FIGURE 3.5. A modified version of the Werry–Weiss–Peters Activity Rating Scale. (From "Development of Activity Level in Children" by D. K. Routh, C. S. Schroeder, and L. O'Tuama, *Developmental Psychology*, 1974, *10*, 163–168. Reprinted by permission of D. K. Routh.)

TABLE 3.5. Norms by Age Level for the Werry–Weiss–Peters Activity Rating Scale for Parents

Age (years)	Mean score[a]	1 SD[b]	2 SD
3	15.20	20.96	26.72
4	12.35	20.25	28.15
5	11.13	16.25	21.37
6	12.40	21.32	30.24
7	9.95	14.50	19.05
8	9.30	13.84	18.38
9	8.08	12.12	16.16

Note. Norms are derived from "Development of Activity Level in Children" by D. K. Routh, C. S. Schroeder, and L. O'Tuama, *Developmental Psychology,* 1974, *10,* 163–168. Norms apply to both sexes of parents and children.

[a]The score on each rating scale is obtained by assigning 1 point for every answer of "some" and 2 points for every answer of "much" and summing the total points.

[b]SD = standard deviation above the mean.

behavior, bedtime/sleep behavior, mealtime behavior, attention seeking, talkativeness, restlessness, and play behavior.

A more recently developed questionnaire for use by parents of hyperactive children is the Achenbach Child Behavior Checklist (CBCL), displayed in Figure 3.6. This is a 113-item rating scale. Parts I–VII consist of questions dealing with children's social and athletic activities and with their household responsibilities. The items in Part VIII are each answered with scores of 0 ("not true"), 1 ("somewhat true"), or 2 ("very true") points. Parts I–VII yield three scales dealing with social competence (activities, social behavior, and school behavior) and Part VIII yields nine scales dealing with specific childhood diagnostic categories (schizophrenia, depression, noncommunication, obsession–compulsion, somatic complaints, social withdrawal, hyperactivity, aggression, and delinquency). The score for each Part VIII scale is obtained by summing the points for those items loading on each scale. Two higher-order factor scales (Internalizing and Externalizing) plus a total score are also obtained. These scores are plotted on two profile sheets, using percentile conversions or standard scores based on the normative sample. The scales were developed by factor-analyzing the responses for 450 disturbed boys. It was initially standardized for boys 6 to 11 years old but will eventually be expanded for children 4 to 16 years of age. The initial standardization report by Thomas Achenbach of the National Institute of Mental Health appeared in 1978; it used a sample of 300 normal children. The norms for the scale are shown in the profiles set forth in Figures 3.7 and 3.8. Socioeconomic status (SES) was noted to affect all scales significantly. Age was not found to affect the scores significantly on any of the nine scales, and thus the data across ages 6 to 11 were collapsed into one profile. The items assigned to each scale are listed at the bottom of each profile. These scores are converted to *t* scores or percentiles on the profile to yield a pattern of internalizing versus externalizing symptoms. The three social competence scores are obtained, as previously noted, from the information provided by parents on Parts I–VII of the scale.

The original report found that clinic-referred children scored higher on all scales than normal children. Test–retest reliability is quite high (.72 to .97), with a significant decrease in scores between the repeated ratings (8-day interval) occurring only on the depression scale. Test–retest correlations over a 15-month period yielded a mean correlation of .63 for the scales, indicating satisfactory stability over time. A comparison of mothers' and fathers' ratings for 37 clinic-referred boys yielded a mean correlation of .74 on the scales, suggesting good interparent agreement.

The CBCL promises to be a useful and well-developed scale for clinical use with hyperactive children. Its advantages lie in its larger item pool, its broader range of symptom scales, its good to excellent test–retest and interrater reliability, and its use of items reflecting both adaptive competence and behavior problems. Studies need to be done correlating the scores on the scales with other measures of important social, adaptive, and academic behavior of clinically disturbed children, both in present and future contexts, to establish their concurrent and predictive validity.

The profile obtained on 60 hyperactive children, ages 5 to 11 years, has been shown in Chapter 1. These results indicated that hyperactive children are likely to score in the clinically disturbed range on more than simply the hyperactive scale. This is consistent with the findings discussed in Chapter 1 that show a variety of social and emotional problems associated with hyperactivity. The highest scores were found on the scales of hyperactivity, aggression, delinquency, and obsessive–compulsive behavior. Thus, the scale reliability discriminates hyperactive from normal children and reveals a number of their associated problems.

Another behavior rating scale of some usefulness in evaluating hyperactive children is the Personality Inventory for Children (PIC), by Robert Wirt, David Lachar, James Klinedinst, and Phillip Seat. In essence, it is the childhood equivalent of the Minnesota Multiphasic Personality Inventory (MMPI), except that it is completed by parents rather than by the children themselves. More than 20 years of research were devoted to its standardization and validation; it is thus one of the most well-developed rating scales for psychologically disturbed children. The scale consists of 600 items which yield 14 clinical subscales and two validity subscale scores, as shown in Figure 3.9. Separate norms and profiles are available for males and females and for ages 3–5 and 6–16 within each sex. A manual for interpreting the profiles is provided with the scale and is published by Western Psychological Services in Los Angeles, California (see Wirt, Lachar, Klinedinst, & Seat, 1977, in "Suggested Reading").

Four clinical subscales are typically elevated in the population of hyperactive children, these being the hyperactivity, delinquency, social skills, and achievement subscales. In older hyperactive children, the subscale for depression may also be clinically elevated. The hyperactivity subscale comprises 36 of the 600 full scale items. These 36 items were chosen for their sensitivity in discriminating a sample of hyperactive children from nonhyperactive children referred to child guidance centers for other problems. A cutoff score of 18 correctly classified 90% of the hyperactive and 94% of the nonhyperactive children. This cutting score also correctly classified 95% of a sample of normal children as part of a cross-validation study. These "hit rates" are as good as or better than those for the other rating scales discussed above. Test–retest reliability for this subscale is .78 to .85—quite satisfactory in comparison with other scales. Interrater agreement between mothers and fathers ranges between .47 and .49, suggesting that mothers and fathers in

CHILD BEHAVIOR CHECKLIST FOR AGES 4-16

CHILD'S NAME

SEX
☐ Boy
☐ Girl

AGE

RACE

CHILD'S BIRTHDATE

TODAY'S DATE

Mo. _____ Day _____ Yr. _____

Mo. _____ Day _____ Yr. _____

PARENT'S TYPE OF WORK (Please be specific—for example: auto mechanic, high school teacher, homemaker, laborer, lathe operator, shoe salesman, army sergeant, even if parent does not live with child.)

FATHER'S
TYPE OF WORK: _____

MOTHER'S
TYPE OF WORK: _____

THIS FORM FILLED OUT BY:

☐ Mother
☐ Father
☐ Other (Specify):

I. Please list the sports your child most likes to take part in. For example: swimming, baseball, skating, skate boarding, bike riding, fishing, etc.

☐ None

Compared to other children of the same age, about how much time does he/she spend in each?

	Don't Know	Less Than Average	Average	More Than Average
a. _____	☐	☐	☐	☐
b. _____	☐	☐	☐	☐
c. _____	☐	☐	☐	☐

Compared to other children of the same age, how well does he/she do each one?

	Don't Know	Below Average	Average	Above Average
	☐	☐	☐	☐
	☐	☐	☐	☐
	☐	☐	☐	☐

II. Please list your child's favorite hobbies, activities, and games, other than sports. For example: stamps, dolls, books, piano, crafts, singing, etc. (Do not include T.V.)

Compared to other children of the same age, about how much time does he/she spend in each?

Compared to other children of the same age, how well does he/she do each one?

	Don't Know	Below Average	Average	Above Average
	☐	☐	☐	☐
	☐	☐	☐	☐
	☐	☐	☐	☐

	Don't Know	Less Than Average	Average	More Than Average
☐ None				
a. _____	☐	☐	☐	☐
b. _____	☐	☐	☐	☐
c. _____	☐	☐	☐	☐

III. Please list any organizations, clubs, teams, or groups your child belongs to.

Compared to other children of the same age, how active is he/she in each?

	Don't Know	Less Active	Average	More Active
☐ None				
a. _____	☐	☐	☐	☐
b. _____	☐	☐	☐	☐
c. _____	☐	☐	☐	☐

IV. Please list any jobs or chores your child has. For example: paper route, babysitting, making bed, etc.

Compared to other children of the same age, how well does he/she carry them out?

	Don't Know	Below Average	Average	Above Average
☐ None				
a. _____	☐	☐	☐	☐
b. _____	☐	☐	☐	☐
c. _____	☐	☐	☐	☐

T. Achenbach, University of Vermont, Burlington, VT 05405

PAGE 1

9-80 Edition

FIGURE 3.6. (*Continued*)

V.

1. About how many close friends does your child have?
☐ None ☐ 1 ☐ 2 or 3 ☐ 4 or more

2. About how many times a week does your child do things with them?
☐ less than 1 ☐ 1 or 2 ☐ 3 or more

VI. Compared to other children of his/her age, how well does your child:

	Worse	About the same	Better
a. Get along with his/her brothers & sisters?	☐	☐	☐
b. Get along with other children?	☐	☐	☐
c. Behave with his/her parents?	☐	☐	☐
d. Play and work by himself/herself?	☐	☐	☐

VII. 1. Current school performance—for children aged 6 and older:

☐ Does not go to school

	Failing	Below average	Average	Above average
a. Reading or English	☐	☐	☐	☐
b. Writing	☐	☐	☐	☐
c. Arithmetic or Math	☐	☐	☐	☐
d. Spelling	☐	☐	☐	☐
Other academic subjects: for example: his- e.	☐	☐	☐	☐

tory, science, foreign
language, geography.

f. _____ ☐ ☐ ☐ ☐

g. _____ ☐ ☐ ☐ ☐

2. Is your child in a special class?

☐ No   ☐ Yes—what kind?

3. Has your child ever repeated a grade?

☐ No   ☐ Yes—grade and reason

4. Has your child had any academic or other problems in school?

☐ No   ☐ Yes—please describe

When did these problems start and end?

FIGURE 3.6. (Continued)

VIII. Below is a list of items that describe children. For each item that describes your child *now* or *within the past 6 months*, please circle the *2* if the item is *very true* or *often true* of your child. Circle the *1* if the item is *somewhat* or *sometimes true* of your child. If the item is *not true* of your child, circle the *0*.

0	1	2	1.	Acts too young for his/her age		16
0	1	2	2.	Allergy (describe): _____		
0	1	2	3.	Argues a lot		
0	1	2	4.	Asthma		
0	1	2	5.	Behaves like opposite sex		20
0	1	2	6.	Bowel movements outside toilet		
0	1	2	7.	Bragging, boasting		
0	1	2	8.	Can't concentrate, can't pay attention for long		
0	1	2	9.	Can't get his/her mind off certain thoughts; obsessions (describe): _____		
0	1	2	10.	Can't sit still, restless, or hyperactive		25
0	1	2	11.	Clings to adults or too dependent		
0	1	2	12.	Complains of loneliness		
0	1	2	13.	Confused or seems to be in a fog		
0	1	2	14.	Cries a lot		
0	1	2	15.	Cruel to animals		30

0	1	2	31.	Fears he/she might think or do something bad		
0	1	2	32.	Feels he/she has to be perfect		
0	1	2	33.	Feels or complains that no one loves him/her		
0	1	2	34.	Feels others are out to get him/her		
0	1	2	35.	Feels worthless or inferior		50
0	1	2	36.	Gets hurt a lot, accident-prone		
0	1	2	37.	Gets in many fights		
0	1	2	38.	Gets teased a lot		
0	1	2	39.	Hangs around with children who get in trouble		
0	1	2	40.	Hears things that aren't there (describe): _____		
0	1	2	41.	Impulsive or acts without thinking		55
0	1	2	42.	Likes to be alone		
0	1	2	43.	Lying or cheating		
0	1	2	44.	Bites fingernails		
0	1	2	45.	Nervous, highstrung, or tense		60

0	1	2	16.	Cruelty, bullying, or meanness to others
0	1	2	17.	Day-dreams or gets lost in his/her thoughts
0	1	2	18.	Deliberately harms self or attempts suicide
0	1	2	19.	Demands a lot of attention
0	1	2	20.	Destroys his/her own things 35
0	1	2	21.	Destroys things belonging to his/her family or other children
0	1	2	22.	Disobedient at home
0	1	2	23.	Disobedient at school
0	1	2	24.	Doesn't eat well
0	1	2	25.	Doesn't get along with other children 40
0	1	2	26.	Doesn't seem to feel guilty after misbehaving
0	1	2	27.	Easily jealous
0	1	2	28.	Eats or drinks things that are not food (describe):
0	1	2	29.	Fears certain animals, situations, or places, other than school (describe):
0	1	2	30.	Fears going to school 45

0	1	2	46.	Nervous movements or twitching (describe):
0	1	2	47.	Nightmares
0	1	2	48.	Not liked by other children
0	1	2	49.	Constipated, doesn't move bowels
0	1	2	50.	Too fearful or anxious
0	1	2	51.	Feels dizzy 65
0	1	2	52.	Feels too guilty
0	1	2	53.	Overeating
0	1	2	54.	Overtired
0	1	2	55.	Overweight 70
			56.	Physical problems without known medical cause:
0	1	2	a.	Aches or pains
0	1	2	b.	Headaches
0	1	2	c.	Nausea, feels sick
0	1	2	d.	Problems with eyes (describe):
0	1	2	e.	Rashes or other skin problems 75
0	1	2	f.	Stomachaches or cramps
0	1	2	g.	Vomiting, throwing up
0	1	2	h.	Other (describe):

Please see other side

FIGURE 3.6. (Continued)

121

0 1 2	57.	Physically attacks people	
0 1 2	58.	Picks nose, skin, or other parts of body (describe): _____	80
0 1 2	59.	Plays with own sex parts in public	16
0 1 2	60.	Plays with own sex parts too much	
0 1 2	61.	Poor school work	
0 1 2	62.	Poorly coordinated or clumsy	
0 1 2	63.	Prefers playing with older children	20
0 1 2	64.	Prefers playing with younger children	
0 1 2	65.	Refuses to talk	
0 1 2	66.	Repeats certain acts over and over; compulsions (describe): _____	
0 1 2	67.	Runs away from home	25
0 1 2	68.	Screams a lot	
0 1 2	69.	Secretive, keeps things to self	
0 1 2	70.	Sees things that aren't there (describe): _____	
0 1 2	84.	Strange behavior (describe): _____	
0 1 2	85.	Strange ideas (describe): _____	
0 1 2	86.	Stubborn, sullen, or irritable	
0 1 2	87.	Sudden changes in mood or feelings	
0 1 2	88.	Sulks a lot	45
0 1 2	89.	Suspicious	
0 1 2	90.	Swearing or obscene language	
0 1 2	91.	Talks about killing self	
0 1 2	92.	Talks or walks in sleep (describe): _____	
0 1 2	93.	Talks too much	50
0 1 2	94.	Teases a lot	
0 1 2	95.	Temper tantrums or hot temper	
0 1 2	96.	Thinks about sex too much	
0 1 2	97.	Threatens people	
0 1 2	98.	Thumb-sucking	55
0 1 2	99.	Too concerned with neatness or cleanliness	
0 1 2	100.	Trouble sleeping (describe): _____	

0 1 2	71.	Self-conscious or easily embarrassed
0 1 2	72.	Sets fires
0 1 2	73.	Sexual problems (describe):
		_____ 30
0 1 2	74.	Showing off or clowning
0 1 2	75.	Shy or timid
0 1 2	76.	Sleeps less than most children
0 1 2	77.	Sleeps more than most children during day and/or night (describe): _____
0 1 2	78.	Smears or plays with bowel movements 35
0 1 2	79.	Speech problem (describe): _____
0 1 2	80.	Stares blankly
0 1 2	81.	Steals at home
0 1 2	82.	Steals outside the home
0 1 2	83.	Stores up things he/she doesn't need (describe):
		_____ 40

PLEASE BE SURE YOU HAVE ANSWERED ALL ITEMS.   PAGE 4

0 1 2	101.	Truancy, skips school
0 1 2	102.	Underactive, slow moving, or lacks energy
0 1 2	103.	Unhappy, sad, or depressed 60
0 1 2	104.	Unusually loud
0 1 2	105.	Uses alcohol or drugs (describe):
0 1 2	106.	Vandalism
0 1 2	107.	Wets self during the day
0 1 2	108.	Wets the bed 65
0 1 2	109.	Whining
0 1 2	110.	Wishes to be of opposite sex
0 1 2	111.	Withdrawn, doesn't get involved with others
0 1 2	112.	Worrying
	113.	Please write in any problems your child has that were not listed above:
0 1 2		_____ 70
0 1 2		_____
0 1 2		_____

UNDERLINE ANY YOU ARE CONCERNED ABOUT.

FIGURE 3.6. The Achenbach Child Behavior Checklist. (From "The Child Behavior Profile: I. Boys Aged 6-11" by T. Achenbach, *Journal of Consulting and Clinical Psychology*, 1978, 46, 478-488. Copyright 1978 by T. Achenbach. Reprinted by permission.)

123

Behavior Problems - Boys Aged 6-11

Internalizing

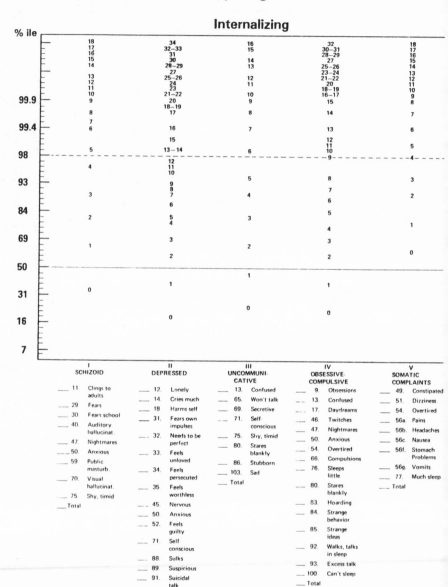

% ile

	I SCHIZOID	II DEPRESSED	III UNCOMMUNICATIVE	IV OBSESSIVE-COMPULSIVE	V SOMATIC COMPLAINTS
	___ 11. Clings to adults	___ 12. Lonely	___ 13. Confused	___ 9. Obsessions	___ 49. Constipated
	___ 29. Fears	___ 14. Cries much	___ 65. Won't talk	___ 13. Confused	___ 51. Dizziness
	___ 30. Fears school	___ 18. Harms self	___ 69. Secretive	___ 17. Daydreams	___ 54. Overtired
	___ 40. Auditory hallucinat.	___ 31. Fears own impulses	___ 71. Self conscious	___ 46. Twitches	___ 56a. Pains
	___ 47. Nightmares	___ 32. Needs to be perfect	___ 75. Shy, timid	___ 47. Nightmares	___ 56b. Headaches
	___ 50. Anxious	___ 33. Feels unloved	___ 80. Stares blankly	___ 50. Anxious	___ 56c. Nausea
	___ 59. Public masturb.	___ 34. Feels persecuted	___ 86. Stubborn	___ 54. Overtired	___ 56f. Stomach Problems
	___ 70. Visual hallucinat.	___ 35. Feels worthless	___ 103. Sad	___ 66. Compulsions	___ 56g. Vomits
	___ 75. Shy, timid	___ 45. Nervous	___ Total	___ 76. Sleeps little	___ 77. Much sleep
	___ Total	___ 50. Anxious		___ 80. Stares blankly	___ Total
		___ 52. Feels guilty		___ 83. Hoarding	
		___ 71. Self conscious		___ 84. Strange behavior	
		___ 88. Sulks		___ 85. Strange ideas	
		___ 89. Suspicious		___ 92. Walks, talks in sleep	
		___ 91. Suicidal talk		___ 93. Excess talk	
		___ 103. Sad		___ 100. Can't sleep	
		___ 112. Worrying		___ Total	
		___ Total			

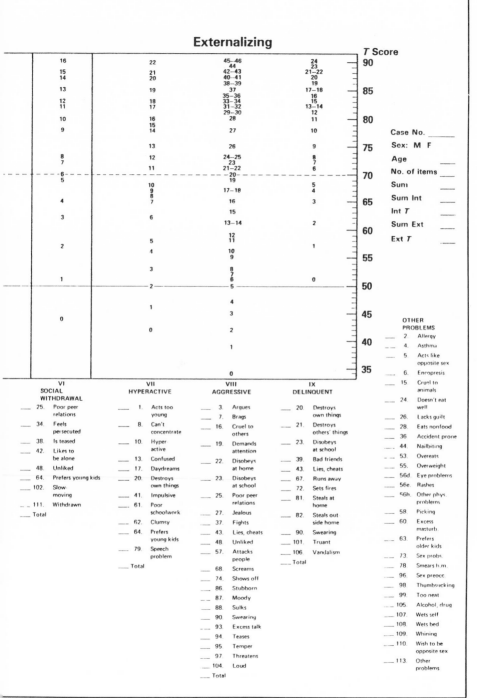

FIGURE 3.7. Profile sheet for displaying the results of the clinical scales of the Achenbach Child Behavior Checklist. (Copyright 1978 by T. Achenbach. Reprinted by permission.)

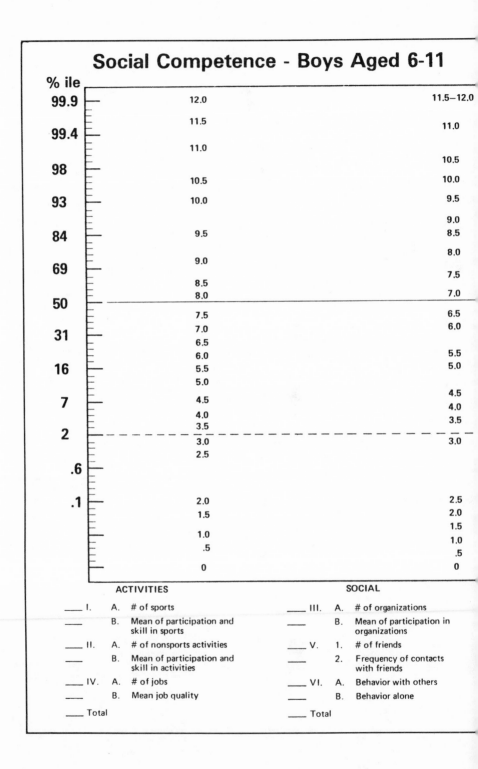

Social Competence - Boys Aged 6-11

% ile

99.9	12.0	11.5–12.0
99.4	11.5	11.0
	11.0	
98		10.5
	10.5	10.0
93	10.0	9.5
		9.0
84	9.5	8.5
		8.0
69	9.0	7.5
	8.5	
50	8.0	7.0
	7.5	6.5
31	7.0	6.0
	6.5	
	6.0	5.5
16	5.5	5.0
	5.0	
		4.5
7	4.5	4.0
	4.0	3.5
	3.5	
2	3.0	3.0
	2.5	
.6		
.1	2.0	2.5
	1.5	2.0
		1.5
	1.0	1.0
	.5	.5
	0	0

ACTIVITIES

____	I.	A.	# of sports
____		B.	Mean of participation and skill in sports
____	II.	A.	# of nonsports activities
____		B.	Mean of participation and skill in activities
____	IV.	A.	# of jobs
____		B.	Mean job quality
____ Total			

SOCIAL

____	III.	A.	# of organizations
____		B.	Mean of participation in organizations
____	V.	1.	# of friends
____		2.	Frequency of contacts with friends
____	VI.	A.	Behavior with others
____		B.	Behavior alone
____ Total			

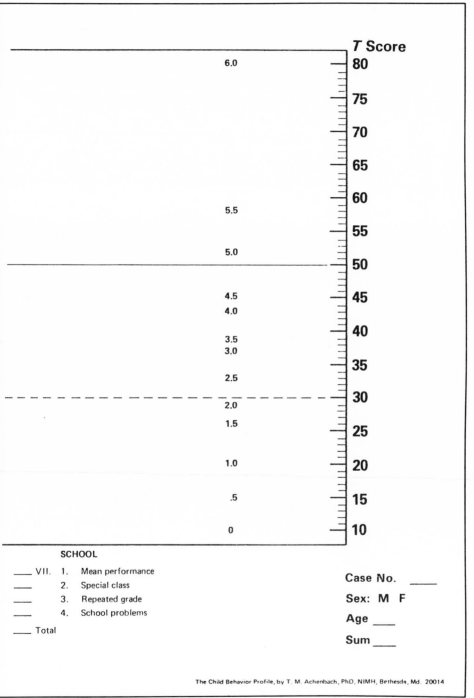

FIGURE 3.8. Profile sheet for displaying the results of the social competence scales of the Achenbach Child Behavior Checklist. (Copyright 1978 by T. Achenbach. Reprinted by permission.)

Personality Inventory for Children

PROFILE FORM

R.D. Wirt, Ph.D.; D. Lachar, Ph.D.; J.K. Klinedinst, Ph.D. and P.D. Seat, Ph.D.

Published by:

WPS WESTERN PSYCHOLOGICAL SERVICES
PUBLISHERS AND DISTRIBUTORS
12031 WILSHIRE BOULEVARD
LOS ANGELES, CALIFORNIA 90025
A DIVISION OF MANSON WESTERN CORPORATION

MALE
Ages 6-16

Child's Name: _____

Birthdate: _____

School Grade: _____

Age: _____

ID: _____

Informant: _____

Relation to Child: _____

Date Tested: _____

T scale: 120 115 110 105 100 95

Scales: LIE, F, DEFENSIVENESS, ADJUSTMENT, ACHIEVEMENT, INTELLECTUAL SCREENING (AGE 6, AGE 7, AGE 8, AGE 9, AGE 10+), DEVELOPMENT, SOMATIC CONCERN, DEPRESSION, FAMILY RELATIONS, DELINQUENCY, WITHDRAWAL, ANXIETY, PSYCHOSIS, HYPERACTIVITY, SOCIAL SKILLS

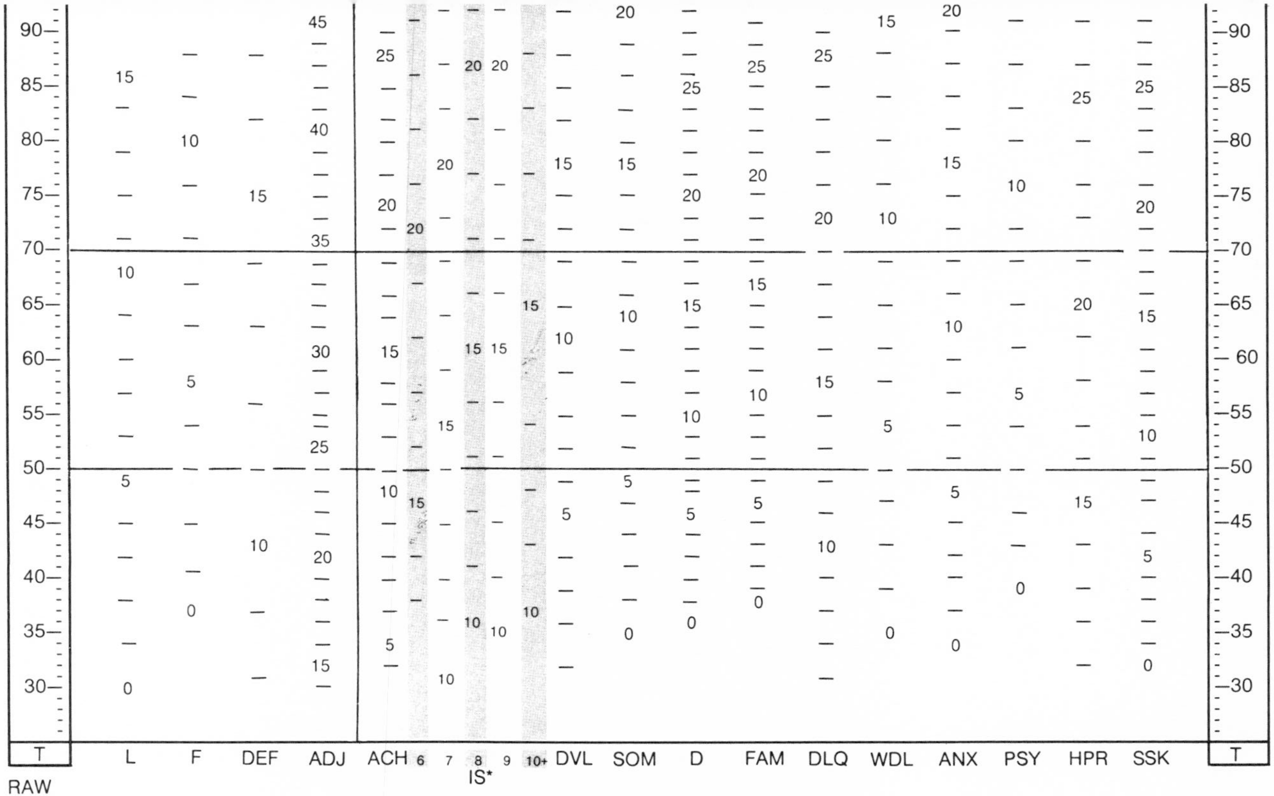
T
L
F
DEF
ADJ
ACH
6 7 8 9 10+
IS*
DVL
SOM
D
FAM
DLQ
WDL
ANX
PSY
HPR
SSK
T

RAW SCORES ___ ___ ___ ___ ___ ___ ___ ___ ___ ___ ___ ___ ___ ___ ___ ___ ___

*This scale is not a substitute for an individual intellectual assessment administered to the child.

W-152C 2 3 4 5 6 7 8 9 Printed in U.S.A.

FIGURE 3.9. (*Continued*)

Personality Inventory for Children

PROFILE FORM

R.D. Wirt, Ph.D.; D. Lachar, Ph.D.; J.K. Klinedinst, Ph.D. and P.D. Seat, Ph.D.

Published by:

WPS WESTERN PSYCHOLOGICAL SERVICES
PUBLISHERS AND DISTRIBUTORS
12031 WILSHIRE BOULEVARD
LOS ANGELES, CALIFORNIA 90025
A DIVISION OF MANSON WESTERN CORPORATION

FEMALE
Ages 6-16

Child's Name: _____ Informant: _____

Birthdate: _____ Age: _____ Relation to Child: _____

School Grade: _____ ID: _____ Date Tested: _____

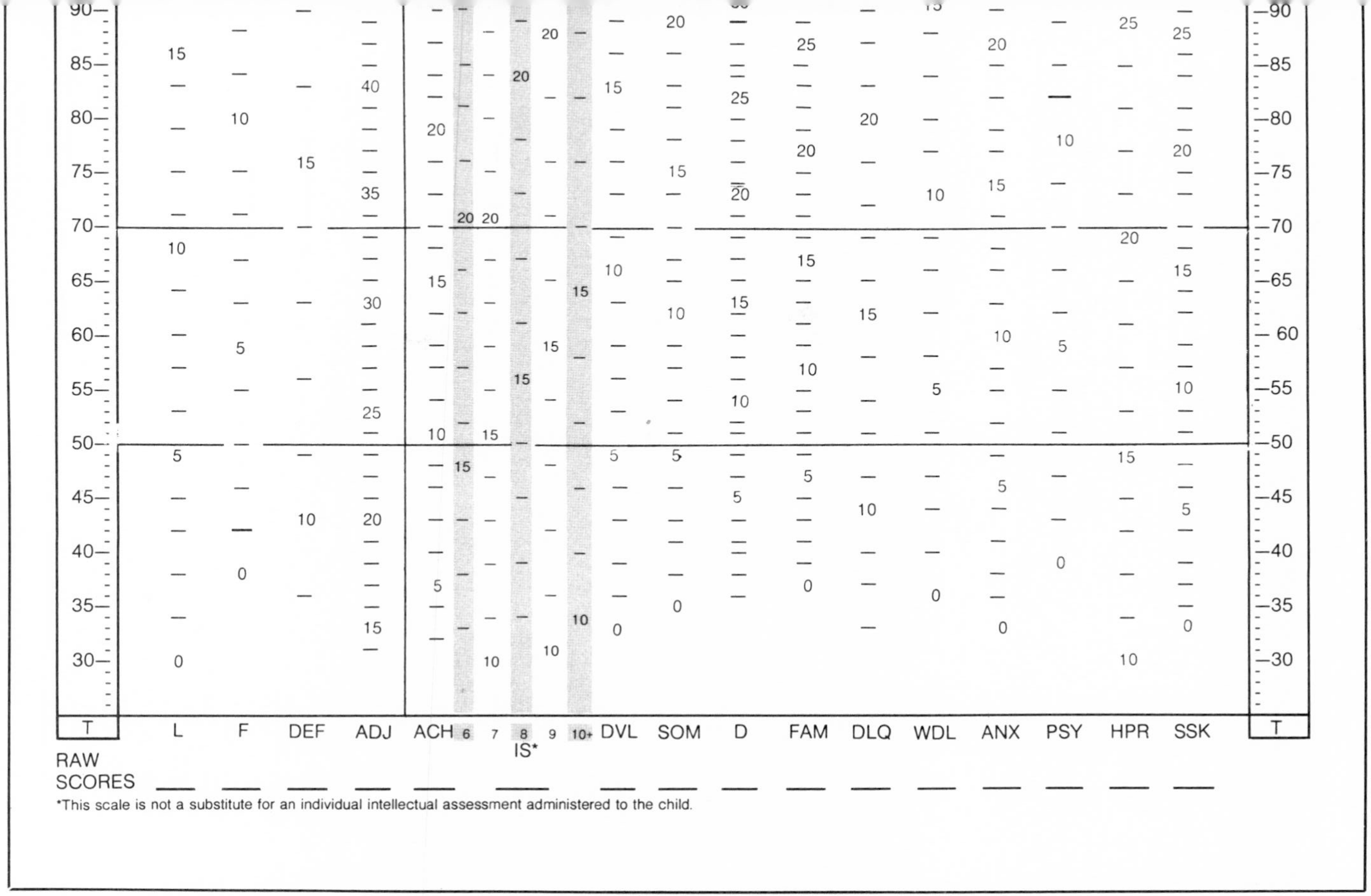
T
L
F
DEF
ADJ
ACH
6
7
8
9
10+
IS*
DVL
SOM
D
FAM
DLQ
WDL
ANX
PSY
HPR
SSK
T
RAW SCORES
*This scale is not a substitute for an individual intellectual assessment administered to the child.

FIGURE 3.9. Profile sheet for displaying the results of the Personality Inventory for Children. (Copyright 1977 by Western Psychological Services. Reprinted by permission. Not to be reproduced in whole or in part without written permission.)

some cases may not agree as to whether or not their children are hyperactive—a problem seen in the other rating scales as well. The authors of the PIC suggest that mothers should serve as informants when possible, considering fathers' greater likelihood of underestimating children's level of problem behaviors.

Despite its awesome ability to question parents about many different problem areas for their children, the PIC has several disadvantages. First, it is an extremely long and cumbersome scale to complete, taking many parents well over an hour. This may not be significant if the parents complete the scale at home before or after their initial appointments or in a waiting room while their children are being tested. Second, its length and wording make it quite threatening if not impossible for parents of low literacy levels. Third, there has been very little research to date on the use of the PIC with hyperactive children, other than in the initial validity studies. Its contribution to assessment of these children beyond that already provided by other methods remains to be thoroughly documented. Fourth, there has been no comparison of the hyperactivity subscale with other, more traditional scales of hyperactivity, such as the Conners scale, to evaluate their degree of agreement. Finally, as with all rating scales, there exists some question as to how useful the PIC is in treatment planning, since it fails to assess the situational variables so instrumental to that task. Nonetheless, when time during the evaluation is not at a premium and when parental literacy level is not a problem, this scale may be of much utility to the evaluation in its ability to raise hypotheses for more detailed pursuit with objective observational methods.

One final scale that I utilize with hyperactive children is the Home Situations Questionnaire (HSQ). This scale is an adaptation of the interview format discussed earlier and is unique in that it deals primarily with the *settings* in which behavior problems occur, rather than with the type of behavior problem, as the other scales do. The scale is shown in Figure 3.10; it consists of 16 different problem situations likely to be mentioned by parents of hyperactive children. The parents indicate whether their children have problems in each setting and then rate the severity of the problems on a scale of 0 to 9. Clinicians can use this scale as a substitute for the part of the interview mentioned earlier that deals with parent–child interactions in various home and public settings. Parents can be questioned about the children's problems in those settings with the highest ratings. The scale nicely complements the others in suggesting which settings are most problematic for the children and hence on which of these settings interventions will have to focus.

The data on a 14-item version of the HSQ for 30 hyperactive and 30 normal children matched in age and IQ are shown in Table 3.6. This table

Name of Child _____

Name of Person Completing This Form _____

Does this child present any behavior problems in any of these situations? if so, indicate how severe they are.

Situation	Yes/No (Circle one)		If Yes, How Severe? (Circle one) Mild Severe								
When playing alone	Yes	No	1	2	3	4	5	6	7	8	9
When playing with other children	Yes	No	1	2	3	4	5	6	7	8	9
When at meals	Yes	No	1	2	3	4	5	6	7	8	9
When getting dressed	Yes	No	1	2	3	4	5	6	7	8	9
When washing/bathing	Yes	No	1	2	3	4	5	6	7	8	9
When you are on the telephone	Yes	No	1	2	3	4	5	6	7	8	9
When watching TV	Yes	No	1	2	3	4	5	6	7	8	9
When visitors are in your home	Yes	No	1	2	3	4	5	6	7	8	9
When you are visiting someone else	Yes	No	1	2	3	4	5	6	7	8	9
When in supermarkets, stores, church, restaurants, or other public places	Yes	No	1	2	3	4	5	6	7	8	9
When asked to do chores at home	Yes	No	1	2	3	4	5	6	7	8	9
When going to bed	Yes	No	1	2	3	4	5	6	7	8	9
When in the car	Yes	No	1	2	3	4	5	6	7	8	9
When with a babysitter	Yes	No	1	2	3	4	5	6	7	8	9
When at school	Yes	No	1	2	3	4	5	6	7	8	9
When asked to do school homework	Yes	No	1	2	3	4	5	6	7	8	9

FIGURE 3.10. The 16-item version of the Home Situations Questionnaire.

shows that hyperactive children are significantly more likely to have problems in virtually every situation measured by the scale and are rated as having more severe problems in each situation than normal children. The greatest problems for most hyperactive children take place when they are playing with other children, when a parent is on the telephone, when visitors are in the home, when they are asked to do chores, and when they go to bed. A child with problems in five or more settings will be two standard deviations above the mean for normal children. Using a cutoff score of seven or more problem settings would correctly identify 100% of the children in each

TABLE 3.6. Percentages of Hyperactive and Normal Children Displaying Behavior
Problems in Each of 14 Settings and Mean Parent-Rated Severity

	Hyperactives ($n = 30$)		Normals ($n = 30$)	
Setting	%	Severity[a]	%	Severity[a]
When playing alone	40	4.3	0	0.0
When playing with other children	90	5.4	10	1.6
When at meals	87	4.7	13	3.0
When getting dressed	73	6.1	10	2.3
When washing/bathing	43	5.1	17	1.2
When parent is on phone	93	6.6	33	1.3
When watching television	80	5.0	3	2.0
When visitors are in home	97	6.1	30	1.6
When visiting others' homes	97	5.4	13	1.5
When in public places	97	5.4	23	2.7
When father is at home	73	3.9	7	2.5
When asked to do chores	87	5.6	37	2.0
When going to bed	83	5.0	20	1.5
When riding in the car	73	4.8	20	1.7

Note. Comparisons are based on a 14-item version of the Home Situations Questionnaire
administered to parents of 30 hyperactive and 30 normal children of normal intelligence, aged 5
to 9.
[a]Parents were asked to rate problem severity on a scale of 0 (no problem) to 9 (severe
problem).

group. This scale is currently undergoing studies to establish its interparent
and test–retest reliability, as well as its correlations with the other rating
scales mentioned above and with objective observations of parent–child
interactions.

In summary, it appears that a thorough assessment of hyperactive
children would include at least the Conners PSQ, the Achenbach CBCL and
the HSQ. These scales assist in establishing the diagnosis of hyperactivity, in
elucidating the associated behavior problems and social competence deficits,
in establishing the statistical deviance of these problems, and in revealing the
specific settings in which they are problematic. Where desirable, these scales
can be supplemented by the WWPARS, though these data would seem to be
redundant, and by the PIC, if a more thorough "personality profile" of a
particular child is of specific interest to the examiner.

Teacher Rating Scales

As noted earlier, teacher ratings of behavior tend to be more reliable and more sensitive to hyperactive behaviors than parent ratings. Such ratings, in addition to personal contacts with teachers and to teacher diaries, form an indispensable part of the evaluation of hyperactive children. Like parent rating scales, however, teacher rating scales are subject to the same criticisms noted earlier in this chapter.

The most widely used scale for teachers is the Conners Teacher Rating Scale (TRS). This is a 39-item scale similar to the PSQ, with items grouped into three general classes: group participation, classroom behavior, and attitude toward authority. Each item is rated "not at all," "just a little," "pretty much," or "very much," with 0, 1, 2, or 3 points assigned to each answer respectively. The scale is set forth in Figure 3.11. Factor analysis of the scale revealed five general item clusters: aggressive conduct, daydreaming–inattention, anxiety–fearfulness, hyperactivity, and sociability–cooperation. Like the PSQ, the TRS can be scored for the hyperactivity index (10 items), with a mean score of 1.5 or higher generally accepted as indicating hyperactivity. Normative data, however, are provided in Table 3.7. It would seem better to use a score of two standard deviations above the mean for age as a more rigorous criteria for defining hyperactivity in the classroom. The scale has shown acceptable test–retest reliability, and it discriminates hyperactive from normal children. It has also been shown to be sensitive to drug and behavioral treatments, with higher scores being predictive of a more positive drug response.

Another scale that clinicians may find helpful for use with hyperactive children is the Behavior Rating Scale (BRS), developed in 1979 by Phillip Kendall and Lance Wilcox of the University of Minnesota. Since hyperactive children are believed to have primary deficits in the development of self-control (rule-governed behavior), this scale would seem to be of some benefit in the clinical assessment of these children. We have found it a useful adjunct to the other scales mentioned above, since they only indirectly assess this dimension of behavior. The full scale is set forth in Figure 3.12; it consists of 33 items dealing with problems of self-control. The scale was standardized using only teacher ratings. Each item is rated on a 7-point continuum, and the total score is based on the sum of these ratings. Norms for children in grades 3 to 6 for males and females are displayed in Table 3.8. Scores for girls were found to decrease significantly with age, while the small decline for boys was not statistically significant. The scale has a high correlation for internal consistency, which suggests that its items all assess a common dimension of behavior. Test–retest reliability over 3 to 4 weeks showed an excellent correlation of .84. The construct validity of the scale was evaluated

Teacher's Questionnaire

Name of Child _____   Grade _____

Date of Evaluation _____

Please answer all questions. Beside *each* item, indicate the degree
of the problem by a check mark (✔)

	Not at all	Just a little	Pretty much	Very much
1. Restless in the "squirmy" sense.				
2. Makes inappropriate noises when he shouldn't.				
3. Demands must be met immediately.				
4. Acts "smart" (impudent or sassy).				
5. Temper outbursts and unpredictable behavior.				
6. Overly sensitive to criticism.				
7. Distractibility or attention span a problem.				

8. Disturbs other children.				
9. Daydreams.				
10. Pouts and sulks.				
11. Mood changes quickly and drastically.				
12. Quarrelsome.				
13. Submissive attitude toward authority.				
14. Restless, always "up and on the go."				

15. Excitable, impulsive.				
16. Excessive demands for teacher's attention.				
17. Appears to be unaccepted by group.				
18. Appears to be easily led by other children.				
19. No sense of fair play.				
20. Appears to lack leadership.				
21. Fails to finish things that he starts.				

22. Childish and immature.				
23. Denies mistakes or blames others.				
24. Does not get along well with other children.				
25. Uncooperative with classmates.				
26. Easily frustrated in efforts.				
27. Uncooperative with teacher.				
28. Difficulty in learning.				

FIGURE 3.11. The Conners Teacher Rating Scale. (Reprinted by permission of C. K. Conners.)

TABLE 3.7.   Norms for the Conners Teacher Rating Scale (TRS)

Age (years)	n^a	(I) Conduct problems		(II) Hyperactivity		(III) Inattention– passivity		Hyperactivity index	
		$\bar{x}$	SD	$\bar{x}$	SD	$\bar{x}$	SD	$\bar{x}$	SD
Males by age									
3–5	13	.45	.80	.79	.89	.92	1.00	.81	.96
6–8	60	.32	.43	.60	.65	.76	.74	.58	.61
9–11	59	.50	.66	.70	.78	.85	.73	.67	.65
12–14	46	.23	.38	.41	.49	.71	.63	.44	.43
15–17	30	.22	.37	.34	.44	.68	.67	.41	.45
Females by age									
3–5	11	.53	.68	.69	.56	.72	.71	.74	.67
6–8	42	.28	.37	.28	.38	.47	.64	.36	.45
9–11	49	.28	.49	.38	.51	.49	.53	.38	.48
12–14	48	.15	.23	.19	.27	.32	.42	.18	.24
15–17	25	.33	.68	.32	.63	.45	.47	.36	.62

Note. Norms are taken from "Normative Data on Revised Conners Parent and Teacher Rating Scales by C. H. Goyette, C. K. Conners, and R. F. Ulrich, *Journal of Abnormal Child Psychology*, 1978, 6, 221–236. Copyright 1978 by Plenum Publishing Corp. Reprinted by permission. The scores are derived by assigning 0, 1, 2, or 3 points to the answers of "not at all," "just a little," "pretty much," and "very much," respectively, for each item. The points for each item assigned to each factor are then summed and divided by the number of items in that factor or category to get the factor score. The items assigned to each factor or category from the original Conners Teacher Rating Scale are as follows:

Conduct problems: questions 4, 5, 6, 10, 11, 12, 23, and 27.

Hyperactivity: questions 1, 2, 3, 8, 14, 15, and 16.

Inattention–passivity: questions 7, 9, 18, 20, 21, 22, 26, and 28.

Hyperactivity index: questions 1, 5, 7, 8, 10, 11, 14, 15, 21, and 26.

[a]n = number of subjects per age group.

by correlating teacher ratings on the scale with behavioral observations in the classroom of off-task verbal and physical behavior, off-task attention, out-of-seat behavior, and interruptions, as well as the Matching Familiar Figures Test, the Porteus Mazes, and a delay-of-gratification task. The correlations were significant, although significance was of a low order, with all measures except the delay-of-gratification task. The BRS failed to correlate with measures of mental age or intelligence; this suggests that it assesses a construct different from general intelligence—a necessary finding for establishing discriminant validity of the scale. Studies with clinic-referred

Name of Child _____ Grade _____

Rater _____

Please rate this child according to the descriptions below by circling the appropriate number. The underlined 4 in the center of each row represents where the average child would fall on this item. Please do not hesitate to use the entire range of possible ratings.

1. When the child promises to do something, can you count on him or her to do it?

    1   2   3   4   5   6   7
   always   never

2. Does the child butt into games or activities even when he or she hasn't been invited?

    1   2   3   4   5   6   7
   always   never

3. Can the child deliberately calm down when he or she is excited or all wound up?

    1   2   3   4   5   6   7
   yes   no

4. Is the quality of the child's work all about the same, or does it vary a lot?

    1   2   3   4   5   6   7
   same   varies

5. Does the child work for long-range goals?

    1   2   3   4   5   6   7
   yes   no

6. When the child asks a question, does he or she wait for an answer, or jump to something else (e.g., a new question) before waiting for an answer?

    1   2   3   4   5   6   7
   waits   jumps

7. Does the child interrupt inappropriately in conversations with peers, or wait his or her turn to speak?

    1   2   3   4   5   6   7
   waits   interrupts

8. Does the child stick to what he or she is doing until he or she is finished with it?

    1   2   3   4   5   6   7
   yes   no

9. Does the child follow the instructions of responsible adults?

    1   2   3   4   5   6   7
   always   never

10. Does the child have to have everything right away?

    1   2   3   4   5   6   7
   no   yes

11. When the child has to wait in line, does he or she do so patiently?

    1   2   3   4   5   6   7
   yes   no

12. Does the child sit still?

    1   2   3   4   5   6   7
   yes   no

13. Can the child follow suggestions of others in group projects, or does he or she insist on imposing his or her own ideas?

    1   2   3   4   5   6   7
   able   imposes
   to follow

FIGURE 3.12. (*Continued*)

14. Does the child have to be reminded several times to do something before he or she does it?

1 2 3 4 5 6 7
never   always

15. When reprimanded, does the child answer back inappropriately?

1 2 3 4 5 6 7
never   always

16. Is the child accident-prone?

1 2 3 4 5 6 7
no   yes

17. Does the child neglect or forget regular chores or tasks?

1 2 3 4 5 6 7
never   always

18. Are there days when the child seems incapable of settling down to work?

1 2 3 4 5 6 7
never   often

19. Would the child more likely grab a smaller toy today or wait for a larger toy tomorrow, if given the choice?

1 2 3 4 5 6 7
wait   grab

20. Does the child grab for the belongings of others?

1 2 3 4 5 6 7
never   often

21. Does the child bother others when they're trying to do things?

1 2 3 4 5 6 7
no   yes

22. Does the child break basic rules?

1 2 3 4 5 6 7
never   always

23. Does the child watch where he or she is going?

1 2 3 4 5 6 7
always   never

24. In answering questions, does the child give one thoughtful answer, or blurt out several answers all at once?

1 2 3 4 5 6 7
one   several

25. Is the child easily distracted from his or her work or chores?

1 2 3 4 5 6 7
no   yes

26. Would you describe this child more as careful or careless?

1 2 3 4 5 6 7
careful   careless

27. Does the child play well with peers (follows rules, waits turn, cooperates)?

1 2 3 4 5 6 7
yes   no

28. Does the child jump or switch from activity to activity rather than sticking to one thing at a time?

1 2 3 4 5 6 7
sticks   switches
to one

FIGURE 3.12. (*Continued*)

29. If a task is at first too difficult for the child, will he or she get frustrated and quit, or first seek help with the problem?	1 2 3 4 5 6 7 seeks help quits
30. Does the child disrupt games?	1 2 3 4 5 6 7 never often
31. Does the child think before he or she acts?	1 2 3 4 5 6 7 always never
32. If the child paid more attention to his or her work, do you think he or she would do much better than at present?	1 2 3 4 5 6 7 no yes
33. Does the child do too many things at once, or does he or she concentrate on one thing at a time?	1 2 3 4 5 6 7 one thing too many

FIGURE 3.12. The Behavior Rating Scale for Children. (From "Self-Control in Children: Development of a Rating Scale" by P. C. Kendall and L. E. Wilcox, *Journal of Consulting and Clinical Psychology*, 1979, *47*, 1020–1029. Copyright 1979 by P. Kendall. Reprinted by permission.)

children find that it discriminates them from normal children to a useful degree.

An additional rating scale, similar to the HSQ for parents, has been developed for teachers. The School Situations Questionnaire (SSQ) is shown in Figure 3.13; like the HSQ, it is concerned with the settings in which behavior problems occur rather than with the type of problems. It therefore serves as a useful supplement to the Conners TRS, which yields no information on setting aspects of behavior problems in school. Studies to develop normative, reliability, and validity data on the scale are now under way.

It is my practice to send out all three questionnaires to teachers of hyperactive children referred to the clinic. In doing so, information on the types of problems the children have, the degree to which self-control is a problem, and the settings most likely to be problematic for the children can be obtained. This, of course, is followed up by phone calls or personal contacts with the teachers to clarify their answers and obtain additional information, as described earlier in the teacher interviews.

TABLE 3.8. Means and Standard Deviations on the Self-Control Rating Scale for Males and Females in Grades 3-6

	Male			Female		
Grade	M	SD	n	M	SD	n
3	120.2	44.5	10	107.5	50.3	12
4	123.6	43.6	16	80.2	27.7	13
5	119.6	45.4	14	70.6	37.2	14
6	107.0	47.9	19	59.7	21.8	12
Total	117.6	49.3	59	79.5	37.2	51

Note. Norms are from "Self-Control in Children: Development of a Rating Scale" by P. C. Kendall, and L. E. Wilcox, Journal of Consulting and Clinical Psychology, 1979, 47, 1020–1029. Copyright 1979 by the American Psychological Association. Reprinted by permission. Higher scores indicate less self-control (more impulsivity).

FIGURE 3.13. The School Situations Questionnaire.

Name of Child _____

Name of Person Completing This Form _____

Does this child present any behavior problems for you in any of these situations? If so, indicate how severe they are.

Situation	Yes/No (Circle one)		If Yes, How Severe? (Circle one) Mild Severe								
While arriving at school	Yes	No	1	2	3	4	5	6	7	8	9
During individual desk work	Yes	No	1	2	3	4	5	6	7	8	9
During small group activities	Yes	No	1	2	3	4	5	6	7	8	9
During free-play time in class	Yes	No	1	2	3	4	5	6	7	8	9
During lectures to the class	Yes	No	1	2	3	4	5	6	7	8	9
During recess	Yes	No	1	2	3	4	5	6	7	8	9
During lunch	Yes	No	1	2	3	4	5	6	7	8	9
While in the hallways	Yes	No	1	2	3	4	5	6	7	8	9
While in the bathroom	Yes	No	1	2	3	4	5	6	7	8	9
During field trips	Yes	No	1	2	3	4	5	6	7	8	9
During special assemblies	Yes	No	1	2	3	4	5	6	7	8	9
While on the bus	Yes	No	1	2	3	4	5	6	7	8	9

Summary

In summary, numerous parent and teacher rating scales are available for use with hyperactive children. Most show problems in one aspect or another of acceptable standardization criteria. Almost all are of little help in establishing the antecedents and consequences of problem behaviors that will be critical to treatment planning. Nonetheless, their utility is in their reference to available normative data; this assists in a true normative approach to assessment, as is noted at the beginning of this chapter. That is, these scales help to indicate whether a child's problems as described by parents are truly deviant for the child's age. They are, however, based on adult opinions, and the limitations of such opinions must be appreciated. These scales should never serve as a substitute for the collection of observational data on the children's problems and on parent–child interactions when facilities and resources permit them to be observed. While the rating scales may be helpful in assessing whether treatment has brought the child's behavior closer to normal, they are of much less help in the actual designing of therapeutic strategies.

It is our custom to require that the following criteria from ratings be met before a child is diagnosed as hyperactive:

1. Score of 1.5 or higher on the hyperactivity index of the Conners PSQ, or

2. A score of 20 or higher on the WWPARS. A score of two standard deviations above the mean for age on either questionnaire would be a more rigorous criterion.

3. Problems with behavior in 50% or more of the situations in the HSQ.

Where a diagnosis of hyperactivity in school is of interest, the following criteria are used:

1. Score of 1.5 or higher on the hyperactivity index of the Conners TRS (or two standard deviations above the mean for age).

2. Problems with behavior in at least 50% of the situations on the SSQ.

These criteria are then used in conjunction with information from the parental interview to reach a diagnosis of hyperactivity. To reiterate, the first of these additional criteria is an onset of symptoms by 6 years of age, or a duration of symptoms for 12 months prior to referral for evaluation for children under 6 years of age. The child must also be of average intelligence, or the symptoms must be deviant in relation to the child's mental age, according to the rating scales and tables of norms provided here. In addition, the presence of gross neurologic, sensory, or motor impairment and of psychosis must be ruled out.

CONCLUSION

This chapter has reviewed two crucial elements in the evaluation of hyperactive children: the clinical interview and the use of standardized behavior rating scales. While problems with reliability and validity exist for each aspect of the evaluation, there is no doubt that their combination can lead to a highly useful approach to assessment, with each partially negating the problems contributed by the other. General approaches to establishing "deviancy" in child behaviors have also been reviewed; it has been suggested that more than one approach is necessary to the evaluation of hyperactive children. Finally, several criteria for achieving the diagnosis of hyperactivity have been drawn from the clinical interview and behavior rating scales. These establish the presence and nature of symptoms, their onset and duration, and their pervasiveness, as well as their statistical deviance in relation to normal children of the same age. Additional rating scales can be used to determine other behavioral or personality problems in addition to the symptoms of hyperactivity. Heavy emphasis in the evaluation is placed on the assessment of adult–child interactions and on a nonjudgmental style of pursuing these procedures. The next chapter discusses those objective psychological methods that can augment these initial components of the assessment process.

SUGGESTED READING

Achenbach, T. M. The child behavior profile: I. Boys aged 6–11. *Journal of Consulting and Clinical Psychology*, 1978, *46*, 478–488.

Benjamin, A. *The helping interview.* Boston: Houghton Mifflin, 1969.

Cairns, R. B., & Green, J. A. How to assess personality and social patterns: Observations or ratings? In R. B. Cairns (Ed.), *The analysis of social interactions.* Hillsdale, N.J.: Erlbaum, 1979.

Edinburg, G. M., Zinberg, N. E., & Kelman, W. *Clinical interviewing and counseling: Principles and techniques.* New York: Appleton-Century-Crofts, 1975.

Furman, W. Promoting social development: Developmental implications for treatment. In B. Lahey & A. Kazdin (Eds.), *Advances in child clinical psychology* (Vol. 3). New York: Plenum, 1980.

Goyette, C. H., Conners, C. K., & Ulrich, R. F. Normative data on revised Conners parent and teacher rating scales. *Journal of Abnormal Child Psychology*, 1978, *6*, 221–236.

Kendall, P. C., & Wilcox, L. E. Self-control in children: Development of a rating scale. *Journal of Consulting and Clinical Psychology*, 1979, *47*, 1020–1029.

Mash, E. J., & Terdal, L. G. (Eds.). *Behavioral assessment of childhood disorders.* New York: Guilford, 1981.

Morganstern, K. P. Behavioral interviewing: The initial stages of assessment. In M. Hersen & A. Bellack (Eds.), *Behavioral assessment: A practical handbook.* New York: Pergamon, 1976.

O'Leary, K. D., & Johnson, S. B. Psychological assessment. In H. Quay & J. Werry (Eds.), *Psychopathological disorders of childhood* (2nd ed.). New York: Wiley, 1979.

Routh, D. K., Schroeder, C. S., & O'Tuama, L. Development of activity level in children. *Developmental Psychology*, 1974, *10*, 163–168.

Wirt, R. D., Lacher, D. Klinedinst, J. K., & Seat, P. D. *Multidimensional description of child personality: A manual for the Personality Inventory for Children.* Los Angeles: Western Psychological Services, 1977.

CHAPTER FOUR

THE EVALUATION OF HYPERACTIVE CHILDREN: OBSERVATIONAL METHODS AND PSYCHOLOGICAL TESTS

General observations drawn from particulars are the jewels of knowledge, comprehending great store in a little room.—*John Locke*

At this point in the evaluation process, interviews and rating scales will have given the examiner some idea of a particular child's problems, the degree of their deviancy from normal behavior, and their settings. These sources of information will assist in narrowing the focus of the evaluation to certain behaviors and their settings so that objective methods of observing the problems are more likely to capture the essence of the parental complaints. Such a narrowing of focus also permits the selection of certain objective instruments or methods most likely to record the child's problems accurately. If one takes the traditional view of hyperactivity, then at this point one would set about making objective measurements of the child's activity level or attention span in various situations to confirm the parental complaints. A variety of measures of hyperkinetic symptoms too numerous to review here exists. The important question is whether or not such measures are of any value in clinical assessment or treatment planning. I do not believe so, and a brief survey of some of these instruments should support this view.

Numerous measures of activity level have been developed for research with hyperactive children (see Ross & Ross, 1976, in "Suggested Reading"). Some researchers have used modified self-winding wrist watches called "actometers" to assess wrist or ankle activity. Other have used pedometers attached to wrists, ankles, or children's belts to measure motion of arms, legs, or trunks, respectively. A few researchers have placed pneumatic pads on the floor to count footsteps or have marked off a playroom floor with tape or electric eyes to measure grid crossings during movement in the room. One early project made use of an ultrasonic generator in a playroom to set up a series of standing sound waves that, when disturbed, were measured by sound wave receivers. Finally, motion-sensitive seat cushions have been developed to assess "seat restlessness" in a lab or classroom situation.

From the standpoint of behavioral assessment, these mesaures have serious limitations. First, the quantitative scores they generate show poor reliability over time, across settings, and between judges when raters must be used. Second, normative data are not readily available on most measures, and thus the meaning of the scores is doubtful. Third, the activities being measured are highly influenced by situational factors, but the scores give few if any clues as to what these important factors may be. Fourth—another important point for the planning of treatment—these measures give no information with respect to the antecedent or consequating events of the activities measured. Finally, research has shown that these measures do not correlate with parent rating scales (see Barkley, 1976, and Barkley & Ullman, 1975, in "Suggested Reading"). Hence, studies making use of these measures are not evaluating those aspects of the child's behavior about which the parents are concerned.

Similar disadvantages plague other objective measures of attention span and impulsivity, making them almost useless in clinic situations. If one takes the view of hyperactivity developed in this text, namely, that hyperactivity is a developmental disorder of social conduct, rule-governed behavior, and self-control, then some assessment of children's social interactions seems critical to thorough evaluation. Measures of social interactions, especially with parents, siblings, and teachers, would seem to be of great value in understanding the nature of the problems which bring families to the clinic to begin with. In particular, measures of maternal commands, child compliance, maternal contingent praise, parent and child negative behavior, and positive interactions would appear to be of great assistance in planning treatment and measuring improvements in response to treatment. Thus, the following discussion emphasizes those observation systems that permit the recording of social interactions and their antecedent and consequent events.

GENERAL CONSIDERATIONS

Where time, finances, or resources do not permit the direct observation of parent–child behaviors at home or in a clinic analogue situation, or of teacher–child exchanges in the classroom, then examiners should take greater care during interviews to have parents and teachers specify the nature of these interactions. Having parents and teachers record child behaviors in diaries or on forms designed for that purpose is an excellent aid in such situations. One such form is shown in Figure 4.1. This form permits a parent to record up to five target behaviors over a 7-day period. A hash mark can be

| Data Sheet | Name: _____ Week of: _____ | | | | | |
Target Behaviors	1.	2.	3.	4.	5.	Comments
Day: Date:						
Day: Date:						
Day: Date:						
Day: Date:						
Day: Date:						
Day: Date:						
Day: Date:						

FIGURE 4.1. A form on which parents can record occurrences of up to five child behaviors over a 7-day period at home.

used to record the occurrence of the target response within a given cell. It is sometimes helpful to have parents use letters in the cells to record their own responses to their children's target behavior. For instance, if a child's target behavior is abusing the family pet, then the parent can place a "C" in the cell for that behavior for the initial command to the child to desist from this behavior and an "R" for each repetition of the command, in addition to the hash mark indicating the occurrence of pet abuse. In using such a procedure, examiners should take care not to overwhelm parents with the responsibility of recording large numbers of child behaviors. At most, parents should be asked to record only two or three behaviors each week, or they may not comply with the request.

In some cases, it is helpful to have parents record problem behaviors in diaries for a week before evaluation. In others, it is better to have such information recorded after evaluation and just before treatment so that the parents can be asked to focus their notes on particularly troublesome parent–child interactions in certain situations. The HSQ (see Figure 3.10) is a useful outline of the more problematic settings about which parents may be asked to collect further information. Such parent diaries have shown adequate correlations with more objectively collected data in home or analogue situations. They are also helpful in establishing baseline levels of behavior problems against which to measure treatment success.

In some cases, parents do not comply with requests to collect behavioral records on their children at home. This may result from examiners' poor explanations of the record-keeping process, excessively busy parental routines or activities, or parental lack of appreciation for the importance of this information. Whether the records are clearly fabricated at the last minute or completely nonexistent, examiners should take time to address the problems tactfully with the parents, instead of overlooking the problem and rushing ahead to treatment. In many cases, the same reasons for parents' failure at keeping records will be those for their failure at implementing treatment suggestions.

If direct observations of problem behaviors are possible at home, at school, or in a clinic playroom setting, then clinicians need to consider other issues. No matter where observations are taken, the possibility that reactivity may distort the observations must be recognized. That is, many people change their behavior when they are aware that others are observing and recording what they do; as a result, such observations may not be representative of what is actually happening when the observers are not around. This makes it imperative that examiners summarize the results of their observations to parents or teachers and ask how similar these are to the problems which have brought the children in for treatment. The observations also need to be compared to the information gathered in interviews and on rating scales. When discrepancies occur, they should be discussed with the parents or teachers before any treatment is begun. When observations in the home or school are to be arranged, they should coincide with the peak problem situations revealed by other aspects of the evaluation. Parents or teachers should be asked to keep to their usual routines and to behave as typically as possible. If clinic playroom observations are to be used, then the rooms should be made to look as homelike as possible, and the tasks the mothers and children are given should be related in some way to the types of problems that the children experience at home. Research has also shown that parent–child interactions will vary as a function of a family's socioeconomic status and the sex of the parent being observed with a child. Thus, a parent of lower SES may give more directives and disciplining than one of middle SES may, but this should not be construed as inappropriate for the social context in which the family lives. Finally, clinicians using direct observations should never attempt to confirm or reject diagnoses solely on the basis of observational data. While such data are extremely helpful for planning treatments and monitoring their effects, they are limited in many respects. Diagnoses should therefore be made through consideration of various types and sources of information, no single one of which is adequate alone for the diagnosis of hyperactivity.

Whichever system is chosen for recording interactions, close attention should be given to compliance and negative interaction from children and to commands and contingent praise from parents, as these have been found to have the greatest generality across settings and the highest association with scores on parent and teacher rating scales. Factors that can lead to command–compliance problems for parents and children are listed in Table 4.1, with some suggestions as to how they might be treated. More specific suggestions on teaching parents ways of managing child noncompliance are given in Chapters 6 and 7.

Assuming direct observations of child behaviors are feasible, where should they occur? Some have argued that observations made in the home or classroom are likely to be the most representative of those behaviors of which parents or teachers are complaining. But such observations are expensive to undertake, and they are just as subject to the problems of observer reactivity and response generality as are clinic playroom observations. While the natural settings of home or school provide the advantage of children's familiarity with them, this is no guarantee that the typical behavior problems will be observed during the brief time in which recording will be taking place. A few clinicians have videotaped behavior in the home or class, using machines operated by a parent or teacher in order to capture more representative samples of conduct problems. The expense of such recording puts it beyond the reach of most clinicians, however, and there is still the family's reactivity to the recording with which to contend. Others have used voice-initiated sound recording systems in the home or class, but these are subject to similar criticisms—as well as to the problem of invasion of privacy, since *all* interactions are recorded.

Observations can be made at less cost in a clinic playroom equipped with a one-way mirror and a sound system. The question here, however, is whether the behaviors seen in the room are typical of those causing problems at home. If the playroom is furnished like a typical room in a home, the likelihood of observing behaviors similar to those seen in the home may be enhanced. (Classroom-like settings are very difficult to duplicate in clinic settings and are not cost-effective. Hence, direct observations in an actual class, when feasible, are the best source of objective information when classroom behavior problems are of interest.) When clinic playrooms are used to code parent–child behaviors, two other factors seem to enhance the likelihood of observing typical child behavior problems. First, the more closely the tasks given in the playroom are to those with which the children have problems at home, the more likely it is that those problems will be seen in the clinic. And, second, the more familiar children are with the playroom, the less inhibited they will be and the more likely they will be to display problems. This suggests that, when possible, interviews with parents can be conducted in the playroom with the children present at least part of the time. This should give the children at least an hour to habituate to the playroom before direct observations of parent–child interactions are recorded.

CLINIC PLAYROOM (ANALOGUE) SETTINGS

Circumstances in the clinic do not often easily permit the use of direct home observations of parent–child interactions for most of the children referred to the clinic. We have therefore developed a clinic playroom with an observation mirror, a two-way communications system, and furnishings similar to a family room or living room. The playroom furnishings consists of a sofa; a cushioned swivel rocking chair; a coffee table; a television set with a portable stand; a smaller table; several chairs; toys; trash cans; wall pictures; and a small child-size broom and dust pan. A cardboard box filled with unfolded clothes is also provided for use during the task period. Magazines are available for reading and are located on the coffee table. A black line of tape is placed across one end of the playroom, and it is also used during the task period.

When the observations of a particular parent–child dyad are to occur, the *mother* and the child are taken to the playroom and told to play as they might do at home if they were not disturbed. Mothers are almost always the parents chosen for these observations, as they are almost always the parents who bring the children to the clinic and probably the ones who are having more trouble managing the children at home. The interactions between

TABLE 4.1.   Problems Leading to Noncompliance

Problem	Corrective action
Parents present vague, ambiguous, or distorted commands.	Instruct parents on presenting clear and concise direct commands.
Parents give commands as questions.	Train parents in use of direct commands without voice inflection implying a question or without direct questions.
Child refuses to initiate compliance to parental command.	Train parents to provide positive attention contingent on episodes where compliance is initiated within 5 seconds and to use brief time-out periods contingent upon noncompliance after 5 seconds.
Child is unable to sustain compliance to a command.	Train parents to provide positive attention for very brief periods of compliance. Then train them to gradually shape or increase the intervals of compliance for which they will give positive attention. When child terminates compliance before task completion, train parents to give one warning for child to return to the task, then apply brief time out.
Duration of child's compliance is excessive.	Train parents to use a kitchen timer with child by setting timer to interval somewhat greater than that eventually desired for the task. Instruct them to make attention and praise contingent on compliance within the interval and time out contingent on failure to do so within interval. Have them gradually reduce the time interval on timer until desired compliance time is achieved; they should gradually remove use of timer.
Child's compliance is of poor quality.	Insure that parents have concisely specified the desired behaviors for the task and desired outcome and that the child has the requisite skills. Parents then model desired behavior, consequate child's behavior for (non)imitation, and specify in writing on a chore card (for children who can read) the desired outcome. Parents then consequate task performance on basis of adherence to modeled or written standards. They should reduce use of written standards as needed.
Parents frequently intrude while child correctly complies with commands.	This problem often results from the child's poor quality of compliance, excessive duration of compliance, or parents' provision of vague commands to the child. If

TABLE 4.1.   (*Continued*)

Problem	Corrective action
	so, then treat as above. Otherwise, the problem may be that the child complies correctly for his or her age, but the parents intrude on compliance because of excessively high or strict expectations for compliance. When this is detected, focus treatment on altering parental expectations to more appropriate levels.
Child's development in language or intellect is delayed.	This can lead to any or all of the above problems. When such a delay is suspected, the child should receive thorough developmental testing. Parents can then be trained in all of above methods, but especially in reducing the number and complexity of commands to the child.
Parents consequate child's (non)compliance inadequately.	This may be observed in conjunction with any or all of the above problems. The parent may ignore the child's appropriate compliance when it does occur, fail to punish noncompliance, or fail to consequate (non)compliance within a short time after its occurrence. Parents can be trained to provide only one command and to consequate (non)compliance within 5 seconds after command.
Stimuli eliciting child behavior that competes with compliance are present (e.g., TV is on while child is doing homework).	Reduce or remove competing stimuli.

Note. From "Hyperactivity" by R. A. Barkley. In E. J. Mash and L. G. Terdal (Eds.), *Behavioral Assessment of Childhood Disorders.* New York: Guilford Press, 1981. Copyright 1981 by Guilford Press. Reprinted by permission.

mother and child are recorded behind the mirror for 20 minutes, either on videotape or by trained behavior coders on the scene. Following this free-play period, the examiner provides the mother with a series of commands to give the child. Two sets of 15 commands each have been developed so that repeated observations using alternate sets of commands can be made in the playroom during treatment. Rarely do behavior problem children get through all 15 commands satisfactorily in the 20 minutes allotted for the task period. This is particularly true if cartoon shows are on the television set, which is left on during both free-play and task periods. The tasks or commands that I have used are listed in Figure 4.2. A third series of five tasks is also provided in this figure, because they are the ones that have been employed most often in my published studies of parent–child dyads with hyperactive children. I have recently changed from using these five tasks to using the longer series of 15 tasks, as the longer series seems more likely to elicit noncompliance from hyperactive children.

Following the free-play and task periods, the examiner discusses the observations with the mother to determine whether the interactions observed are representative of those the mother feels are problematic at home. When they are not, more time is spent in discussing the ways in which the interactions at home are different from those in the playroom. Where noncompliance has been elicited in the playroom, mothers are often embarrassed or apologetic to examiners. It is frequently necessary to reassure such mothers that their children's misbehavior is fortunate because it provides firsthand evidence of their problems. Clinicians are also likely to find that parents attribute greater credibility to evaluations when playroom observations are employed, perhaps because they believe the clinicians are truly interested in understanding their plight with their children.

Several problems exist in using playroom observations, however. One problem is the limitations placed on them by some children's age. Generally, children 12 years of age or younger respond well to the playroom setting, especially when age-appropriate activities are provided. Older children, however, are likely to find a playroom insulting to their maturity level, and data collected in such settings can be quite suspect or unrepresentative. In such instances, a different set of activities can be used with adolescents and their parents. I have adolescents and parents go into the playroom; the parents have been given a list of situations that are often potential sources of conflict for parents and teenagers. This list is provided in Figure 4.3. The parents are then requested to discuss each situation with their children and to attempt to come to some agreement if initial disagreement on the item is found. When this procedure is used, no free-play period is implemented. In other cases, home observations or parent diaries may be useful alternatives for helping to elucidate problem interactions.

A second problem is some children's reactivity to the mirror. We attempt to preclude this by simply not drawing attention to or discussing the mirror when the children are first placed in the room. Sometimes children persist in playing with or trying to see through the mirror. Observers are then told not to respond to the children if they are seen by them, as a response may encourage further play at the mirror. Often such play serves a useful purpose; command–noncompliance exchanges between a parent and a child can develop over this situation and provide further data on the ways in which the dyad deals with noncompliance.

Finally, clinicians need to consider whether or not other family members should be permitted to observe the mother–child interactions from behind the mirror. In most cases, I do not permit this during the evaluation, as it often enhances the apprehension of the parent being observed. It also leads

SET #1	SET #2
1. Stand up, please.	1. Come here and let me fix your shirt (dress).
2. Open the door.	2. Close the door.
3. Give me one of those toys.	3. Put this toy in the box (mother holds box of Legos or Tinker Toys).
4. Put all of the toys back in their boxes.	4. Put all of the toys on the coffee table.
5. Put the chairs under the table.	5. Empty that waste basket into the other one.
6. Pick up the paper behind the black line.	6. Fold the clothes and put them back in the box neatly.
7. Walk the black line slowly, heel to toe.	7. Walk the black line slowly, heel to toe.
8. Put all of the toys on the coffee table.	8. Take off your shoes.
9. Take off your shoes.	9. Draw the designs three times (a set of geometric designs is provided).
10. Sit over there at the work table.	10. Do all the math problems (problems are provided).
11. Draw these designs three times.	11. Do the Purdue Pegboard (provided and explained to parent).
12. Do all the math problems.	12. Move everything off the coffee table and dust it.
13. Bring the black line through the maze on the Etch-A-Sketch.	13. Stack the magazines neatly on the coffee table.
14. Move all the toys off that table and dust it.	14. Put the toys back on the table.
15. Put your shoes on.	15. Put your shoes on.

SET #3

1. Pick up all the toys and put them in their boxes.
2. Sit down here and draw these geometric designs.
3. Sit down here and do all the math problems.
4. Let's draw a line through the maze on the Etch-A-Sketch (mother gets one knob and child gets the other).
5. Let's build a house together out of the Lego blocks.

FIGURE 4.2.   Three sets of commands for a mother to give a child during observations in a clinic playroom.

Instructions to parent: You and your teenager should try to discuss each of the areas listed below and whether or not you have any disagreements about them.

1. Accomplishing homework on time
2. Completing chores when requested
3. The friends your son/daughter chooses
4. The clothes or style of dress your son/daughter wears
5. Bedtime on weekends
6. Bedtime on school nights
7. The television programs your son/daughter watches
8. Use of the telephone by your son/daughter
9. The type of music your son/daughter likes to listen to
10. The places your son/daughter likes to go during free time
11. The allowance your son/daughter should receive
12. Your son's/daughter's eating habits
13. Your son's/daughter's curfew for dates or other outings
14. Use of family car
15. Response to authority (parent/teacher) at home or school

FIGURE 4.3. Situations to be discussed by a parent and an adolescent child during playroom observations.

to conversations in the observation room that can disrupt attempts at coding the interactions. During individual parent training, however, having each parent alternate as observer of and participant in the playroom can be useful in later discussions of differences in management styles between the parents and of the degree to which the interactions seen in the playroom are typical of those occurring at home.

IN-HOME OBSERVATIONS

If clinicians have the luxury of being able to observe behaviors between a particular parent and child in the home, several precautions and considerations are necessary. The observation period should be planned in advance, and experienced observers should be used. The time at which the observation occurs should coincide, where possible, with that of one or more of the peak problem behaviors identified by the HSQ. Often a parent has trouble with a child when the parent is talking on the telephone. It would therefore be useful to have a spouse, a family friend or relative, or a clinic secretary place a call to the mother while the home observations are occurring. It is quite likely that more than one visit to the home will be necessary before useful data are collected, since the child being observed is initially likely to spend much of the time interacting with the "new visitor." The tasks to be used should be identified beforehand and should be those that the parent feels are most likely to provoke behavior problems. Some of the tasks listed in Figure 4.2 may be useful in this regard. The participants to be observed will have to be restricted to one room or a few rooms of the home so as to maximize their contact during the observation period. Finally, within these constraints, the parent should be requested to act as naturally as possible.

Because of many of these precautions and limitations, I have not found home observations any more useful than those made in the clinic playroom. The transportation time is often lengthy, adding to the expense of the evaluation, and health insurance carriers will rarely pay for this type of evaluation procedure. Reactivity to the recording by the parents and children is likely to be equal to, if not worse than, that seen in a playroom analogue setting, and observations in these cases are seldom representative of the children's real problems. Finally, videotaping equipment may be available, useful, and unobstrusive in the clinic, but it is often expensive, unwieldy, and highly obtrusive when taken into the home.

CLASSROOM OBSERVATIONS

As with observations made in a clinic playroom or at home, those made in the classroom are subject to problems with observers reactivity, representativeness of child behavior problems, generality of observations to other times and school situations, and cost-effectiveness of the procedures. Teachers should be contacted in advance so that visits can be arranged at times convenient to their schedules yet likely to catch the children during the peak problem times suggested by the School Situations Questionnaire that the teachers have completed. When observing the children, care should be taken to protect their identity from their classmates—a point that should be made with teachers as well before visits are made. Failure to do so can often subject the target children to much teasing and harassment from their classmates over the fact that mental health professionals have come to observe them. The class routine should remain as natural as possible during the observations. As with home observations, those made in the classroom will probably require several visits before representative behavior problems will be observed. Again, insurance carriers are unlikely to cover the expenses of these observations, which should be kept as affordable as possible to the families who must bear the brunt of their expense. Whatever recording method is used, observers should give attention to those events that precede or consequate the target child behaviors, as these will likely be the events that will require alteration during treatment.

OBJECTIVE BEHAVIORAL RECORDING METHODS

Where time and resources permit the direct observation of parent–child interactions, clinicians will have to make several decisions; they must select the behaviors they believe are most important for recording, the methods of recording they will use, and the setting in which the observations will take place. Issues related to the setting of the observations have already been discussed. In addition, it has already been noted that command–compliance interactions are probably the most important for gaining additional information about hyperactive children and their social behavior. The coding systems or methods that are best suited to accomplishing these observations remain to be discussed.

Before reviewing several useful methods, it is worthwhile to mention the prerequisites of an adequate behavioral coding procedure for clinical practice. First, the method chosen should have categories of behavior that are relevant to the problems a particular child is experiencing. In most cases, these will involve command–compliance interactions between a parent or a teacher and a hyperactive child. However, in some cases clinicians may be interested in recording such behaviors as disrespectful language toward adults, temper tantrums, destructiveness, aggression to peers or siblings, and so on. The coding system to be used in these instances can be chosen from those already employed in the scientific literature or can be designed by clinicians themselves to suit their particular needs. Second, the clinician or other observers should obviously have some familiarity with the method to be used. Third, some decision will have to be made as to the length of time the observations are to last. Frequently occuring behaviors, such as tics or noncompliance, will require much shorter periods of observation for a representative sample than will less frequently occurring behaviors, such as aggression. And, fourth, the behaviors to be recorded should be clearly defined so as to permit reliable recording yet should also be clearly related to or representative of the primary referral complaints. Recording the number of times a child is out of his or her chair in class, for instance, may have little relevance in the case of a child for whom the major concern is aggression to peers at recess or in the hallways at school.

General Types of Recording Procedures

Behavioral scientists typically divide their recording methods into four general classes: recording of behavioral products; event recording; duration recording; and interval recording or sampling. Probably the easiest recording method is that which relies on the results or products of the desired behavior, since these are often easy to specify, reliable in terms of agreement between observers, and clinically relevant to the referral complaints. For example, recording the number of problems a child completes during a 10-minute math assignment is a very straightforward measure of academic productivity or achievement, should this be a major problem for the child undergoing evaluation. The products of other behaviors, such as littering, stealing toys, pilfering food, or failing to do a chore (e.g., to empty trash or wash dishes) can all be simply and reliably recorded in clinicial situations, either by clinicians or by parents or teachers, with little if any training.

The second method is known as event or frequency recording. This consists simply of recording each occurrence of the behavior of interest. The method is often used with relatively discrete, well-defined behaviors that are of brief duration, such as the number of profanities a child says, the number of tics emitted in a certain period, or the number of times a child pushes or hits another child. Parental behaviors, such as commands, praise, criticism, or physical disciplining, can also be recorded via this method. To use the method properly, a time interval or duration for observing the behavior should be specified, and the behavior should not occur so frequently as to impede the ability of an observer to count its occurrences.

The third general class of recording methods consists of those that note the *duration* of particular behaviors, as opposed to their frequency. Compliance to commands, whining, crying, temper tantrums, or even physical complaints such as headaches are often best recorded by this method because of their longer duration of occurrence, somewhat more ambiguous nature, and perhaps higher frequency of occurrence. Typically, behaviors that are not discrete or brief in their occurrence or that occur at high rates are best recorded by this or the following method. The data in this case would be the lengths of time for which these behaviors occur during each observation session.

The final method is known as interval recording or sampling. In this case, an observation session is divided into equal intervals of time, and the observer merely indicates whether or not the behavior occurs in that interval, not necessarily how frequently it occurs or how long the behavior lasts. For instance, the observer wishing to record out-of-seat behavior for 10 minutes in a classroom divides this period into 15-second intervals. Using a stopwatch or a tape-recorded signal, the observer places an X or O in the box on the recording form for each 15-second interval to indicate whether or not the child is out of his or her seat during that interval. Since most child behaviors are not especially discrete occurrences and are often difficult to define in terms of beginning and ending points, interval recording is a frequently employed method for assessing behavior disorders in children.

Command–Compliance Coding

In many situations, clinicians are interested only in obtaining direct observations of a child's ability to comply with parental commands. Here, a relatively simple coding system will suffice to capture the frequency of maternal commands, repetition of repeated commands, and child compliance. Such a coding system is set forth in Figure 4.4. The observer using this form is going to watch a parent and a child interact for 10 minutes. The period is broken down into 1-minute intervals on the left side of the form. Across the top horizontal axis is the number of new commands given by the parent. Obviously, then, this form can record a maximum possibility of six new commands per minute of observation. Each new command that is given is recorded as follows. When the parent gives the first command during the first minute of observation, the coder places a circle around the letter "C" under the "Parent" subheading for the first command. If the mother should repeat this command, a circle is placed around the letter "R" in that sub-column for each repetition of that command. Under the "Child" subheading for the first command, the observer notes whether or not the child complies with the command *within* 10 seconds after it is *first* given. The coder monitors this by watching the stopwatch for the time that elapses after the first command is given. If the child cries, whines, kicks, throws a temper tantrum, swears, screams, or yells at the mother, then a circle is placed around the letters "Neg" to indicate this. If the mother should give a second *new* command during this first minute of observation, the coder moves to the second "Command" column and records again as above. This procedure is followed for each new command given in that minute of observation until six new commands are given or the 1-minute interval expires. When the first minute is over, the coder moves to the second "Minutes" row and starts recording commands and compliance in the first "Command" column again. The observer can continue the session for more than 10 minutes, if need be, by merely using a second recording form.

This form yields several important measures of parent–child interactions. The number of parent commands given and their rate per minute can be computed. In addition, the percentage of times the child complies within 10 seconds of a new command can also be obtained. Further, the average number of times a command is repeated can be derived, as can the percentage of times a new command provokes negative behavior in the child.

I frequently use this system in the clinic by placing a parent and a child in a playroom for a few minutes of free play. After this, the mother is given a list of commands to give the child, and the interactions are observed for 10 minutes from behind a one-way observation mirror. The free-play period is used to permit habituation to the room and to allow the child time to get involved in a desired play activity before the mother begins the list of commands. After the observation, the results are discussed with the mother to see how representative they are of problems with compliance at home.

The Response Class Matrix

The Response Class Matrix system for recording parent–child interactions was developed by Eric Mash, Leif Terdal, and Kathryn Anderson at the

University of Oregon Health Sciences Center (1973; see Appendix A). The system uses two coders; one scores the mother's behavior as an antecedent and the child's response to her, while the other codes the child's behavior as an antecedent and the mother's response to it. This permits the evaluation of contingent reciprocal interactions in which one person's behavior can be recorded as an antecedent to another's or as a consequence for it. The matrices used by the coders, the definitions of the behavior categories, and more details on the use of the system are set forth in Appendix A.

The coders use a procedure in which they first watch the interaction for a 10-second interval. A tape-recorded signal sounds the end of this interval, at which point the coders record the number signaled by the tape recorder in the cell corresponding to the last completed interaction. They are permitted 5 seconds to record, and then the tape recorder sounds a "ready" signal to prompt the coders to observe the interactions for another 10 seconds.

Observations usually cover at least 15 minutes of free play and 15 to 20 minutes of task accomplishment.

The scores of interest are derived by computing the percentage of occurrence of each antecedent category in relation to the total number of intervals in which recordings were made (see Appendix A). In addition, the coders can compute the conditional probabilities of each person's responses to the other's behavior. For instance, on the mother-antecedent matrix, a coder can derive the percentage of intervals in which commands are given, as well as the probability that the child will respond to these commands with compliance. Coder reliabilities are at least 75% or higher in most studies using the system, and the measures derived from the system correlate significantly with the WWPARS and the Conners PSQ. This intimates that these measures, when taken in clinic playroom situations, assess dimensions of child behaviors that are important to the parents and underlie their referral complaints.

This system is highly useful because of its assessment of reciprocal effects between parents and children and of more behaviors than simply commands and compliance. Like the coding system discussed earlier, this one yields information of value to further understanding of the interactions of hyperactive children with their mothers and to treatment planning using behavioral methods. It has also been shown to be sensitive to changes in parent–child interactions as a result of parent training or stimulant drug treatment. Test–retest stability in the clinic playroom has been quite good, making the system useful for repeated assessment of interactions throughout treatment phases. The system can be used in home, clinic, or classroom settings.

The Response Class Matrix, however, has several disadvantages in clinical settings. First, it requires two observers if the full system is to be used. This can be circumvented by videotaping the interactions for later reanalysis using either matrix. Or the clinician can choose to use only that matrix

Minutes	1		2		3		4		5		6	
	Parent	Child	Parent	Child	Parent	Child	Parent	Child	Parent	Child	Parent	Child
1	C R R R R R	Cpy Ncpy Neg	C R R R R R	Cpy Ncpy Neg	C R R R R R	Cpy Ncpy Neg	C R R R R R	Cpy Ncpy Neg	C R R R R R	Cpy Ncpy Neg	C R R R R R	Cpy Ncpy Neg
2	C R R R R R	Cpy Ncpy Neg	C R R R R R	Cpy Ncpy Neg	C R R R R R	Cpy Ncpy Neg	C R R R R R	Cpy Ncpy Neg	C R R R R R	Cpy Ncpy Neg	C R R R R R	Cpy Ncpy Neg
3	C R R R R R	Cpy Ncpy Neg	C R R R R R	Cpy Ncpy Neg	C R R R R R	Cpy Ncpy Neg	C R R R R R	Cpy Ncpy Neg	C R R R R R	Cpy Ncpy Neg	C R R R R R	Cpy Ncpy Neg
4	C R R R R R	Cpy Ncpy Neg	C R R R R R	Cpy Ncpy Neg	C R R R R R	Cpy Ncpy Neg	C R R R R R	Cpy Ncpy Neg	C R R R R R	Cpy Ncpy Neg	C R R R R R	Cpy Ncpy Neg
5	C R R R R R	Cpy Ncpy Neg	C R R R R R	Cpy Ncpy Neg	C R R R R R	Cpy Ncpy Neg	C R R R R R	Cpy Ncpy Neg	C R R R R R	Cpy Ncpy Neg	C R R R R R	Cpy Ncpy Neg
6	C R R R R R	Cpy Ncpy Neg	C R R R R R	Cpy Ncpy Neg	C R R R R R	Cpy Ncpy Neg	C R R R R R	Cpy Ncpy Neg	C R R R R R	Cpy Ncpy Neg	C R R R R R	Cpy Ncpy Neg

Figure 4.4 — coding system grid (rotated on page)

7	C R R R R R R R R	Cpy Ncpy Neg	C R R R R R R R R	Cpy Ncpy Neg	C R R R R R R R R	Cpy Ncpy Neg	C R R R R R R R R	Cpy Ncpy Neg	C R R R R R R R R	Cpy Ncpy Neg	C R R R R R R R R	Cpy Ncpy Neg	C R R R R R R R R	Cpy Ncpy Neg	C R R R R R R R R	Cpy Ncpy Neg
8	C R R R R R R R R	Cpy Ncpy Neg	C R R R R R R R R	Cpy Ncpy Neg	C R R R R R R R R	Cpy Ncpy Neg	C R R R R R R R R	Cpy Ncpy Neg	C R R R R R R R R	Cpy Ncpy Neg	C R R R R R R R R	Cpy Ncpy Neg	C R R R R R R R R	Cpy Ncpy Neg	C R R R R R R R R	Cpy Ncpy Neg
9	C R R R R R R R R	Cpy Ncpy Neg	C R R R R R R R R	Cpy Ncpy Neg	C R R R R R R R R	Cpy Ncpy Neg	C R R R R R R R R	Cpy Ncpy Neg	C R R R R R R R R	Cpy Ncpy Neg	C R R R R R R R R	Cpy Ncpy Neg	C R R R R R R R R	Cpy Ncpy Neg	C R R R R R R R R	Cpy Ncpy Neg
10	C R R R R R R R R	Cpy Ncpy Neg	C R R R R R R R R	Cpy Ncpy Neg	C R R R R R R R R	Cpy Ncpy Neg	C R R R R R R R R	Cpy Ncpy Neg	C R R R R R R R R	Cpy Ncpy Neg	C R R R R R R R R	Cpy Ncpy Neg	C R R R R R R R R	Cpy Ncpy Neg	C R R R R R R R R	Cpy Ncpy Neg

C = command   Ncpy = noncomply

R = repeat command   Neg = negative behavior by child

Cpy = comply in 10 seconds

FIGURE 4.4. A coding system for recording aspects of command–compliance interactions between a parent and a child over a 10-minute period.

which will yield the more useful data for a particular clinic case. Second, the system requires at least 30 to 40 hours of training for an observer to become proficient and reliable in its use. Third, the wealth of measures and their derivation from each matrix require a minimum of 20 to 30 minutes of scoring, making it more time-consuming in clinical situations than the first system discussed above. In the clinic, when time is an important consideration in evaluations, the simpler system is used in our clinic playroom under the task conditions described earlier. When more time is available, we use the Response Class Matrix with one or two coders and observe children and their mothers for at least 20 minutes of free play and 20 minutes of task accomplishment.

The results for one 4-year-old hyperactive child evaluated in our clinic are shown in Table 4.2; they are compared to the results for 20 normal children in the same situation. As can be seen from this table, this particular child in free play responded significantly less to his mother's interactions, complied less with her commands, and initiated more questions to his mother than normal children in similar situations did. His mother proved significantly more commanding and directive, as well as less responsive to his interactions, during this period. Obviously, the majority of exchanges in free play were of a command–noncompliance nature, whereas with normal children many more of the social exchanges consisted of positive interactions and play. During the task period, this child complied with only 44% of his mother's commands, which is less than half the rate of compliance seen in normal children. The ability of the child to sustain his compliance without further parental commands was six to seven times less than that of normal children. This measure is associated with the child's attention span and reflects the considerable problems this child had in this area. When compliance did occur, this mother was much less encouraging of it than mothers of normal children were. This intimates that the mother was either not very attentive to ongoing positive behaviors or that she found the child's quality of compliance so poor as to be hardly worthy of praise and encouragement. This case suggests a number of treatment recommendations for use in a parent training program. Briefly, this parent obviously needed to be more attentive and responsive to this child's positive interactions and more encouraging of appropriate compliance when it occurred. Decreases in the number of commands (often repeated ones) and increases in punishment contingent upon noncompliance would also have been desirable.

The Stony Brook System

The previous coding systems all assess adult–child social interactions, whether they are observed at home, in the clinic, or in the classroom. Clinicians, however, may wish to record hyperactive, off-task behaviors in the classroom, rather than teacher–child interactions in particular. In this case, the classroom

TABLE 4.2. Observation Measures for the Mother–Child Interactions of a 4-Year-Old Hyperactive Boy Compared to Means and Standard Deviations for Normal Children

Interaction measure	Percentage of interactions for 4-year-old child	Mean (*SD*) for 20 normal children	
During free play			
Mother initiates interaction	32	54	(13)
Child responds	42	84	(16)
Child initiates interaction	52	68	(18)
Mother responds	65	92	(8)
Child plays independently	20	30	(19)
Mother controls play	17	6	(8)
Mother encourages play	58	53	(11)
Mother commands	45	10	(12)
Child complies	48	90	(16)
During task period			
Mother commands	53	21	(11)
Child complies	44	95	(9)
Child compliance duration[a]	1.3	9	(4)
Mother encourages compliance	18	30	(14)

Note. From "Hyperactivity" by R. A. Barkley. In E. J. Mash and L. G. Terdal (Eds.), *Behavioral Assessment of Childhood Disorders.* New York: Guilford Press, 1981. Copyright 1981 by Guilford Press. Reprinted by permission. Measures are derived from the Response Class Matrix (see Appendix A). These measures are further defined in "The Effects of Methylphenidate on the Mother–Child Interactions of Hyperactive Children" by R. A. Barkley and C. E. Cunningham, *Archives of General Psychiatry,* 1979, *36,* 201–208. Means and standard deviations are derived from "A Comparison of the Interactions of Hyperactive and Normal Children with Their Mothers in Free Play and Structured Task" by C. E. Cunningham and R. A. Barkley, *Child Development,* 1979, *50,* 217–224.

[a]All measures are expressed as percentages except for this measure. The total number of intervals of compliance divided by the number of commands given by the parent equals the mean duration of compliance per command.

observation code developed by K. Daniel O'Leary and his colleagues at the State University of New York at Stony Brook may be helpful. This system has been modified somewhat by Howard Abikoff, Rachel Gittelman-Klein, and Donald Klein (1980) at the Long Island Jewish–Hillside Medical Center in New York, and has been validated in studies with hyperactive and normal children.

This coding system uses a 15-second-interval recording procedure and 14 behavioral categories. Only the initial occurrence of each type of behavior during each 15-second interval is recorded, with the exception that off-task behavior, noncompliance, out-of-seat behavior, verbalization, and day-dreaming are scored only if they occur for more than 15 consecutive seconds. The nontimed categories are interference; solicitation; minor motor movement; gross motor movement—standing; gross motor movement—vigorous; physical aggression; threat or verbal aggression to children; threat or verbal aggression to teacher; and absence of behavior. A copy of the manual for using this system is available from Dr. Rachel Gittelman-Klein, Director, Child Development Center, Long Island Jewish–Hillside Medical Center, P.O. Box 38, Glen Oaks, N.Y. 11004.

Research with this coding system has shown it to be highly sensitive to differences in behavior between hyperactive and normal children. Mean intercoder reliability is at least .76—satisfactory for such a complex coding system. The most frequently occurring categories were found to be interference, off-task behavior, minor motor and gross motor movements, and solicitation; interference (disruptiveness) was the category that discriminated most sharply between hyperactive and normal children. The coding system has also shown excellent test–retest stability over five different assessment occasions; its use as a repeated measure during treatment is thus quite satisfactory. It is suggested that if clinicians are to use this system, they omit the categories of extended verbalization and daydreaming because of their very low rate of occurrence.

One of the major disadvantages of this coding system is its failure to record antecedent and consequent events surrounding the coded behaviors. This limits its utility in planning behavioral interventions in the classroom, since there is no indication of what served to cue the behaviors and what consequating events are controlling them. In this respect, the previously discussed systems are more useful in classroom observations. A second problem, which applies to all of the coding systems, is the current lack of normative data for various age levels of children on this classroom coding system. This precludes drawing conclusions as to whether and how deviant a child's behavior in the classroom is, if at all, in relation to that of same-age peers. One method for addressing this problem is to select, with teacher assistance, an average child of the same sex in the same class and make several observations of his or her behavior while visiting the class. These observations can then be used as normal control comparisons for the hyperactive child.

Whichever system is selected for class observations, it is essential that the information so obtained be discussed with teachers to determine its representativeness of typical classroom behavior for the hyperactive children. This will also serve to reveal important information about the children or their backgrounds that was not obtained in the observational data. In addition, as with parents, this discussion will enhance the credibility of the evaluation from the teachers' perspective and thus make it more likely that they will adopt the recommendations stemming from the evaluations.

Other Coding Systems

Several other systems have been widely used in research on deviant child behavior. Probably the best researched and developed of these is the observational system designed by Gerald Patterson and his associates at the Oregon Research Institute (1969). The code consists of 29 behavior categories that capture antecedent–response–consequence sequences in social interactions between a child and other family members. Its intercoder reliability averages 74%, which is excellent for so complex a system. The disadvantage of the system is the need for highly trained coders familiar with its use and the rather lengthy training time needed to become familiar with it.

A second observational system with a sound basis in research is that developed by Robert Wahler at the University of Tennessee (1975). The code uses 18 behavior categories which are objectively defined and yield intercoder agreements of at least 80%; again, the reliability is quite satisfactory for a coding system with this many categories. Like the Patterson procedure, its major drawback is the time required to learn the system and its greater than necessary complexity for use in clinical circumstances with hyperactive children.

PSYCHOMETRIC TESTING

It is not the intent of this chapter to review the basic procedures involved in the psychometric assessment of children. Clinicians should have substantial training and experience in the most frequently used tests before undertaking the evaluation of hyperactive children. Clinicians who do not have this experience should refer such children to an experienced psychometrician for that part of the evaluation involving the assessment of intellectual and achievement skills. It is also not the intent of this chapter to review the scientific literature on learning disabilities; suggested readings in this area are provided at the end of this chapter. However, since hyperactive children are very likely to have specific learning disabilities, psychological tests must often be made a part of the evaluation process. It is therefore the intent of this section to discuss a useful conceptual framework from which to view learning disabilities and to select from among those tests available the ones most useful in the assessment of these disabilities. When there is no evidence suggesting that a child is performing poorly on academic subjects, psychometric tests obviously need not be done, as they only unnecessarily inflate the cost of the evaluation to the family.

Definition and Conceptualization of Learning Disabilities

Children with a specific learning disability are defined by Public Law 94-142 as follows:

Those children who have a disorder in one or more of the basic psychological processes involved in understanding or in using language, spoken or written, which disorder may manifest itself in imperfect ability to listen, think, speak, read, write, spell, or do mathematical calculations. (Federal Register, *41*, [No. 252], Thursday, December 30, 1976, pp. 56966–56998)

This definition excludes children whose problems in learning are primarily the result of visual, hearing, or motor handicaps; mental retardation; emotional disturbance; or environmental, cultural, or economic disadvantage. In other words, these are children who, despite seemingly adequate intelligence or opportunity, show significant deficits in reading, writing, speaking, or mathematical calculations. It is left to each state to determine the size of the deficit necessary to qualify for exceptional educational services in public schools. The definition is not intended to be a scientific one, but only to assist in describing the kinds of problems that would be eligible for treatment and in placing a limit on the number of children who could receive special educational services for learning disabilities in the public schools. Currently, services of this kind are limited to one-sixth of the total population of children requiring exceptional educational services (usually 12% of the school-age population).

It is therefore imperative that clinicians who work with hyperactive children with specific learning disabilities be familiar with their state's criteria for placing children within a learning disabilities program. Some states require that children have deficits that place them 50% or more below those academic achievement levels expected for their age and intelligence. Others require them to be two grade levels below those expected for their age and intelligence, and still others require deficits in two or more academic areas. There are numerous problems with these criteria that are outside the scope of this chapter. Suffice it to say here that some children have learning problems sufficient to impair their classroom performance but that they are not necessarily eligible for special assistance within the public schools.

The following guidelines are offered as suggestions to those who must work within this area of childhood disorders:

1. Where federal, state, or local guidelines exist, these must be consulted and followed.

2. Where no legal guidelines exist, the learning-disabled (LD) child can be considered one who scores at or below the 20th percentile on well-standardized tests of reading, spelling, math, and handwriting.

3. The child should have an IQ score on a well-standardized test that falls within the normal range (IQ > 70) in *either* verbal or nonverbal abilities.

4. The clinician should rule out primary sensory deficits and should assess whether the child has had adequate exposure to and opportunity for formal schooling.

5. Disorders such as psychosis, depression, anxiety, and hyperactivity should be ruled out as *primary* causes of the learning disorder. Such disorders may often be associated with or secondary to a learning problem but do not, in themselves, result in *focal* deficits in only one or a few areas of academic achievement while leaving other areas normal or better.

What, then, causes learning disabilities in children? The research shows a striking parallel to the causes of hyperactivity. Familial–genetic factors seem to play a major role; other etiologies include obstetrical–pregnancy complications; head trauma; neurologic disorders, such as infections, strokes, or tumors; and exposure to toxic substances, such as lead. Environmental theories have proven inadequate in accounting for focal deficits in academic learning. All etiologies, in one way or another, imply some inefficiency, immaturity, dysfunction, or damage to select areas of the cerebral hemispheres. Thus, it would seem that some acquaintance with the literature in neuropsychology is virtually essential to those who would attempt to understand, diagnose, and treat learning disabilities; such an acquaintance is not often found in actual practice. (The reader is directed to Gazzaniga, 1979; Golden, 1978; Hecaen & Albert, 1978; Heilman & Valenstein, 1979; and Luria, 1973, in "Suggested Reading.")

From this perspective, it is important to understand that complex cognitive processes such as reading, spelling, or math do *not* involve simply one or two areas of the brain, but in fact involve numerous areas at various points in the sequence of executing these skills. Difficulties in any particular brain location will interfere with the function of that area, producing one of several possible types of deficits in the academic skill that requires that function. For instance, reading disorders are now believed to be of at least four or five different types, depending on which cognitive function has been impaired. It is therefore inadequate to say that a child has a reading disability without going further to specify the type of reading problem that is occurring.

Current literature in child neuropsychology and learning disabilities suggests that several cognitive functions must develop normally and in relative equilibrium with each other if proper academic skills are to be learned later in childhood. Deficits in or gross inequalities among these functions seem to lead to different types of learning disabilities from those produced by deficits in other functions. These important cognitive or neuropsychological functions appear to be linguistic–conceptual skills; sequential–analytic skills (the ability to hold information in short-term memory for further analysis of its sequence of information); visuospatial–constructive skills; and fine motor planning, execution, and regulation skills (graphomotor skills) especially in the dominant hand. Other important cognitive functions for academic skills that are less likely to be a problem for the LD child include memory, primary sensory perception, motor coordination and agility, and adequate sustained attention and impulse control.

NEUROCOGNITIVE FUNCTIONS	ACADEMIC ACHIEVEMENT SKILLS				
	READING	SPELLING	MATH	WRITING	OTHER
LANGUAGE SKILLS	* * *	* *	*	?	• • •
VISUOSPATIAL SKILLS	*	* *	* * *	* *	• • •
SEQUENTIAL-ANALYTIC SKILLS	* * *	* * *	* * *	* *	• • •
MOTOR PLANNING & EXECUTION	?	- - -	- - -	* * *	• • •
OTHER	• • •	• • •	• • •	• • •	• • •

FIGURE 4.5. Conceptual matrix of the relationship between cognitive–developmental functions and academic achievement skills. The stronger the association between the functions and skills, the greater the number of asterisks in the cell. Dots or dashes imply little, if any, relationship. "?" indicates that the relationship requires further research.

This view of learning disabilities can be depicted in a matrix like the one shown in Figure 4.5. Because our understanding of neuropsychological functions and their role in academic skills is incomplete, so then is this matrix. Nonetheless, it provides some understanding of the ways in which deficits seen on intellectual and neuropsychological tests can lead to scholastic achievement problems in the classroom. In this matrix, neuropsychological functions are shown on the vertical (left) axis, while achievement skills are shown on the horizontal (top) axis. Virtually all of the neuropsychological functions play some role in each achievement skill, yet some play a more important role than others in particular skills. A deficit in one function will therefore lead to a more severe impairment in one academic skill than in another, with the severity of impairment indicated by the number of asterisks in each cell of the matrix. While the situation is certainly more complex than that shown here, this model is adequate to give most clinicians an idea of the LD child's difficulties. One thing from this model seems clear; not only are LD children not a homogeneous group, as was once thought, but even children with difficulties in a particular academic skill are not homogeneous in terms of the manner in which that skill is impaired.

Clinical Implications

If one assumes this conceptualization of specific learning disabilities, then certain implications for assessing these disabilities become apparent:

1. The testing of the child must include well-standardized measures not only of math, reading, and spelling, but also of the four critical neuropsychological functions noted earlier.

2. The interpretation of the scores on these tests should involve a *profile analysis* in which each score is judged in relation to the others, especially the four neuropsychological functions. Remember, it is the relative discrepancy among these functions, and not their individual levels of performance, that seems to create learning disabilities in the classroom.

3. The clinician must pay close attention to the nature and quality of errors on academic testing to understand more thoroughly what cognitive deficits are contributing to the learning problem.

4. The fact that a deficit in a neurocognitive function in *relation* to other functions creates the learning disability underscores an important implication for interpreting test results. A child's score on a single test, even if below normal, does not mean that the child has a "learning disability" as the term is defined here. It is the *discrepancy* between this function and the other three functions that seems to create the academic deficit. Thus, a child who is above average on three of the four prerequisite functions but only average on the fourth will probably have achievement skill problems, despite the fact that none of his scores are below average. This point is often overlooked by psychologists, who conclude that the achievement skill deficits in such a child are due to an "emotional" disorder and that the child is "underachieving." On the other hand, a child can have below-average scores on all of the four neuropsychological functions and have achievement skills all consistently below average. Yet this child would not be called "learning-disabled," because all of the achievement skill levels are consistent with generally below-average intellect.

5. Learning disabilities as defined here are not caused by emotional disorders, as many people seem to believe. However, learning disabilities often lead to the development of secondary emotional disorders, such as depression, anxiety, low self-esteem, aggression, and poor classroom conduct. The direction of effects in this relationship should not be confused.

Selecting Psychometric Tests

Nowhere in the assessment process are opinions likely to differ so much than on the issue of what tests and measures should be employed with LD children.

Each school of thought on the causes and remediation of these disorders has its own favored test batteries, some of which take as long as 6 to 8 hours to administer over 2 or 3 days. Certainly, testing cannot be dispensed with altogether, as some would suggest, for many legal definitions of these disorders rely heavily on test data, if only in the measurement of general intelligence. It is not within the scope of this chapter to evaluate all possible tests that have or could be used with these children. General areas of cognitive development requiring assessment have already been mentioned, and tests should be selected on the basis of their efficiency in assessing these skills. Whatever tests are selected, they should have acceptable standardization data (see APA, 1974, in "Suggested Reading"), adequate "floors" and "ceilings" for the various ages of interest here (ages 5 to 18 years), and some data supporting their predictive, concurrent, and prescriptive validity (see Anastasi, 1976, and Cronbach, 1970, in "Suggested Reading").

Tests of Intelligence

Several tests of intelligence have been used with LD children. The most commonly employed are the Stanford–Binet Intelligence Scale, the Wechsler Intelligence Scale for Children (WISC) and its revised version, the McCarthy Scales of Children's Abilities, and the Slosson Intelligence Test (see *Stanford–Binet Intelligence Scale,* 1973; Wechsler, 1974; McCarthy, 1972; and Slosson, 1963, in "Suggested Reading"). The two most useful among these are the Weschler Intelligence Scale for Children—Revised (WISC-R) and the McCarthy Scales of Children's Abilities. Both tests are quite psychometrically sophisticated and are the best standardized instruments of children's intelligence. The reader should consult Sattler (1974; see "Suggested Reading") for an overview of the issues surrounding the use of these and other widely used intellectual tests with children. The older WISC is to be avoided in evaluating children because of its considerably older normative data; research has also shown that it tends to overestimate IQ by an average of 7 to 10 points, and by as much as 30 points in some cases, in comparison with the WISC-R (see Barkley & Murphy, 1978, in "Suggested Reading").

Of greatest importance to the present discussion is that both the WISC-R and the McCarthy Scales yield data on most or all of the neuropsychological functions subserving the acquisition of more complex achievement skills. Those using the WISC-R should read Kaufman (1980; see "Suggested Reading") for suggestions on its interpretation. The WISC-R yields scores for verbal–linguistic skills, visuospatial–constructive skills, and sequential–analytic skills. At the very least, the Verbal and Performance Scale IQs on this test should be examined for possible hypotheses as to the cognitive deficits contributing to the learning diability. It has been shown that children who show discrepancies greater than 15 points on the WISC-R are likely to have different performance profiles and deficits on the Wide Range Achievement Test (WRAT), depending on which scale IQ is higher or lower, especially in older children. While the significance that should be attributed to this verbal–performance discrepancy is in doubt, large discrepancies can often generate hypotheses on the possible nature of the type of learning disability a child experiences when such discrepancies are coupled with results of the achievement tests.

One subtest pattern that appears to occur with unusual frequency in children with hyperactivity and learning disorders is the ACID pattern. This refers to especially low performances on the arithmetic, coding, information, and digit span subtests of the WISC-R. Many investigators believe that these subtests evaluate the sequential analysis of symbolic information; this suggests that problems in this cognitive ability underlie the learning disability. At present, the utility of this pattern for prescribing particular interventions has yet to be demonstrated.

Like the WISC-R, the McCarthy Scales yield not only a general IQ score, but various subscale scores for different cognitive–perceptual–motor skills. Scaled scores for memory, motor, perceptual organization, verbal, and numerical reasoning abilities are provided; these can serve to generate hypotheses about the nature of children's learning disabilities that are worthy of closer scrutiny.

Both tests show relatively high correlations with measures of reading, spelling, and math, depending on the subscales examined and the nature of the achievement tests. The McCarthy is more appropriate for children 3 to 8 years of age, while the WISC-R should not be used with children under 6½ to 7 years of age because of the relatively few items in each subtest such children can pass and thus the insensitivity of these subtests to subtle deficits. I find the WISC-R preferable for children 8 years of age or older because of the wealth of data it yields, the greater amount of research that has been conducted with it, and its higher upper age limits (16 years, 11 months) compared to the McCarthy. These factors permit more consistent test–retest data to be collected during the repeated evaluations likely to occur over the academic careers of these children.

Achievement Tests

A number of achievement tests exist; the most commonly used of these are listed in Table 4.3. I am most comfortable with using the Peabody Individual Achievement Tests (PIAT), the WRAT, and the Gray Oral Reading Test (see Dunn & Markwardt, 1970; Jastak, Bijou, & Jastak, 1978; and Gray, 1967, in "Suggested Reading"). Where significant problems in reading or math are revealed, these can be pursued more thoroughly with the Gates–McKillop Reading Tests or the Key Math Tests (see Table 4.3). Since the

TABLE 4.3. Achievement Tests Commonly Used with Learning-Disabled Children

Test	Publisher
Classroom Reading Inventory	William C. Brown
Doren Diagnostic Reading Test	American Guidance Service
Durrell Analysis of Reading Difficulty	Harcourt Brace Jovanovich
Follett Individual Reading Test	Follett
Gates–McKillop Reading Diagnostic Tests	Teachers College Press
Gilmore Oral Reading Test	Harcourt Brace Jovanovich
Gray Oral Reading Test	Bobbs-Merrill
Key Math Diagnostic Arithmetic Test	American Guidance Service
Peabody Individual Achievement Test	American Guidance Service
Sequential Tests of Educational Progress	Educational Testing Service
Spache Diagnostic Reading Scales	California Test Bureau
Wide Range Achievement Test	Jastak Associates
Woodcock Reading Mastery Tests	American Guidance Service

Note. From "Learning Disabilities" by R. A. Barkley. In E. J. Mash and L. G. Terdal (Eds.), *Behavioral Assessment of Childhood Disorders.* New York: Guilford Press, 1981. Copyright 1981 by Guilford Press. Reprinted by permission.

PIAT and the WRAT contain higher similar reading recognition (word pronunciation) subtests, only one of these subtests should be given for cost-efficiency of testing.

It is recommended that all three tests (PIAT, WRAT, and Gray) be given when appropriate to a child's age; they assess somewhat different types of academic achievement, and comparisons among them are likely to generate valuable hypotheses as to target problems and planning for intervention. The PIAT yields both age- and grade-level equivalents and percentiles for children at any grade level from kindergarten through grade 12. Subtests assess mathematics, reading recognition (single-word pronunciation), reading comprehension (silent reading of sentences), spelling (recognition), and general information (factual knowledge). Except for reading recognition and general information, the subtests provide multiple-choice answers. Hence, neither an oral explanation of the answer nor a written response is required—only an *indication* of the answer.

The WRAT also evaluates children at any grade level. It yields scores (grade levels or percentiles) in arithmetic, spelling, and reading recognition. As noted above, this last subtest should not be given if the full PIAT is administered. Since the math and spelling subtests require timed written responses, its results can be contrasted with the scores of the PIAT on math and spelling, which are untimed and involve no writing. Children doing substantially more poorly on the WRAT subtests than on the PIAT subtests in these areas would appear to have greater difficulties with written expression than with actual skill knowledge. Furthermore, the written spelling sample from the WRAT provides essential suggestions of possible subtypes of reading problems.

Neither the PIAT nor the WRAT go beyond single-word level in assessing oral reading. Hence, some test of oral reading, such as the Gray Oral Reading Test, is imperative in the assessment of oral reading of paragraphs, as well as of comprehension. For example, a child with a visuospatial type of reading problem is likely to perform at near-normal levels on the PIAT reading subtests (both recognition and comprehension), as the child has near-normal phonetic–analytic (word attack) skills. However, when more protracted reading is involved—especially under timed circumstances, as on the Gray Test—problems in reading will emerge. The child's reading is likely to be word-by-word, slow, and laborious, filled with multiple partial mispronunciations. The Gray Test permits some breakdown of oral reading error types critical to understanding the nature of the reading problem; need of aid in reading, gross and partial mispronunciations, omissions, insertions, substitutions, repetitions, and inversions. Scores on paragraph comprehension are also yielded by this test.

Tests of Tactile Perception

Two tests of tactile sensory perception have shown consistent reliability in predicting reading problems in children. These are the finger localization and fingertip symbol writing tests from the Halstead–Reitan Neuropsychological Test Battery (see Reitan & Davison, 1974, in "Suggested Reading"). These tests are likely to be used more often with children 8 years of age or younger, as the direct assessment of reading at this age may reveal only minor problems. In cases where significant deficits (greater than 1.5 standard deviations from normal) are seen on the two tests, I am likely to identify such children to the school as being at high risk for later reading failure. In evaluating children 9 years of age or older, these tests are of limited utility; many, though not all, reading deficits are fairly apparent by this age.

Other Clinical Measures

In addition to giving the Halstead–Reitan tests noted above, examiners should assess children's handwriting further by having them write their names as many times as possible in 1 or 2 minutes, as well as to write sentences to dictation. The latter test is given by selecting two sentences above and below a child's failure level on the WRAT spelling test and dictating these to the child. Obviously, both of these unstandardized tests assess handwriting skill, as well as providing another sample of written spelling ability.

In addition to standardized tests, examiners should not hesitate to use more nonstandardized tests or to use tests in nonstandardized ways to pursue hypotheses as to the nature of children's problems. If a motor planning problem (apraxia) is suspected as a basis for deficits in written expression, then simply asking the child to *demonstrate* the use of commonly encountered items (pencil, key, drum, rifle, etc.) in the absence of such items can be helpful in revealing such problems.

A variety of neuropsychological tests and tests of mental skills have been used with LD children. Some clinicians advocate the use of the full Halstead–Reitan Neuropsychological Test Battery in evaluating learning disabilities. The Luria–Nebraska Neuropsychological Test Battery (see Golden, Hammeke, & Purisch, 1980, in "Suggested Reading") is also being standardized for use with children. While these and other tests may be helpful when questions of neurologic impairment, recovery of skills following impairment, or degree of deficits in cases of litigation are raised, they are not likely to be cost-effective in assessment and treatment planning with most LD children. Not only are they extremely time-consuming to administer, but they tend to be highly redundant with intellectual tests such as the WISC-R or the McCarthy Scales in most of the skills they assess. Furthermore, they are not any more likely to yield information that is useful to treatment planning than are the recommended tests of intelligence and achievement already discussed. The reader is referred to Baron (1978; see "Suggested Reading") for a further discussion of the use of these tests with children.

General Testing Considerations

Examiners are interested not only in the scores children obtain on the above tests, but also in the quality of their performance and the nature of the errors made. In addition, note should be taken of the children's awareness of and reaction to errors, general demeanor during testing, and sustained performance or concentration on the tasks as they increase in level of difficulty. LD children are more likely to express aversion to the task, to ask for greater feedback on their performances, and often to give up more readily as difficult items are reached. These should serve to raise hypotheses for further assessment during direct classroom observation.

I believe that examiners should make every effort to motivate children to perform at their best possible levels. Hence, great amounts of encouragement, praise (noncontingent on correctness of performance) and generally positive feedback are provided. The goal of testing is not so much to achieve a representative sample of in-class performance, but to see exactly what the children can do when motivation is heightened. It is assumed that this approach yields information about cognitive deficits less confounded by motivational deficiencies than is to be found in classroom observations of these children.

It can be useful to vary the presentation of test items from the manner in which they were standardized, once the standardized version has been given and the score obtained. For instance, a child with poor phonetic reading is likely to achieve a score on the reading comprehension subtest of the PIAT that is as poor as if not poorer than the low score achieved on the reading recognition subtest. Is the child's understanding of word meanings as poor as his or her word pronunciation skills in this case? This cannot be answered on the basis of the test scores, as the child's poor silent reading may preclude the correct identification and hence correct comprehension of a word. If in doubt of this, I return to the PIAT at the end of testing and repeat the reading comprehension subtest. However, on this occasion, the examiner reads the sentences to the child and has the child point to the picture that best describes what has been read. In most cases, the child's comprehension score improves dramatically; this suggests that the problem is one of word pronunciation, not of comprehension. In the few cases in which the score fails to improve, a problem in sentence comprehension in addition to the one noted in word pronunciation has been demonstrated more definitely.

In summary, the purpose of testing is to raise hypotheses about areas of academic performance problems in the learning disabled child rather than to provide definitive conclusions about the problems. Only when the test data, observations of behavior, and analyses of error patterns are combined with interview and classroom observation data can an examiner be at all confident about the nature of a child's problems and the best approach to habilitation or retraining.

Case Illustration

In order to demonstrate the utility of psychometric testing with hyperactive children, the following case study is offered. Greg was 11 years and 8 months old and had a history of hyperactive behavior since the age of 2. He was referred for evaluation of difficult behavior at both home and school. The interview with his parents and his teacher, as well as the behavior rating scales, were all consistent with the diagnosis of hyperactivity. The parents were also concerned about his poor grades on his report card and his apparent problems with and aversion to reading and spelling. Greg was in the fourth and final quarter of his sixth-grade year at a public school, and there was some question as to whether he would be passed to a seventh-grade program. Both the parents and the teacher felt that Greg could achieve at grade level if he would simply pay attention and complete his assignments. In view of the failing marks on his third-quarter report card, as well as his reported difficulties with reading and spelling, it was decided to conduct psychometric testing of his intellectual and academic skills.

Greg was given the WISC-R, the PIAT, the WRAT, and the Gray Oral Reading Test. In addition, he was asked to write several sentences to dictation and to print a series of numbers. The results of the formal tests are shown in Table 4.4. Here it can be seen that Greg is a boy of generally above average intelligence whose verbal intelligence level is approximately 15 points below that of his nonverbal, visuospatial skills. This discrepancy is significant for a boy of this age, as only 18% of same-age boys would be expected to show such a discrepancy, according to the standardization sample for the WISC-R (see Kaufman, 1980, in "Suggested Reading"). Given this discrepancy, it was expected that Greg would show some problems with reading and spelling, despite the fact that his verbal IQ was average. (As noted earlier, it is not the child's level of performance on any single test that determines a learning disability, but the pattern of *relative* deficits.) It was also expected that problems in arithmetic performance might also occur; this expectation was based upon the relatively poor scores on the arithmetic and block design subtests. A substantial body of research supports the relationship between performance on spatial tasks and math ability. The block designs subtest is believed to be the "purest" measure of visuospatial ability on the WISC-R.

The grade-level and percentile scores on the PIAT show that Greg was at grade level in his math skills on this test but was 1 to 1½ grades below his expected grade level (6.7 to 7.0) in his reading recognition (word pronunciation) and his reading comprehension. The comprehension subtest was later given with the examiner reading the sentences to Greg; the only response required of him now, as noted earlier, was to pick out the picture that correctly showed what was read. His performance improved to a 6.9 grade level, suggesting that his verbal comprehension was not impaired. Instead, this boy's poor phonetic reading skills, as seen in his reading recognition, probably prevented him from pronouncing words correctly so that they could be accurately comprehended. For instance, in the reading recognition subtest, Greg pronounced the word "exercise" as "excuse"; this indicates his poor word attack (phonetic) skills and also shows that if Greg made similar mistakes on the reading comprehension subtest, they would change the entire meaning of sentences he read. Thus, a low comprehension score would result. Greg did most poorly in the spelling skills subtest on the PIAT, being at least three grade levels below his expected grade placement and below the 10th percentile for his age. Greg's score on the general information test was 5.5, or 1 to 1½ grades below that expected for his grade placement.

Greg's performances on the WRAT were substantially below normal; both scores were at least two to three grades below expected grade level. The poor performance on spelling here is consistent with the poor spelling score

TABLE 4.4. Psychological Test Scores for an 11-Year-Old Hyperactive Boy with Learning Disabilities

WISC-R

Subtest	Scaled scores	
Information	10	
Similarities	12	
Arithmetic	9	*Verbal IQ:* 105
Vocabulary	12	*Performance IQ:* 120
Comprehension	11	*Full-scale IQ:* 112
Picture completion	14	*Gray Oral Reading Test:* 2.0 grade level
Picture arrangement	18	
Block design	8	
Object assembly	11	
Coding	13	

PIAT

Subtest	Grade level	Grade percentile
Mathematics	7.0	58
Reading recognition	5.4	29
Reading comprehension	5.2	27
Spelling	3.6	12
General information	5.6	30

WRAT

Subtest	Grade level	Grade percentile
Spelling	3.7	16
Arithmetic	4.7	13

on the PIAT, indicating that Greg does equally poorly with spelling, whether the examination format is a multiple-choice test (PIAT) or a written test of recall (WRAT). This fact suggests that Greg's major problems are not in graphomotor skills *per se*; a WRAT spelling score lower than a PIAT spelling score would be expected if this were the case, as would a lower score on the coding subtest of the WISC-R. Some of the spelling errors made by Greg are shown in Figure 4.6. Analysis of these errors shows that most of the spelling mistakes were due to poor phonetic skills. That is, Greg could not write the correct grapheme (written symbol) to match the phoneme (auditory word sound) of the word to be spelled. This was partly indicated by the types of errors Greg made on the PIAT reading recognition test. Children with

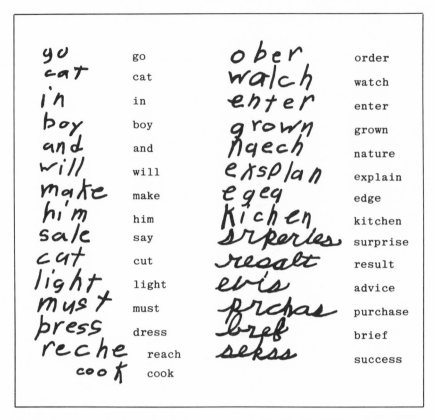

FIGURE 4.6.   Spelling errors for Greg, an 11-year-old hyperactive boy with learning disabilities.

other types of reading–spelling problems may misspell words on this test in ways that are at least phonetically correct, as in "nachur" for "nature" and "woch" for "watch." These errors tell us that such children have problems with visual imagery for words, not with phonetic skills. That is, the children cannot accurately recall the correct "pictures" of what words should look like, so they rely on phonetic skills alone in spelling the words. Accurate spelling, however, requires both normal phonetic and visual memory for written words. With Greg, one sees that most of his misspellings, if pronounced, do not sound even close to the spoken words. This distinction is very important in providing educators with directions to pursue in remediating this spelling *and* reading problem. It is virtually a truism that children's spelling errors will typically tell you their reading errors as well.

It is surprising to see that Greg's written math score on the WRAT (4.7) was two grades below expectation, since he performed normally on the

PIAT math test. Since the PIAT test is multiple-choice, requires no writing, requires very little setting up for the math problems and their operations, and is a test in which children are read the questions, it is primarily a test of math concepts. There are several reasons why Greg might do less well on the WRAT math test, which is timed (10 minutes), is not read to children by examiners, involves some writing and spatial skills, and is not a multiple-choice test (recognition) but one of recall and problem solving. First, Greg might do poorly because of a problem in graphomotor skills. This is unlikely in view of the spelling test results compared earlier. Second, Greg had considerable problems with concentration; these would most likely show up on the WRAT math test, during which he received no interaction with the examiner. Again, the good coding performance on the WISC-R might mitigate against this hypothesis, as it is similarly structured and timed. Yet, because its time limit is only 2 minutes, it may not be as reflective of attentional deficits as a 10-minute test. This hypothesis, then, is still tenable. Third, Greg showed a somewhat poor performance in the block design section of the WISC-R, a highly spatial subtest. Poor spatial skills do correlate with poor performance in written math of the sort seen on the WRAT, so math performance of this sort could be a result of poor abstract spatial perception. Examining the actual errors made on the test produces two further possible hypotheses for poor math performance. Greg made all of his errors by faulty operations. That is, Greg added instead of subtracted and vice versa, and he did not know how to multiply numbers of two digits or more. Second, Greg attempted very few problems beyond those he could solve quickly. Thus, poor knowledge of operations and poor concentration and persistence contributed to Greg's failure on this test. Neither problem would show up on the PIAT math test. All of these hypotheses were discussed with the classroom teacher for further treatment planning.

The score on the Gray Oral Reading Test indicates that Greg's worst skill is reading of complex paragraphs under timed circumstances. This test most closely approximates classroom reading, and Greg is at least 4.7 grade levels behind that expected for his grade placement. Greg's greatest mistakes here were in wild guessing of words, slow and laborious reading, and partial mispronunciations, all common to readers with poor phonetic skills. Greg's inattention also showed here in his frequent loss of place while reading because of other low-level distractions in the room.

Greg's handwriting samples revealed problems similar to those already noted—poor phonetic spelling with omission of syllables, and careless, inattentive penmanship.

To summarize, Greg is a boy of average to above-average intelligence with relatively poor performances on verbal tasks and tasks involving abstract spatial perception. Greg is 1 to 1½ grades below grade level in single-word reading, 3 grades below grade level in spelling and *written* math, and

4½ grades behind in oral reading of paragraphs. Wisconsin law—the state law applicable in this case—requires a child to be 50% below that grade level expected for his age and intelligence in at least two areas of academic achievement before he or she can be placed in a program for learning disabilities. The learning problems of poor verbal ability, dysphonetic reading–spelling, and poor written math therefore qualified Greg for exceptional educational services. It is obvious that Greg's hyperactivity would certainly have exacerbated his disabilities further in a regular classroom setting.

The remediation of learning disabilities is not the subject of this text and will not be addressed here. Clinicians working with such children should be thoroughly acquainted with the literature on this subject before undertaking assessment or treatment of these children.

MEDICAL EXAMINATION

Hyperactive children are often referred for medical and neurological evaluations because of their generally immature physical appearance, motor clumsiness, mildly dysmorphic features, neurologic "soft" signs, allergies, and problems with learning, enuresis, and encopresis. Yet these exams are rarely of help in assessment toward rational treatment planning; in fact, they are often the bane of physicians' existence, either because the problems they see are untreatable or because they lack experience with those problems that are treatable (e.g., behavior and learning disorders). Therefore, referral for medical evaluation should be the exception, not the rule, with hyperactive children.

Under some circumstances, the medical exam may be useful. Obviously, if medication is to be used, then a physical exam and periodic medical follow-ups are essential. Where allergies are common, as they often are, a referral to an allergist can be useful in alleviating these further irritants to already difficult child behavior and affect. It should not be concluded, however, that the allergies are the primary cause of the hyperactivity, as is often believed. Where enuresis or encopresis occur, the physical exam is needed to detect—or, more frequently, to rule out—medical causes of these problems. Once physical causes are ruled out, more appropriate behavioral programs can be implemented, sometimes with pharmacologic agents as adjuncts (e.g., Tofranil for enuresis). Some hyperactive children although probably less than 10%, do have seizures. When this is known or suspected, referral to a neurologist is essential. In such cases, anticonvulsants may exacerbate hyperactivity, making it imperative that greater than usual care be taken in choosing anticonvulsants for these children. Many hyperactive children are clumsy, some to such a degree that attention from a physical or occupational therapist might be desirable. Referral to a physician is often required to obtain these services. Finally, when the hyperactivity is of acute onset and is associated with changes in affect, orientation, or decreases in developmental–cognitive skills, this may suggest a very rare neurological disease that is treatable, making referral to a neurologist essential. When all of these problems are absent, referral to the physician should not be initiated.

COST-EFFECTIVENESS OF ASSESSMENT

One often-overlooked issue in evaluating children is the typically exorbitant expense the families and/or insurance carriers have to bear for the evaluations. Professionals tend to become quite cavalier in this regard when insurance coverage or other third-party reimbursement is available to patients. In deciding which procedures to use in the evaluation, examiners should take care to select only those that will yield information useful to decision making about the particular case. A period of 2 to 4 hours is adequate for evaluation of the hyperactive child with perhaps an additional 2 hours being added when psychometric testing is needed to elucidate possible learning disabilities.

Professionals operating outside public school systems are professionally and ethically obligated to inform families that the psychometric evaluations of intelligence, achievement, speech and language, and even motor development are provided to them *without cost* under Public Law 94-142 through their public schools upon request. Some parents will choose not to ask for this assistance because of the frequent delays (some as long as 3 months) in getting the evaluations done, their desire for outside professional consultations or second opinions if schools have already evaluated the children, or their need for treatment programs for *home* behavior problems. In any case, the parents should always be given the option to request this free evaluation.

Expensive medical procedures, excessive or highly technical direct observation methods, excessive psychological testing, and overly detailed interviewing all inflate the expense of the evaluation; such professional largesse generally produces extensive yet useless data. If evaluations of hyperactive children are to remain credible, useful, and available or affordable to all who require them, clinicians must make economically intelligent decisions in conducting evaluations.

CONDUCTING THE PARENT FEEDBACK CONFERENCE

Once an evaluation has been completed, the examiner must then review the findings with the parents. This is a critical phase in the assessment process, since the way in which the parents are made to perceive their child's problems and possible treatments for these will determine not only their degree of acceptance of the results, but also their motivation for subsequent treatment approaches. The examiner should allot sufficient time for this conference, usually at least an hour, and should not rush through or hastily present the findings and recommendations. In this discussion, the examiner should adjust the level of his or her vocabulary to fit that of the parents' background and educational level. Periodically throughout the explanation, it is helpful to stop and question the parents briefly as to their feelings and understanding of the findings so far. Do they agree or disagree with what has been said? Are they depressed, guilty, or angry over the conclusions? Finally, the parents should be asked about any questions or concerns they have about the results.

It is important to remember the perspective which the parents are likely to bring to this conference. Up to this point, they have probably felt responsible for the child's problems and guilty over their causal role in them. The mother is especially likely to feel depressed, incompetent, and generally low in self-esteem. It is professionally irresponsible for the examiner to overlook these feelings or to contribute to them by directly or indirectly telling the parents what they have done wrong. Instead, an objective description of the problem and its possible causes, coupled with occasional acknowledgment of the parents' feelings about living with a difficult-to-manage child, is important.

At the outset, it is important to reiterate the list of concerns that originally brought the parents to the clinic and to see whether they wish to add any other concerns to this list. Sometimes, after progressing through the evaluative procedures, parents will remember a concern about the child that they did not initially verbalize. This is especially likely after they have answered all of the items on the questionnaires they have filled out. At this point, it should be mentioned to the parents that many of the difficulties they are having with the child are consistent with the diagnosis of hyperactivity. The examiner should then explain how the diagnosis has been reached (see the criteria listed at the beginning of Chapter 3) and what it essentially means. It is important to demonstrate to the parents how the supporting information leads to the conclusion of hyperactivity and influences the treatment recommendations that will come later.

Subsequently, it is important to discuss the possible causes of hyperactivity and, when possible, which of these may have played a role in this child's case. It is helpful to the parents to admit the uncertainty about etiology in most cases and yet to reassure them that the child's condition does not stem from anything they have necessarily done. However, it can be pointed out that while the problem is part of the child's temperament or disposition, it can be improved or exacerbated by the ways in which the parents choose to manage the child and by other problems which may exist within the family, such as parental psychiatric or marital disorders.

This discussion with the parents then leads to one on the long-term outcome and prognosis of such children, the factors that predict prognosis, and the ways in which this information pertains to their child. It should be stressed that, if left untreated, the child is likely to have innumerable problems in later childhood and adolescence. Yet it should also be emphasized that there are no "cures" for hyperactivity. Instead, several methods are available to facilitate effective coping with the child, in some cases reducing symptom severity by as much as 70% to 80%. But the parents must be prepared for the fact that this child is more prone to behavior problems than one who is not hyperactive, and that this is likely to be the case until the child is into his late adolescent years. I believe that this is a realistic appraisal of the prognosis of hyperactive children, based on current research literature.

For those children in whom academic learning problems have been suspected and for whom testing has been done, care in the explanation of the tests and their results is necessary in this area that so often proves confusing to parents. Test jargon is to be thoroughly avoided. Parents should be given brief, elementary explanations of each test and its results, and interpretations of them in layman's terms. If learning disabilities have been found, then a discussion of their nature, likely etiology, and prognosis should occur. Explain the description of learning disabilities in Public Law 94-142 to the parents, and make it clear that it mandates free exceptional educational services to their child if they so desire them. A conference with school personnel is almost always required to review these findings, and parents should be informed of this and their permission sought. In many cases, one or both parents may themselves have had a learning disability during their schooling—a fact that can be used in explaining to them how their child must now feel in trying to master the demands of schooling. Like hyperactivity, learning disabilities can be improved but can rarely be cured, and this point should be made clear to parents lest they assume the goal of special educational services is to "normalize" their child.

The most appropriate treatments for the child's problems are reviewed with the parents, and their feelings about each are elicited. When parent training in child management is indicated, as it usually is, then the examiner should take care to explain that the parents are not necessarily doing anything wrong with the child. Instead, it is explained that the methods most parents employ to handle children are not the most effective ones to use with hyperactive children. The purpose of the parent training, then, is to teach the parents the most effective management methods for hyperactive children. This explanation has been quite well received by parents I have seen, and it may further motivate them to attend the training sessions. If drugs are to be used, a detailed explanation of the rationale for such therapy, its intended effects, and its known side effects should be presented (see Chapter 5). Parents often have many misconceptions about medication that must be confronted and dispelled when drug therapy seems indicated.

Finally, the parents are reassured of the availability of professional services throughout the child's development, should future problems emerge after treatment is over. Parents have often remarked that they feel they can cope with the child's problems, once they understand their nature, chronicity, and malleability and know that professional support services are available when needed in the future. At this point, reading material on hyperactivity may be given to the parents to take home, and they are encouraged to call if there should be any questions. The treatment sessions are then scheduled at the close of the conference.

CONCLUSION

The clinical evaluation of hyperactive children is a complex process that should not be undertaken by those who do not have sufficient time or knowledge to do it properly. The evaulation has been shown to consist at least of parent, child, and teacher interviews and completion of standardized rating scales by the target child's parents and teachers. Heavy emphasis in the evaluation is given to assessing the social interactions of the child with parents and teachers. When direct observations of these are feasible, several behavior coding systems are useful in clinical settings. When they are not, parent and teacher diaries should be used to collect information on those interactions occurring in problem situations. When learning disabilities are suspected, then the child should receive appropriate testing of cognitive–developmental functions and academic achievement skills by an experienced psychometrician. When treatable maladies are revealed, the child should be referred for medical/neurological examination. In most cases, however, medical exams are not likely to be useful and hence should not be undertaken without serious consideration. Whichever procedures are chosen, the examiner must always critically evaluate the cost-effectiveness of such procedures. Throughout the evaluation and the parent feedback conference, the attitude of the examiner toward the parents should be nonjudgmental; blaming or fault-finding should be avoided. Regardless of the specific findings, it is quite likely that long-term, periodic interventions will be needed to help the parents and school to cope with (not to cure) the problems of the hyperactive child.

SUGGESTED READING

Abikoff, H., Gittelman-Klein, R., & Klein, D. F. Classroom observation code for hyperactive children: A replication of validity. *Journal of Consulting and Clinical Psychology,* 1980, *48,* 555–565.

American Psychological Association. *Standards for educational and psychological tests.* Washington, D.C.: Author, 1974.

Anastasi, A. *Psychological testing* (4th ed.). New York: Macmillan, 1976.

Barkley, R. A. The effects of methylphenidate on various measures of activity level and attention in hyperkinetic children. *Journal of Abnormal Child Psychology,* 1977, *5,* 351–369.

Barkley, R. A., & Cunningham, C. E. Do stimulant drugs improve the academic performance of hyperactive children?: A review of outcome research. *Clinical Pediatrics,* 1978, *17,* 85–92.

Barkley, R. A., & Murphy, J. Pseudodeterioration of intelligence in children. *Annals of Neurology,* 1978, *4,* 388.

Barkley, R. A., & Ullman, D. A comparison of objective measures of activity level and distractibility in hyperactive and nonhyperactive children. *Journal of Abnormal Child Psychology,* 1975, *3,* 213–224.

Baron, I. S. Neuropsychological assessment of neurological conditions. In P. Magrab (Ed.), *Psychological management of pediatric problems* (Vol. I). Baltimore: University Park Press, 1978.

Cronbach, L. J. *Essentials of psychological testing* (3rd ed.). New York: Harper & Row, 1970.

Cunningham, C. E., & Barkley, R. A. A comparison of the interactions of hyperactive and normal children in free play and structured task. *Child Development,* 1979, *50,* 217–224.

Dunn, L. M., & Markwardt, F. C. *Peabody individual achievement test.* Circle Pines, Minn.: American Guidance Service, Inc., 1970.

Gaddes, W. H. *Learning disabilities and brain function: A neuropsychological approach.* New York: Springer-Verlag, 1980.

Gazzaniga, M. S. *Neuropsychology* (Vol. II of *Handbook of behavioral neurobiology*). New York: Plenum, 1979.

Golden, C. J. *Diagnosis and rehabilitation in clinical neuropsychology.* Springfield, Ill.: Charles C Thomas, 1978.

Golden, C. J., Hammeke, T. A., & Purisch, A. D. *The Luria-Nebraska neuropsychological battery.* Los Angeles: Western Psychological Services, 1980.

Gray, W. S. *Gray oral reading test.* New York: Bobbs-Merrill, 1967.

Hecaen, H., & Albert, M. L. *Human neuropsychology.* New York: Wiley, 1978.

Heilman, K. M., & Valenstein, E. *Clinical neuropsychology.* New York: Oxford University Press, 1979.

Hughes, H. M., & Haynes, S. N. Structured laboratory observation in the behavioral assessment of parent–child interactions: A methodological critique. *Behavior Therapy,* 1978, *9,* 429–447.

Jastak, J. F., Bijou, S. W., & Jastak, S. *Wide range achievement test.* Wilmington, Del.: Jastak Associates, 1978.

Kaufman, A. S. Issues in psychological assessment: Interpreting the WISC-R intelligently. In B. Lahey & A. Kazdin (Eds.), *Advances in child clinical psychology* (Vol. 3). New York: Plenum, 1980.

Kinsbourne, M., & Caplan, P. J. *Children's learning and attention problems.* Boston: Little, Brown, 1979.

Luria, A. R. *Higher cortical functions in man.* New York: Basic Books, 1973.

Mann, R. A. Assessment of behavioral excesses in children. In M. Hersen & D. Barlow (Eds.), *Handbook of behavioral assessment.* New York: Pergamon, 1976.

Mash, E. J., Terdal, L. G., & Anderson, K. The Response Class Matrix: A procedure for recording parent–child interactions. *Journal of Consulting and Clinical Psychology,* 1973, *40,* 163–164.

McCarthy, D. *McCarthy scales of children's abilities.* New York: The Psychological Corporation, 1972.

Patterson, G. R., Ray, R. S., Shaw, D. A., & Cobb, J. A. A manual for coding family interactions. New York: Microfiche Publications, 1969.

Reitan, R. M., & Davison, L. A. (Eds.). *Clinical neuropsychology: Current status and applications.* New York: Wiley, 1974.

Roberts, M. W., & Forehand, R. The assessment of maladaptive parent-child interaction by direct observation: An analysis of method. *Journal of Abnormal Child Psychology,* 1978, *6,* 257-270.

Ross, D. M., & Ross, S. A. *Hyperactivity.* New York: Wiley, 1976.

Sattler, J. M. *Assessment of children's intelligence.* Philadelphia: W. B. Saunders, 1974.

Slosson, R. L. *Slosson intelligence test for children and adults.* New York: Slosson Educational Publications, 1963.

Stanford-Binet intelligence scale. Boston: Houghton Mifflin, 1973.

Wahler, R. G. Some structural aspects of deviant child behavior. *Journal of Applied Behavior Analysis,* 1975, *8,* 27-42.

Wechsler, D. *Manual for the Wechsler Intelligence Scale for Children—Revised.* New York: The Psychological Corporation, 1974.

CHAPTER FIVE

DRUG MANAGEMENT OF HYPERACTIVITY

To help the young soul, to add energy, inspire hope, and blow the coals into a useful flame; to redeem defeat by new thought and firm action; this, though not easy, is the work of divine men.—Ralph Waldo Emerson

Stimulant drugs are now the most common treatment for hyperactive children. Over 600,000 children annually, or between 1% and 2% of the school-age population, take these medications for management of their behavior. This is a 400% increase over the 150,000 children estimated to be taking these medications in 1970. Most of these children are between 6 and 10 years of age, and they frequently discontinue the use of medication after about 3 years or upon reaching puberty. As Rachel Gittelman-Klein and her colleagues have noted (1980), the short-term efficacy of these drugs in improving the behavior of hyperactive children is indisputable. No other form of therapy for hyperactivity has received as much research as the stimulant drugs, especially methylphenidate. To those who have worked with hyperactive children before and after medication is begun, no other treatment currently known can produce such dramatic improvements in hyperactivity in so short a time as these medications. Yet drug treatment remains controversial, for it is not without its problems and precautions.

Despite their widespread use, these drugs are often improperly prescribed and even less properly monitored. Gerald Solomons reported in a study at the University of Iowa Hospitals (1973) that only 55% of the hyperactive children receiving stimulants were "adequately" monitored—the minimal criteria for "adequacy" being only two telephone contacts between family and physician in a 6-month period. Furthermore, many families were permitted to adjust the medication dosage on their own without consulting their physicians. Some improvements in this situation have occurred since this study was made; many states have now passed legislation requiring that prescriptions for certain stimulants (typically the amphetamines and methylphenidate) only be written for a 1-month supply and that each prescription be renewed in writing. Such measures eliminate the ease with which prescriptions for these drugs can be simply called in to neighborhood pharmacies. In Wisconsin, the prescription must also indicate the diagnosis for which such a drug is being prescribed, must be filled within a week of the date on the prescription, and is generally not honored in pharmacies in neighboring states. These restrictions have been placed on the prescription of these drugs more for the purposes of restricting illegal traffic in them and overuse of them for dietary management than for controlling the use of them with hyperactive children in particular. They have nonetheless produced this latter effect by compelling monthly contacts between physicians and families of such children. It is to be hoped that these contacts are used to review the children's drug responding and possible side effects.

The effectiveness of these medications, in any case should not be mis-judged or impugned because of the inadequacies in their prescription and monitoring. Such misjudgments are often seen in the demands of certain special interest groups that these drugs be taken off the market. As this chapter shows, the stimulant drugs are quite effective in the day-to-day management of many of the problem behaviors presented by hyperactive children. When used properly, they are beneficial to many of these children and are often more cost-effective than their psychoeducational alternatives. Nevertheless, they are not a panacea for treating hyperactivity, and it is now widely recognized that they should never be used as the sole form of therapy for these children. As the previous chapters have shown, hyperactive children present with a wide variety of physical, cognitive, academic, behavioral, and social problems, and it would be ludicrous to expect any drug to manage all of these problems effectively. It is the purpose of this chapter to sum-marize the research findings on the use of stimulant drugs with hyperactive children and to suggest guidelines for their clinical use. In doing so, the author readily acknowledges the guidance provided in the excellent reviews of this area by Dennis Cantwell, Alan Sroufe, C. Keith Conners and John Werry, and Richard Safer and Daniel Allen (see Cantwell, 1980; Sroufe, 1975; Conners & Werrry, 1979; and Safer & Allen, 1976, in "Suggested Reading"). This information, however, is liberally mixed with observations from my own published reviews on stimulant drug research as well as from my clinicial and scientific work with hundreds of hyperactive children over the past 7 years.

HISTORY OF STIMULANT DRUG USE WITH CHILDREN

The first reported use of stimulant drugs with behavior problem children is typically credited to Charles Bradley in 1937, although, in an earlier issue of another journal, there is a report by Matthew Molitch and August Eccles (1937) on the use of stimulant drugs with a similar group of children. Bradley employed amphetamine (Benzedrine) with children on an inpatient resi-dential care ward and noted dramatic improvement in their conduct and school performance. There are few further studies of stimulant drug use with children until the late 1950s and early 1960s, when Bradley's work seems to have been rediscovered by clinicians working with children. This increase in drug use at this time probably corresponds to the discovery, marketing, and wisespread use of the phenothiazines with adults, as well as to the release of methylphenidate for commerical use in 1957.

The use of these drugs with hyperactive children was given impetus by the positive reports of Eisenberg, Laufer, Denhoff, Solomons, and later Conners on the efficacy of the stimulant drugs in improving children's behavior, measured primarily through parent and teacher opinion and rating scales. Becuase of these positive reports and the lack of information on any long-term deleterious effects, the use of these medications increased to such an extent that over 150,000 children were taking them for behavior management by 1970. At this point, a major controversy developed over a report in the *Washington Post* stating that 5% to 10% of the children in the Omaha, Nebraska, school system were being given stimulant drugs to control their classroom behavior. The report was erroneous, but it prompted a Congressional investigation that served indirectly to spawn numerous scientific investigations into the specific effects of stimulants on various measures of cognitive, academic, and behavioral parameters of children. Although these papers revealed many positive effects of these drugs, they also began to suggest that there were both short-term and long-term side effects about which clinicians ought to be concerned.

Today, despite several highly critical books and articles appearing in the lay literature, stimulant drugs are widely dispensed and are seen as the drugs of choice, if not the treatment of choice by some, for hyperactive children. This multimillion-dollar-a-year pharmaceutical market saw the entry of pemoline into the marketplace in 1975 for use specifically with hyperactive children. To date, between 400 to 500 articles on stimulant drug use with hyperactive children have appeared; this is more research than has been done on any other group of psychotropic drugs used with children. The fact that fewer than 20 of these papers deal in any way with long-term drug effects (beyond 1 year of treatment) does not seem to have decreased the use of these drugs with children for as long as 7 to 10 years in some cases. While there has been a corresponding increase in research on psychological and education alternatives to medication, stimulant drugs remain a stable, commonplace mode of therapy for hyperactive behavior.

PHARMACOLOGICAL ASPECTS OF STIMULANT DRUGS

The stimulant drugs are so named because of their ability to increase the arousal or alertness of the central nervous system (CNS). Because of their structural similarity to certain brain neurotransmitters, they are considered sympathomimetic agents. The three most commonly used stimulant drugs are *d*-amphetamine (Dexedrine), methylphenidate (Ritalin), and pemoline (Cylert). Other stimulant compounds, such as caffeine or deanol, are not discussed here because of their lack of demonstrated efficacy for hyperactive children. Later in this chapter, the use of certain antidepressant drugs having some efficacy with hyperactive children is also briefly discussed.

The primary mode of action of racemic amphetamine (Benzedrine) and *d*-amphetamine (Dexedrine) is believed to be that of increasing catecholamine activity in the CNS, probably by increasing the availability of the catecholamines at the synaptic cleft, although this is still a matter of debate. Both dopamine and norepinephrine are believed to be affected by these drugs. The site or mode of action of methylphenidate is less clearly understood, though it is believed to be similar to that of the amphetamines. It may be that methylphenidate has more effect on dopamine activity than on other neurotransmitters, but this remains a speculation at this time. The mechanism of the action of pemoline is not understood at this time, mainly because of its fairly recent release for commercial use and the paucity of studies conducted on it to date. The actual locus of action within the CNS is also not well studied for these medications. Some have suggested that brain stem activation is the primary locus, while others postulate midbrain or frontal cortex involvement. Obviously, further research on these parameters is necessary.

All of the stimulant drugs are easily taken by mouth, are rapidly absorbed from the gastrointestinal tract, and cross the blood–brain barrier easily. In their exceptional chapter on these medications, Cantwell and Gabrielle Carlson (1978; see "Suggested Reading") cite evidence suggesting that 30% to 50% of the dose of amphetamines is excreted unmetabolized in the urine, having a plasma half-life of approximately 6.54 ± 2.54 hours (depending upon urinary pH levels). The amphetamines appear to reach their peak effects on behavior between 1 and 2 hours after ingestion and to dissipate in their behavioral effects within 4 to 5 hours after ingestion. Methylphenidate has a plasma half-life of between 2 and 7 hours and is entirely metabolized within 12 hours, with almost none of the drug appearing in the urine. As with amphetamines, the peak behavioral effects occur within 1 to 2 hours and are dissipated within 3.5 to 5 hours after oral ingestion. Pemoline has not been as well studied but appears to have a half-life of 12 hours, with 50% of it being excreted unmetabolized in the urine. Within 24 hours, 75% of the dose seems to be excreted in urine.

DRUG RESPONSE RATES

In 1977, I reported a review of the literature on more than 110 stimulant drug studies of hyperactive children (see "Suggested Reading"). In this review, 31 studies were found to report rates of clinical improvement, often ambiguously defined, in response to medications. These studies appear in Table 5.1. A total of 14 studies of methylphenidate reported an average improvement rate of 77% among patients given the drug, with the conditions of 23% remaining unchanged or worsened. Of 15 studies of amphetamines, an average of 74% of the children given the drugs improved, while the conditions of 26% were unchanged or worsened. At that time, only two studies of pemoline reported improvement rates, but these rates are quite similar to those of the other drugs—73% of the children taking it improved, while 27% were unaffected or showed worse behavior on the drug. Finally, 11 studies reported improvement rates in response to placebo treatments; the average, however, was 39%, although four studies found rates of 50% or more. Clearly, then, the stimulant drugs are judged by parents, teachers, and physicians to produce effects on behavior much greater than the effects of placebos. A problem here, however, is the manner in which "improvement" was assessed. In most cases, the measures of "improvement" were merely the opinions of those who worked with the children; few, if any, objective measures were employed to support the impressions. Sufficient studies have been conducted to reveal the specific effects of stimulants on children's behavior, although more certainly need to be undertaken to evaluate the long-term efficacy of these drugs.

CLINICAL EFFECTS: SHORT-TERM

There are many excellent scientific reviews of the clinical effects of stimulant drugs on hyperactive children, some of which are listed at the end of this chapter. It is not my intent here to review the studies in detail or to debate their methodological inadequacies. As noted earlier, there are probably more than 400 studies of stimulant drugs with children; many of these reports contain one flaw or another in their definitions of hyperactivity, procedures, experimental designs, dependent measures, and data analyses. Nonetheless, the general trends in these studies can be mentioned here and their implications for clinical practice assessed.

Physiological–Psychophysiological Effects

These studies are thoroughly reviewed in a paper by James Hastings and myself (1978; see "Suggested Reading"). Very little research has been done on the physiological or metabolic effects of stimulants with hyperactive children. What has been done suggests that amphetamines may decrease growth hormone, at least temporarily, while methylphenidate may increase growth hormone. Amphetamines may also increase the amount of free fatty acid in plasma. There is so little research in this area that these results must remain speculations until their findings are further tested and replicated.

TABLE 5.1. Drug Response Rates by Drug Type

Author(s)	Number of subjects	Judge	Percentage improved	Percentage unchanged or worsened
Amphetamines				
Bradley (1937–1938)	30	Hospital staff	76	24
Bradley (1950)	275	Hospital staff	73	27
Bradley & Bowen (1941)	100	Hospital staff	79	21
Comly (1971)	40	Teacher	78	22
Conners (1972)	81	Clinician	96	4
Conners et al. (1967)	37	Teacher	81	19
Conners et al. (1972)	27	Clinician	96.3	3.7
	22	Teacher	77.3	22.7
Epstein et al. (1968)	10	Parent	70	30
	10	Clinician	70	30
Knopp et al. (1973)	22	Clinician	64	36
	22	Parent	67	33
Rapoport et al. (1971)	16	Teacher	69	31
Steinberg et al. (1971)	46	Teacher	79	21
Weiss et al. (1968)	26	Parent	85	15
Winsberg et al. (1972)	32	Parent	44	56
Winsberg et al. (1974)	18	Teacher	78	22
Zrull et al. (1963)	91	Clinician	57	43
Total: 15 studies	915	18 judges	74 (mean)	26 (mean)
Methylphenidate				
Comly (1971)	134	Parent	88	22
Hoffman et al. (1974)	34	Physician	84	16
	34	Parent	77	23
Knights & Hinton (1969)	40	Teacher	88	12
	40	Parent	73	27
Knobel (1962)	150	Clinician	90	10
Lytton & Knobel (1959)	20	Clinician	75	25
Rapoport et al. (1974)	27	Psychologist	69	31
	29	Physician	94	6
Satterfield et al. (1973)	57	Teacher	68	32
Schain & Reynard (1975)	98	Parents and teachers	79	21
Schnackenberg & Bender (1971)	10	Parent	60	40

TABLE 5.1. (*Continued*)

Author(s)	Number of subjects	Judge	Percentage improved	Percentage unchanged or worsened
Methylphenidate (*Continued*)				
Seger & Hallum (1974)	29	Parent	86	14
	29	Teacher	90	10
Weiss *et al.* (1971)	26	Parent	94	6
Werry & Sprague (1974)	37	Physician	51	49
Winsberg *et al.* (1974)	18	Teacher	61	39
Zimmerman *et al.* (1958)	54	Clinician	65	35
Total: 14 studies	866	18 judges	77 (mean)	23 (mean)
Magnesium pemoline				
Conners (1972)	81	Clinician	77	23
Conners *et al.* (1972)	26	Clinician	77	23
	22	Teacher	63.7	36.4
Total: 2 studies	105	3 judges	73 (mean)	27 (mean)
Placebo				
Conners (1972)	81	Clinician	30	70
Conners *et al.* (1972)	27	Clinician	29.6	80.4
	23	Teacher	30.4	69.6
Knights & Hinton (1969)	40	Teacher	67	33
	40	Parent	54	46
Rapoport *et al.* (1971)	18	Psychologist	38	61
	18	Physician	33	66
Schain & Reynard (1975)	48	Parents and teachers	8	92
Weiss *et al.* (1968)	12	Parent	50	50
Weiss *et al.* (1971)	26	Parent	50	50
Zrull *et al.* (1963)	84	Clinician	37	63
Total: 8 studies	417	11 judges	39 (mean)	61 (mean)

Note. From "A Review of Stimulant Drug Research with Hyperactive Children" by R. A. Barkley, *Journal of Child Psychology and Psychiatry*, 1977, *18*, 137–165. Copyright 1977 by Pergamon Press. Reprinted by permission. References within table to other sources are detailed in original source.

Many more studies have evaluated the effects of the stimulants on various psychophysiological measures, but many of the results are still inconclusive. Heart rate, as well as systolic and diastolic blood pressure, may be increased by the stimulants. At average doses, heart rate increases 8 to 15 beats per minute and blood pressure by 4 to 10 mm Hg. Both changes are considered mild and are probably outweighed by other daily physiologic stresses, such as those of digestion. Whether there is habituation to these effects is not known, but they are clearly dose-related. Heart rate variability is reduced by methylphenidate, as is heart rate deceleration to a reaction time task. The latter result is consistent with changes in cognitive functions such as attention span or concentration. The stimulants appear to heighten the background electrical activity of the CNS and to increase its sensitivity to stimulation as measured in studies using electroencephalograms (EEGs) and audio- and visual-evoked potentials. These findings may be loosely construed as suggesting that the stimulants heighten excitatory brain mechanisms while enhancing those responsible for inhibition. This probably results in the improvements in concentration, motor coordination, and impulse control often seen with these drugs. No evidence exists to suggest that these drugs have any significant effects on various aspects of sleep other than the fact that they produce mild insomnia, to be discussed later.

Cognitive Effects

Numerous studies have been conducted on the effects of stimulants on measures of intellect, memory, vigilance, attention, concentration, and learning. To date, a majority of the studies finds that the drugs primarily affect measures of attention span, concentration, and impulsivity. Positive drug effects have also been observed on measures of short-term memory and learning of paired verbal or nonverbal material. Measures of more complex cognitive skills, such as those assessed by intelligence tests, have generally not been affected by these drugs. The drug effects on various tasks are particularly salient in situations that require children to restrict their behavior and to concentrate on assigned tasks. Drug effects in free-play situations are less certain. Measures of complex learning, problem solving, and reasoning do not appear to be improved by these medications.

Some studies have suggested that stimulants may result in state-dependent learning. That is, what children learn while on the medication may not be as easily recalled when they are off the medication, or vice versa. These effects are not well established and are of small magnitude where they are found. This has, however, led some investigators to suggest that hyperactive children should remain on medication during weekends, holidays, and summer vacations so that their learning or retention will not be disrupted. Such a conclusion seems premature, given the paucity of studies and the inconsistencies in their results.

Scholastic Effects

In 1978, Charles Cunningham and I reviewed 17 studies that measured the effects of stimulants on the academic achievement or productivity of hyperactive children (see "Suggested Reading"). These studies appear in Table 5.2. Of the 55 dependent measures used, 83.6% were unaffected by the drugs. Those types of measures that were improved showed no consistency in the types of abilities affected, leading us to conclude that these drugs have almost *no* effect on scholastic achievement. We then reviewed six follow-up studies, covering periods from 1 to 10 years, which showed results highly consistent with this conclusion. Hence, neither short-term nor long-term studies support any utility of the stimulants in improving academic performance. As Cantwell has rightfully suggested, these studies suffer from various methodological flaws; this aspect of the issue is thus inconclusively studied at this time. Nonetheless, the burden of proof is on those who would suggest that such positive effects do, in fact, occur.

Behavioral Effects

There have been numerous studies of the effects of stimulant drugs on various behaviors of hyperactive children. These drugs have been shown to have positive effects, related to the improvements seen in attention span noted earlier, on the ability of such children to remain with assigned tasks longer and to reduce their task-irrelevant restlessness and motor activity. These conclusions were substantiated in a review of this literature by Charles Cunningham and myself, the results of which appear in Table 5.3. As Table 5.3 shows, the stimulants are found to reduce a variety of types of activity level significantly, especially in structured, task-oriented situations. Problems with aggression, impulsive behavior, noisiness, noncompliance, and disruptiveness have all been shown to improve with these drugs.

We have recently completed a series of studies on the effects of stimulants on the parent–child interactions of hyperactive children (see Barkley & Cunningham, 1980, in "Suggested Reading"). More recent studies of teacher–child interactions bear out our original findings that the stimulant drugs improve compliance to commands to hyperactive children and increase their responsiveness to the interactions of others. Negative and off-task behaviors are also reduced. In turn, parents and teachers reduce their rate of commands and degree of supervision over these children, and increase their praise and positive responsiveness to the children's behavior. Some children on medication appeared to show reductions in their initiation of interactions with others, but this has not been replicated in a more recent study of ours using 68 hyperactive boys. Cunningham has recently reported positive effects of the stimulant drugs on the interactions of hyperactive children with their peers in free-play and task situations—results already shown to occur in

TABLE 5.2. Review of Stimulant Drug Studies Using Objective Measures of Academic Achievement

Author(s)	Drug and daily dose	Measures used	Results
Ayllon et al. (1975)	Ritalin (10–20 mg)	Laidlaw Series Workbooks (math); Merrill Linguistic Readers.	No change in percentage of math or reading problems correctly completed.
Blacklidge & Ekblad (1971)	Ritalin (20 mg)	Wide Range Achievement Test (WRAT) math subtest, Gray Oral Reading Test.	No change in scores.
Bradley & Bowen (1940)	Benzedrine (20–30 mg)	Number of pages of math and spelling done per month.	Significant improvement in math only.
Christensen (1975)	Ritalin (.3 mg/kg)	Percentage of math problems completed and percentage done correctly.	No significant changes.
Conners (1972)	Ritalin (up to 30 mg) Dexedrine (up to 15 mg)	WRAT: reading, math, and spelling tests.	No significant changes.
Conners et al. (1972)	Dexedrine (5–25 mg)	WRAT: reading, math, and spelling tests.	Significant improvement in math only.
Conners et al. (1972)	Dexedrine (5–40 mg) Cylert (25–125 mg)	WRAT: reading, math, and spelling tests; Gates Diagnostic Reading Test; Gray Oral Reading Test.	Significant improvement in WRAT spelling and Gray Oral Reading Tests.
Conrad et al. (1971)	Dexedrine (10–20 mg)	WRAT: reading and math tests.	No significant changes.
Finnerty et al. (1971)	Dexedrine (5–15 mg)	WRAT: reading, math, and spelling tests.	No significant changes.

Study	Drug (dose)	Measures	Results
Gittelman-Klein & Klein (1976)	Ritalin (10–60 mg)	WRAT: reading, math, and spelling tests; Gray Oral Reading Test.	No significant changes.
Hoffman et al. (1974)	Ritalin (20–80 mg)	WRAT: reading, math, and spelling tests.	No significant changes.
Knights & Viets (1975)	Cylert (mean dose of 73 mg)	WRAT: reading, math, and spelling tests.	No significant changes.
Rapoport et al. (1974)	Ritalin (30 mg)	WRAT: reading, math, and spelling tests.	No significant changes.
Rie et al. (1976)	Ritalin (5–40 mg)	Iowa Test of Basic Skills: vocabulary word analysis, reading, spelling, math 1, and math 2 tests.	Significant improvement only in word analysis.
Rie et al. (1976)	Ritalin (5–20 mg)	Iowa Test of Basic Skills: vocabulary, word analysis, reading, spelling, math 1, and math 2 tests.	Significant improvement only in vocabulary test.
Wolraich et al. (1978)	Ritalin (.3 mg/kg)	Accuracy in copying a paragraph and number of correct responses made in reading assignments.	No significant changes.
Weiss et al. (1971)	Ritalin (up to 50 mg)	Durrell Analysis of Reading Difficulty Test.	Significant improvement on tests of oral reading, silent memory, and spelling subtests.
Werry & Sprague (1974)	Ritalin (.1–1 mg/kg)	Burt Reading Test.	No significant changes.

Note. From "Using Stimulant Drugs in the Classroom" by R. A. Barkley, *School Psychology Digest*, 1979, *8*, 412–425. Copyright 1979 by National Association of School Psychologists. Reprinted by permission. References within table to other sources are detailed within original source.

TABLE 5.3. Review of Stimulant Drug Research on Activity Levels in Hyperactive Children

Author(s)	Measure	Type of activity	Nature of significant drug effects
		Structured settings	
Barkley (1977)	Actometer	Wrist and ankle	Both decreased.
Millichap et al. (1958)	Actometer	Wrist	Trend to decrease.
Millichap & Johnson (1974)	Actometer	Wrist	Decreased.
Rie et al. (1976)	Actometer	Wrist and ankle	Wrist activity declined. Trend for ankle to decline ($p < .054$).
Barkley (1977)	Grid-marked floor	Locomotor	Trend to decrease.
Barkley (1977)	Stabilimetric chair	Seat	Decreased.
Christensen & Sprague (1973)	Stabilimetric chair	Seat	Decreased.
Sprague et al. (1970)	Stabilimetric chair	Seat	Decreased.
Sprague & Sleator (1973)	Stabilimetric chair	Seat	Decreased.
Sroufe et al. (1973)	Stabilimetric chair	Seat	Decreased.
Werry & Aman (1975)	Stabilimetric chair	Seat	Decreased.
		Free-play settings	
Barkley (1977)	Actometer	Wrist and ankle	Both decreased.
Barkley & Cunningham (1978)	Actometer	Wrist and ankle	Both decreased.
Rapoport et al. (1971)	Actometer	Torso	Trend to decrease.
Barkley (1977)	Grid-marked floor	Locomotor	Decreased.
Rapoport et al. (1971)	Grid-marked floor	Locomotor	Decreased.
Montagu & Swarbrick (1975)	Pressure floor mats	Locomotor	Decreased.
Montagu & Swarbrick (1975)	Ultrasonic generator	Total body	Decreased.
Ellis et al. (1974)	Three measures of activity level taken from analysis of filmed observations	Locomotor and "energy units"	No change.

Note. From "Stimulant Drugs and Activity Level in Hyperactive Children" by R. A. Barkley and C. E. Cunningham, *American Journal of Orthopsychiatry*, 1979, 49, 491–499. Copyright 1979 by American Orthopsychiatric Association, Inc. Reprinted by permission. References within table to other sources are detailed within original source.

classroom interactions between hyperactive children and their classmates by Carol Whalen and her associates (1978).

The aforementioned findings are important, for they demonstrate that medication not only affects hyperactive children, but indirectly affects the behavior of important adults and other children to those children. This point was brought forcefully home to Charles Cunningham and myself in a single case study of two hyperkinetic twin boys and their mother (see Chapter 2). Objective observations were made of various behaviors of both mother and children in a clinic playroom during free-play and task periods. Observations were made during alternating drug and placebo phases, with dramatic results. These were shown in Figure 2.1. It is obvious that when the children received medication, their rates of independent play increased. This suggests that the mother found the play much more acceptable during medication phases. In the graphs at the bottom of the figure, it can be seen that the compliance of these boys improved substantially each time they were placed on medication. In response, their mother became more rewarding of their compliance. When changes such as these occur in parental behaviors, they obviously contribute further to a positive drug response in the child.

In the classroom, hyperactive children on medication show reduced rates of off-task and out-of-seat behavior, disruptiveness, noisiness, and general motor activity in comparison with their behavior on placebos. These changes have been found to be equal to, and in some cases greater than, those achieved by various forms of behavior modification; this suggests that the combined effects of these treatments are not much greater than either alone. As Chapter 7 makes clear, however, behavioral approaches can produce remarkable improvements in academic achievement and produc-tivity—something that remains to be demonstrated for the stimulant drugs.

Effects on Mood and Emotion

Despite the finding that adults generally report elevations in mood and euphoria when taking stimulant drugs, these effects are rarely seen in chil-dren. In my 1976 review of this literature, I found only one paper that reported such effects, and they occurred for only a few of the children in the study. In a more recent paper, Judith Rapoport and her colleagues at the National Institute of Mental Health (1978) compared the effects of Dexe-drine on adults and children. Here, again, adults reported feelings of euphoria, while few if any of the children reported such feelings. The children did report feeling "funny," "different," or, in some cases, dizzy. As Rapoport suggests, it may be that actual developmental differences in re-sponse to stimulant medication make adults more likely to experience tem-porary elevations in mood. However, it is also possible that children are not as adept at labeling their feelings and thus underreport euphoria, simply labeling it as feeling "funny."

In contrast, numerous papers have found that children experience various negative moods or emotions in reaction to stimulant drugs. These are discussed under "Side Effects," below. Many of these mood changes are reported to occur as the drugs are "washing out" of the body in late morning or late afternoon. However, no studies have objectively evaluated these reactions during the time course of stimulant drug therapy.

CLINICAL EFFECTS: LONG-TERM

Few studies using rigorous methodology have evaluated the long-term efficacy of stimulant medications. Those that have examined the issue have generally found negative results. Hyperactive children who had been on drugs but were off at the time of follow-up were not found to differ in any important respect from those who had never received the medications. Hence, no enduring effects of up to 5 years of drug treatment were observed in these studies. While this might be due to possible habituation to the effects of the drugs, this seems unlikely, since, even after 5 years of drug therapy, teachers were found to be able to tell when the children were removed from their medication.

THE PARADOX OF STIMULANT DRUG THERAPY

The observations that stimulant drugs improve attention, simple learning, and classroom behavior, but do not substantially alter academic achievement and productivity, are both surprising and paradoxical. There are several reasons why academic improvement might not occur. First, hyperactive children may be placed on medication too late in their schooling to affect their classroom learning. The fact that hyperactive children often begin medication by first or second grade would seem to contradict this hypothesis. Second, it is possible that the tests used to evaluate achievement are simply not sensitive to the subtle effects that the stimulants might have in the short term on actual classroom performance. While possible, this explanation also seems inadequate in the face of the results of long-term drug studies. The third and most likely explanation is that the stimulant drugs simply cannot affect those factors that contribute to the academic problems of hyperactive children. That is, it seems likely that the underachievement of these children is due to more than simply the children's poor attention or off-

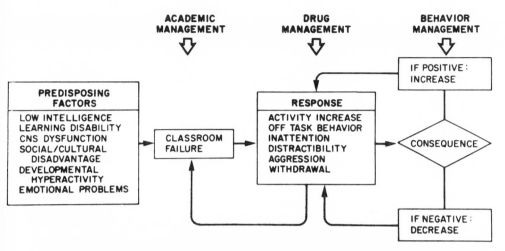

FIGURE 5.1 A model for the development and maintenance of hyperactive behavior in response to classroom failure. (From "The Role of Academic Failure in Hyperactive Behavior" by C. E. Cunningham and R. A. Barkley, *Journal of Learning Disabilities,* 1978, *11,* 15–21. Copyright 1978 by Professional Press, Inc. Reprinted by permission.)

task behavior. Hyperactive children are frequently shown to have specific learning disabilities, to be from lower socioeconomic groups and thus to be more educationally disadvantaged than normal children as a whole, to have generally lower IQ scores than children from similar neighborhoods, and to be more physically immature and to have more emotional problems than normal children. All of these factors can predispose children to classroom failure, over and above those contributed by their developmental hyperactivity.

This situation is depicted in Figure 5.1, which also shows where the various treatments for hyperactive behavior in school can intervene in the process. Factors that predispose a child to fail at school are shown on the left in the diagram. The effects of failure in school are increased restlessness, off-task behavior, aggression, and in some cases withdrawal. Whether these behaviors are further exacerbated depends on their environmental consequences. Behavioral therapies that focus on the consequences of hyperactive behaviors may well reduce the behaviors, but they do not affect scholastic failure. Stimulant drugs modify the neurologic substrate for hyperkinetic behaviors, but they similarly fail to improve classroom achievement. Only educational therapies that directly address children's level of productivity and success in the classroom can produce changes in achievement. Interestingly, as this figure suggests, such therapies produce the indirect effect of improving classroom behavior without being specifically planned to accomplish such changes. In the classroom, then, it will take more than medication to improve the underachievement of hyperactive children.

PREDICTING THE CLINICAL RESPONSE TO STIMULANTS

In 1976, I reviewed a total of 36 previous research reports that attempted to distinguish the hyperactive children who would respond favorably to these drugs (responders) from those who would not (nonresponders). The types of predictors used in these studies were classified as follows: psychophysiological factors, neurological factors, familial factors, demographic/sociological factors, diagnostic categories, adult rating scales, psychological factors, and behavioral profiles. Those behavioral and psychophysiological measures related to attention span were found to be the best and most reliable predictors of improvement during stimulant drug treatment. In other words, the greater the inattention of children, the better their reaction to medication. Such a finding is hardly surprising, in view of the fact that the stimulants have their primary mode of action on attention span. This area, however, is far from being adequately or conclusively researched.

Some studies also found that the type of relationship between parent and child was a good predictor of drug response (see Barkley, 1976, in "Suggested Reading"): the better the mother–child relationship, the better the response to medication. This is similar to the findings in my studies of mother–child interactions reported earlier (see Barkley & Cunningham, 1980, in "Suggested Reading"). In many children, the drugs produce positive changes in the behavior of both the children and their mothers. It may be that mothers who are more appreciative and rewarding of these initial positive changes in their children's behavior while on stimulants produce further positive reactions to drug treatment. In support of this, Cunningham and I obtained results that suggested that mothers who were more interactive with their children and more rewarding of child compliance prior to drug therapy had children who showed greater positive changes in behavior as a result of drug treatment.

Many studies report that higher ratings of hyperactivity on child behavior rating scales predict better responding to medication. This may simply reflect regression to the mean, or it may relate to the earlier conclusion that children with more problems with attention span are better drug responders. These studies and several clinical reports suggest, however, that children who are more anxious or who are rated as such by their parents and teachers on questionnaires such as those developed by Conners have a poorer response to the stimulant drugs. At this time, it seems as if the only useful clinical information to be gained from this research is that the more inattentive or less anxious children are, the better their response to medication will be. The Conners rating scales seem useful in assessing these parameters (see Chapter 3).

DOSE EFFECTS OF MEDICATION

There are very few studies from which to draw any firm conclusions on the effects of different doses of stimulant drugs on hyperactive children. The results of these few studies are generally consistent, however, and permit some useful clinical suggestions to be made. Perhaps the most widely known study of this issue was published by Robert Sprague and Esther Sleator at the University of Illinois (1977). They evaluated the effects of methylphenidate at two dose levels on classroom behavior and on ability to perform a simple learning task. The doses of medication were .3 mg/kg and 1 mg/kg. Classroom behavior was assessed through the Conners TRS, while learning was assessed through the use of a short-term memory task. In this task, a child is shown a matrix of children's pictures and than a few seconds later is shown a single picture which the child must identify as one of those in the matrix or a different one. The difficulty level of the task is varied by increasing the number of pictures in the matrix from 3 to 9 or to 15.

The results of this study are shown in Figure 5.2 and suggest some rather controversial interpretations. It can be seen that learning on the laboratory memory task peaks at a dose of .3 mg/kg, declining thereafter as the dose reaches 1 mg/kg. Teacher ratings, on the other hand, do not reach their peak of improvement until the 1 mg/kg level. These results have been translated into theoretical dose curves (see Figure 5.3) and interpreted as showing that the dose necessary to improve classroom conduct will prove detrimental to learning. Since most physicians rely on parent or teacher opinion to titrate dose levels, the obvious implication is that we are over-medicating hyperactive children if the true goal of medication is improved learning in the classroom. Indeed, the doses being used might well be detrimental to classroom learning. Another interpretation is possible, however, from these results. It may well be that the TRS is less sensitive to drug effects on classroom conduct than the laboratory memory task is to changes in learning produced by the drug. That is, it may be that the ideal dose for classroom social conduct is also .3 mg/kg but that this would not be detected by an insensitive rating scale. The problem may be not only in using the rating scale but in using teacher opinion, which itself may be less sensitive to drug effects than direct observations of classroom behavior may be. The best conclusion from this study would appear to be that it takes a higher dose to change a *teacher's opinion* of a child's conduct than it does to change either actual short-term memory or actual classroom behavior.

The results of my research using direct observations of social inter-

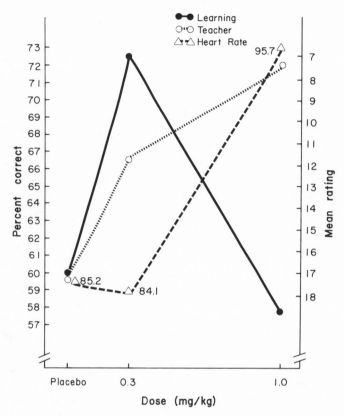

FIGURE 5.2. Three different dose-response curves produced by three different target behaviors. The learning curve is the same as the accuracy curve from matrix 15 of the laboratory learning task. The teacher curve represents social behavior as rated by the teacher, who used a scale on which the numbers become smaller as the child improves. The heart rate curve indicates the number of beats per minute. (From "Methylphenidate in Hyperkinetic Children: Differences in Dose Effects on Learning and Social Behavior" by R. Sprague and E. Sleator, *Science*, 1977, *198*, 1274–1276. Copyright 1977 by the Association for the Advancement of Science. Reprinted by permission.)

actions between parents and hyperactive children seem to bear this out. For the past 2 years, I have studied the effects of two doses (.3 and .7 mg/kg) of methylphénidate on parent–child interactions; these are observed during both free play and task accomplishment. The findings show that the .3 mg/kg dose produces optimal changes in these interactions in terms of child compliance, play, interaction, and responsiveness to parents, while the .7 mg/kg dose may interfere with compliance, increase children's irritability and negativism, and decrease their responsiveness to their parents. I have most often recommended the use of the lower dose to pediatricians referring children for this evaluation. Hence, from this standpoint, doses between .3

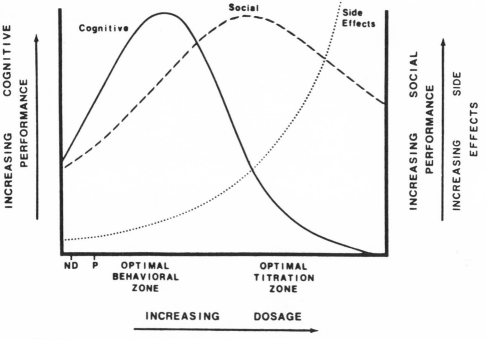

FIGURE 5.3. Theoretical dose–response curves for learning and classroom behavior for methylphenidate. (From "Drugs and Dosages: Implications for Learning Disabilities" by R. Sprague and E. Sleator. In R. Knights and D. Bakker (Eds.), *The Neuropsychology of Learning Disorders.* Baltimore: University Park Press, 1976. Copyright 1976 by University Park Press. Reprinted by permission.)

and .5 mg/kg are the best for maximizing improvements in social conduct and learning in hyperactive children. While higher doses may in some cases produce equivalent results, they also increase side effects; they are therefore unnecessary for most hyperactive children.

SIDE EFFECTS

A variety of studies have reported on the occurrence of short-term and possible long-term side effects of stimulant drug use in children.

Short-Term Side Effects

In my 1977 review of the literature on stimulant drugs, I found 29 studies that reported the side effects of stimulant drug use with their subjects. The number of studies reporting each side effect is set forth in Table 5.4. Here it can be seen that the most common side effects are insomnia and decreased

TABLE 5.4.   Stimulant Drug Side Effects

Author(s)	Side effects								
	Insom.[a]	Decr. app.[b]	Wt. loss[c]	Irrit.[d]	Abd. pain[e]	Head.[f]	Drows.[g]	Sad.[h]	Other
Arnold et al. (1976)	X	X			X	X			
Arnold et al. (1972)	X	X							Proneness to crying; euphoria.
Bradley (1937–1938)	X		X						
Bradley (1950)	X	X	X	X	X				Anxiety; tic-like behavior; proneness to crying; fine hand tremor.
Bradley & Bowen (1941)	X	X							Dizziness; nausea; fine hand tremor.
Claghorn et al. (1971)	X								
Comly (1971)	X		X						
Conners (1972)	X	X							Dazed appearance; nail biting; facial tics.
Conners et al. (1969)	X	X							
Conners et al. (1972)	X	X		X					
Epstein et al. (1968)	X	X	X	X	X	X		X	Proneness to crying.
Garfinkel et al. (1975)		X	X	X					
Greenberg et al. (1972)	X	X	X		X	X			Depression; 1 case of induced psychosis.
Hoffman et al. (1974)	X	X	X	X	X	X			
Knights & Hinton (1969)	X	X		X	X				Bedwetting; 1 case of induced psychosis.
Knobel (1962)	X	X				X			
Lucas & Weiss (1971)	X			X	X	X			3 cases of induced psychosis.

Study	Insomnia[a]	Decreased appetite[b]	Weight loss[c]	Irritability[d]	Abdominal pain[e]	Headaches[f]	Drowsiness[g]	Sadness[h]	Other
Mackay et al. (1973)	X								Euphoria.
McConnell et al. (1964)			X						Excessive clinging to others. (X)
Millichap & Boldrey (1967)	X	X				X			
Montagu & Swarbrick (1975)		X				X			
Rapoport et al. (1971)	X	X	X						
Rapoport et al. (1974)	X	X	X		X	X			Nausea; dizziness; constipation; dry mouth. (X)
Rie et al. (1976)									Decreased humor, range of emotion, and responsiveness to the environment.
Schain and Reynard (1975)			X	X					Lethargy. Increased solitary play.
Schleifer et al. (1975)	X	X	X		X				
Schnackenberg & Bender (1971)	X	X							
Schnackenberg (1973)	X	X							
Seger & Hallum (1974)	X	X			X				
Steinberg et al. (1971)	X	X							
Weiss et al. (1971)	X	X	X	X	X	X			
Werry & Sprague (1974)	X	X	X	X	X	X	X		Nausea and many others (see article). (X)
Winsberg et al. (1972)				X					Anxiety; 1 case of induced psychosis. (X)
Winsberg et al. (1974)	X	X					X		Dizziness; nightmares; tremor.
Zimmerman et al. (1958)	X	X							
Total: 29 studies	26	23	12	13	11	10	4	4	4 — 6 cases of induced psychosis; many others.

Note. From "A Review of Stimulant Drug Research with Hyperactive Children" by R. A. Barkley, *Journal of Child Psychology and Psychiatry*, 1977, *18*, 137–165. Copyright 1977 by Pergamon Press. Reprinted by permission. References within table to other sources are detailed within original source. [a]Insomnia. [b]Decreased appetite. [c]Weight loss. [d]Irritability. [e]Abdominal pain. [f]Headaches. [g]Drowsiness. [h]Sadness.

appetite, reported in 90% and 79% of the studies, respectively. Irritability and weight loss were the next most frequent side effects, though they were reported in fewer than half of those studies reviewed. Headache and abdominal pain occurred in slightly fewer studies, while the remaining side effects were relatively uncommon. It is worth noting that several of the side effects deal with negative mood changes, such as sadness, proneness to crying, and irritability. As observed previously, adults are more likely to report euphoria, not dysphoria, as a side effect of these drugs.

One side effect that should receive serious attention from clinicians is the increase in nervous tics produced by the stimulant drugs, especially the cases (at least 10 reported to date) of irreversible Gilles de la Tourette syndrome in children receiving stimulant drugs. Tourette syndrome is a neurologic disorder comprised of multiple, persistent motor tics and compulsive vocalizations. In 60% of the cases, involuntary and compulsive use of obscenities also develops. The disorder typically arises between 4 and 7 years of age; it begins with facial tics and progresses over a period of months or years to tics of the neck, shoulders, arms, trunk, and legs in some cases. This cephalocaudal progression may be somewhat different in each case. Shortly after the initial tics develop, repetitive sniffing, throat clearing, coughing, or vocalizations may develop (e.g., guttural sounds, high-pitched noises, barking sounds). The presence of the multiple and persistent tics with the vocalizations is considered diagnostic. It is speculated that the disorder is the result of a hypersensitivity to dopamine within the basal ganglia of the brain. The disorder cannot be cured, but the symptoms can be treated with the tranquilizer haloperidol (Haldol). The disorder worsens through adolescence, after which 30% or more of the children may show improved symptomatology during young adulthood. The rest remain unchanged or show mild worsening of the symptoms. Stress, excitement, anxiety, or the ingestion of stimulant compounds such as caffeine can temporarily worsen the symptoms.

The important point to be made here is that some hyperactive children can develop tics or even Tourette syndrome in response to methylphenidate and perhaps to the other stimulant drugs as well. In some of the 10 cases reported in the literature and in two cases in my own clinic, hyperactive children with a prior history of tics developed Tourette syndrome after being treated for only a few weeks to a few months with methylphenidate. In these cases, the Tourette syndrome did *not* disappear after withdrawal from the stimulant drug. The children are now being given haloperidol for symptom control. I also know of several cases where children given Cylert developed irreversible facial tics. Both children receiving Cylert were highly anxious hyperactive boys. It is therefore recommended that, until these effects are further clarified, hyperactive children who have a prior history of nervous tics or who are rated as highly anxious by parents or teachers should not be treated with any stimulant drug. When drugs are used with hyperactive children without these risk factors and tics develop, *the medication should be discontinued immediately.* In either case, the parents should be forewarned not to have their children treated with stimulant drugs in the future, should they consult other professionals for the children's hyper-activity.

Another side effect, and one that has been inconsistently reported, is that of reduced social interactions with others while children are on medi-cation. My own research and clinical experience suggest that this pheno-menon tends to occur at doses of .5 mg/kg or higher. At first glance, some might assume that this is a desirable effect, since hyperactive children display high rates of negative interactions that may be reduced by these drugs. However, my own research tends to show that the total rate of social interactions can be reduced to 50% of normal rates with the stimulant drugs. This effect, combined with the occasional negative mood changes, often results in requests from parents that the drugs be discontinued, despite positive changes in other child behaviors. Some parents comment that the child is no longer "spontaneous" or childlike in his behavior, but is too controlled or socially aloof.

Each stimulant drug also seems to produce unique side effects. For instance, I have found that a few children develop allergic skin rashes after a few weeks or more of treatment with pemoline. Ceasing the drug seems to eliminate the rash. Conners and Eric Taylor (1980) recently reported a similar phenomenon but found that they could return the children to pemo-line after the rash had resolved with no recurrence of the rash. I have also found that pemoline tends to increase lip-licking, lip-biting, and light picking of the finger tips (not the nails). Reducing the dose seems to eliminate the problem. With methylphenidate, we have found that some children show heightened emotional sensitivity and proneness to crying, particularly in late morning or late afternoon as the dose is beginning to diminish in effective-ness. All of the drugs can produce symptoms of psychosis at high doses, or even at small doses in very young children (below 3 or 4 years of age).

All of these side effects are clearly dose-related. Many of them diminish within 1 to 2 weeks of beginning medication, and all, except possibly the nervous tics, disappear upon ceasing the medication. Where side effects persist beyond 1 to 2 weeks of treatment initiation, they can be made more tolerable by a slight lowering of the dose. It has been estimated that 1% to 3% of hyperactive children cannot tolerate any dose of stimulant medication.

Long-Term Side Effects

The deleterious effects of using stimulant drugs (over several months to several years) with children has not been well studied. Parents are often quite concerned about possible addiction to these drugs or increased risk of abusing other drugs as teenagers. There are no reported cases of addiction or serious drug dependence to date with these medications. Several studies have examined the question of whether children on these drugs are more likely to abuse other substances as teenagers than those not taking them. The results suggest that they are not, although more research is needed to rule this out conclusively. Nonetheless, the possibilities are viewed as remote by most investigators in this area. In fact, there is some clinical evidence to suggest that the children on medication frequently dislike it and wish its discontinuance as soon as possible, especially if they are older children or adolescents. Hence, the use of medication in childhood may actually predispose children to avoid other medications in later years.

One possible long-term side effect that has been of concern to many clinicians and scientists is the suppression of height and weight gain. Early reports by Safer and Allen and their associates at Johns Hopkins University Medical School (1972, 1973) indicated that both methylphenidate and d-amphetamine produced this effect. Later studies found it to be dose-related and to occur primarily within the first year of drug treatment. A rebound in growth or habituation to this effect seems to occur thereafter, and there is no appreciable effect on eventual adult height or weight. This side effect is felt to be secondary to appetite suppression effects of the drugs, although a recent paper suggests that the drugs may have some direct effect on growth hormone levels in the blood. Presently, it is the conclusion of the committee of the Food and Drug Administration established to review the issue (see Roche, Lipman, Overall, & Hung, 1979, in "Suggested Reading") that the suppression in growth is a relatively transient side effect of the first year or so of treatment and has no significant effects on eventual adult height or weight. Nonetheless, it behooves the clinician to monitor growth periodically in children receiving stimulant drugs.

While there is no evidence available on either side of the issue, there is some concern as to the effects of chronic stimulant drug use on the development of the cardiovascular system in children. All of the drugs reviewed here have some effects on heart rate and blood pressure, although they are relatively mild. The concern, however, is that these children might be at an increased risk for cardiovascular problems in middle to late life. At present, most of the drugs have not been on the market long enough to permit such research.

CLINICAL IMPLICATIONS OF CURRENT RESEARCH

This brief survey of the clinical effects and side effects of stimulant drugs suggests the following conclusions about drug use with hyperactive children.

1. Up to 75% of hyperactive children appear to show a positive response to these drugs. The major effect seems to be the improvement of attention span and the reduction of disruptive, inappropriate, and often impulsive behavior.

2. While the drugs are helpful in the day-to-day management of hyperactivity, they produce few, if any, enduring positive changes after their cessation. Academic achievement and productivity are not appreciably improved by the drugs, despite the positive effects on classroom conduct.

3. The side effects, both short- and long-term, are mild, are often transient, and diminish with reduction or discontinuation of medication. Children who have a prior history of tics or who are highly anxious should not be given these medications, as the development of tics, Tourette syndrome, or psychotic behavior may be more likely in this group of children.

4. Despite their lack of effects on achievement or long-term outcome, the stimulant drugs are useful in managing the behavior of hyperactive children. The issue of controlling the behavior of children with drugs is an important yet highly controversial one. The difficulties these children present to others who must live with, work with, or attend school with hyperactive children cannot be overlooked. Not only do these children frustrate parents and teachers, but the effects of their disruptive behavior on the ability of their classmates to receive adequate instruction is at times considerable. If drugs can remove these difficulties while reducing the level of ostracism, censure, and punishment that hyperactive children receive, then they are worthwhile in the treatment of these children.

5. Nonetheless, the drugs are not a panacea for hyperactivity and should generally not be the sole treatment for hyperactive children. Other therapies focusing on the myriad of social, psychological, educational, and physical problems these children often display will be needed. Drugs teach nothing; they merely alter the likelihood of occurrence of behaviors already in the children's repertoire. The numerous skill deficits of these children will still require attention. Since the drugs are used primarily for classroom misconduct, and since they are relatively short-acting, it is the school that reaps their beneficial effects while families must tolerate the side effects. Families will need child management training and other forms of counseling to cope with the children during periods when medication cannot be used. Each professional must therefore be knowledgeable about the resources within the community that will be needed to treat the "total child" with hyperactivity.

FACTORS INFLUENCING STIMULANT DRUG USE

It is naïvely idealistic to assume that stimulant drugs use is based entirely upon an objective assessment of children's needs and their response to medication. A closer look at the clinical use of these drugs suggests that several other factors influence decisions about their use with hyperactive children. A major factor seems to be the availability of other treatments within a given community. Are there other resources for family counseling, training in child management, special educational assistance, and follow-up support during development? What are these resources, are they affordable to the family in question, and how long will the family have to wait to receive them? Are the professionals providing the services both reputable and effective? The answers to these questions often influence the decision as to whether or not to prescribe drugs. A second obvious factor is the degree to which the professional whom a family first contacts knows about and respects these other resources. It is surprising how many physicians, psychologists, psychiatrists, social workers, and educators are skeptical about or blatantly unaware of the services provided by the other professions in their community for the care and management of hyperactive children. Another issue influencing drug treatment is the educational and socioeconomic level of the parents and hence their amenability to nonpharmacologic treatments. Many forms of counseling and parent training require literate, well-motivated clients who can afford the services. When parents are relatively uneducated, are poor, and/or belong to a minority group, alternatives to medication may be severely limited, regardless of the fairness of the situation. Poor and uneducated parents also tend to view children's health and psychological problems in terms of dealing with crises rather than in terms of prevention. As a result, they are likely to seek help only after a child's problems have become quite serious and may only use treatments that temporarily reduce the "crisis." Thus, when such parents are encountered, drugs may be the only viable approach or the only one the parents will utilize for a hyperactive child. Finally, the severity of a problem at the time of referral may dictate a need for immediate treatment that only drugs can effectively provide. Obviously, it requires a well-informed clinician to address these factors adequately and to prevent the overuse of medication with children simply for the sake of convenience or because of an overscheduled clinic caseload.

THE CLINICAL USE OF STIMULANT DRUGS

Suggestions for ways in which to medicate and monitor stimulant drug use with hyperactive children vary widely. What is offered here is an amalgamation of suggestions from my clinical practice and research, and the advice of other respected scientist–practitioners in this area.

When to Use Medication

Probably the most difficult decision to make in clinical practice is that of when to use medication. The simple diagnosis of a child as hyperactive is not an automatic recommendation for drug treatment. Several rules can be followed as aids in this decision, although they are meant only as suggestions that should remain flexible to the needs of the individual case.

1. How old is the child? As will be shown later, drug treatment is often not recommended below 4 years of age, except in unusually severe cases.

2. Have other therapies been used? If this is the family's first contact with the physician or other professionals, drugs should be avoided if possible until other therapies have been tried. I typically ask that the parents go through the child management course (see Chapter 7) before medication is prescribed, if this is their first effort at seeking help. However, when the child's behavior is a severe problem and the family cannot participate in the child management course or that of any other professional in the community, drugs may be the only useful alternative.

3. How severe is the child's current behavior? In some cases, the child's behavior is so unmanageable or distressing to a family that drugs may prove the fastest and most effective way of dealing with the crisis until other forms of treatment can begin. Once the other therapies are making sufficient progress, some effort can be made to reduce or discontinue the medication.

4. Can the family afford the medication, follow-up visits, and so on?

5. Are the parents sufficiently intelligent to supervise the use of the medication adequately and guard against its abuse? Solomons has suggested that some parents will juggle the dose of medications, despite cautions to the contrary, while others may in fact abuse a child through overmedication.

6. In spite of "prodrug" answers to all of the foregoing questions, some parents are simply "antidrug," and such parents should never be coerced into agreeing to try medication. Such parents will often sabotage the drug trial through underuse of the drug or underreporting of its efficacy, just to prove the physician wrong.

7. Is there a delinquent sibling or drug-abusing parent in the household? If so, Solomons suggests that medication not be prescribed as it may be redirected for illicit use or sale.

8. Does the hyperactive child have any history of tics, psychosis, or thought disorder? If so, the stimulant drugs are contraindicated.

9. Is this child highly anxious, fearful, or more likely to complain of psychosomatic disturbances? Again, medication is contraindicated.

10. Does the physician have the time to monitor these medications properly? Unlike many other drugs, the stimulants require judicious prescribing and careful monitoring, for which the physician must allot sufficient time. If this is not possible, the family should be referred to another physician who can monitor the medication.

11. How does the child feel about medication and its alternatives? With older children, it is important that the use of drugs be discussed with them and its rationale sufficiently explained. In cases where children are "antidrug," they may sabotage efforts to use it by not swallowing the pill when it is given or by other means. Carol Whalen has also shown that children's views on origins of their problems and their ability to control them can affect drug responding (see Whalen & Henker, 1976, in "Suggested Reading").

12. Has the child had an adequate physical and psychological evaluation? Stimulants should never be prescribed if the child has not been seen or if the child has only been briefly examined in the office, except in very rare instances when a crisis in the behavior of the child or in family relations has occurred. At the very least, those procedures suggested in Chapter 3 should be used to evaluate the child; in addition, a thorough physical exam, particularly of heart rate, pulse, blood pressure, and growth patterns in height and weight, should be administered before treatment is initiated.

Prescribing and Titrating

As just noted, a child should have a thorough evaluation before the use of stimulants is considered. Even then, very young children should probably not be given these drugs, despite hyperactivity and lack of contraindicated factors. Many investigators have found that the response rate to methylphenidate and *d*-amphetamine in children under 3 years of age is so poor as to rule these drugs out for this age group. With children between 3 to 5 years of age, these two drugs probably have only a 50% response rate. At 6 years or later, the response rate is 75% or higher. With pemoline, I have found children under 5 years to do so poorly that I suggest avoiding the drug's use with this age group. Often, the side effects are quite serious, with little to no positive response. In contrast, I have observed all three drugs to be useful well into the teenage years of older children. In fact, I am likely to recommend a shift to pemoline during the adolescent years because of its greater convenience for prescribing, the fact that it can be taken in only one dose before school to avoid any social stigma attached to drug taking, and the fact that the "street value" of this drug within the community is considerably less than that of methylphenidate and *d*-amphetamine.

If a child is 4 years or older, the first choice of medication seems to be methylphenidate (except in adolescence) because of its greater documentation in research, proven efficacy, and greater dose response information. If a poor response occurs, I will suggest pemoline. If the child fails to respond to pemoline, then I will suggest that the physician switch to the antidepressant imipramine (Tofranil), to be discussed later in this chapter. If this too fails, then drug use may be postponed for at least a year, if not altogether eliminated from consideration. In this case, psychoeducational treatments will have to suffice.

The drugs, their available tablet sizes, and their typical therapeutic ranges are listed in Table 5.5. With methylphenidate, the child will be started at .3 mg/kg b.i.d., and the dose will be adjusted every 3 days by 2.5 mg until a generally therapeutic effect is achieved. The doses to be used rarely exceed

TABLE 5.5. Stimulant Drugs, Tablet Sizes, and Dose Ranges

Brand name	Manufacturer	Generic name	Tablet sizes	Dose range
Ritalin	CIBA	Methylphenidate	5 mg 10 mg 20 mg	.3–1 mg/kg
Dexedrine	Smith, Kline, & French	d-Amphetamine	5 mg (tablet and spansule) 10 mg (spansule) 15 mg (spansule)	.15–.5 mg/kg
Cylert	Abbott	Pemoline	18.75 mg 37.5 mg 75 mg	.5 –2 mg/kg

.7 mg/kg b.i.d. because of the severity of side effects, and the physicians with whom I work have never prescribed more than 1 mg/kg b.i.d. for any child. Once adequate improvement occurs, the physician may need to increase the dose slightly after several weeks or months, possibly because of habituation or because of weight gain by the child that reduces the amount of drug available to the CNS. If the drug is used primarily for classroom management, I suggest that it be discontinued on weekends, holidays, and summer vacations. When beginning use of the drug each Monday produces a renewal of side effects seen only at the start of each week, I suggest that the child be kept on one-half or less of the regular dose during the weekend to maintain habituation to the side effects. If the child is as much of a problem at home as at school, I suggest keeping the child on the medication 7 days a week and try to discontinue the drug only over the school vacation months of the summer, when possible.

I have sometimes found it necessary to recommend the use of a three-times-a-day dose schedule with methylphenidate, primarily because the drug may last 3 hours or less with some children. This problem is often discovered in contacts with a child's teachers, who may observe that the morning dose has essentially worn off by 10:30 or 11:00 A.M. and that the child isn't due for a second dose until noon. I will then suggest the use of this schedule: a breakfast dose at 7:00–8:00 A.M., a second dose at 10:30–11:00 A.M., and a third dose at 2:00–3:00 P.M. While some parents have inquired about using a dose at the dinner hour, we recommend against it in all but a few rare cases because of the insomnia problems associated with doses late in the day.

As Table 5.5 indicates, d-amphetamine is typically given in doses about half those of methylphenidate, though its use in other respects is identical to that of the latter drug. Pemoline is prescribed and titrated quite differently. It is generally given only once a day, in the morning. Its recommended dose is .5 to 2 mg/kg. The dose is titrated upward every 3 to 5 days by 18.75 mg until a therapeutic effect is achieved. On occasion, a second dose, often half that of the morning dose, may be given at 2:00 P.M. if the morning dose is proving ineffective during the afternoon. This, however, will likely increase insomnia problems at bedtime. Recent papers suggest that pemoline is slower in achieving its peak effects and in "washing out" of the body than the other stimulants are; in some cases, its effects may last 2 to 3 days after its discontinuation.

A child's failure to respond to one drug does not preclude a positive response to other stimulants. As many as 20% of those who respond poorly to one stimulant are believed to show a positive response to a second one. I often suggest that Ritalin be used first and then Cylert if a poor response to Ritalin develops. However, Dexedrine spansules in some cases have proven an excellent alternative to Ritalin when Ritalin fails to produce behavioral improvement.

No matter which drug is used, some common principles (and common sense!) apply. The dose should be the lowest possible and should be given only as many times per day as necessary to achieve adequate management of the child's behavior. The drugs should be discontinued on weekends, holidays, and summer vacations, unless, they are necessary during these times. Titration should involve the lowest convenient increments, and adequate time (a minimum of 3 to 5 days) should be given for the effectiveness of the increased dose to be judged before the dose is increased again. When possible, both parents and teachers should be consulted during the titration period for their opinions as to which dose seems most beneficial. Parents should never be given permission to adjust the dose of medication as they see fit. This often leads to overmedication of a child, as the parents may increase the dose every time the child is temperamental, noncompliant, or obstinant. Such occurrences are usually better treated by the altering of parent management styles.

Monitoring Response to Medication

This is probably the weakest link in the chain of procedures followed in medicating hyperactive children. State laws now make it more likely that parents and physicians will have regular contact in the course of continuing drug treatment, although such contact can often be avoided unless physicians take some care to make the meetings genuinely useful in the monitoring of drugs. Once the seemingly appropriate dose level is achieved during the titration period, then several questionnaires used in the initial evaluation can be completed again by the parents and teachers to establish the degree of change in hyperactive behaviors. I use the Conners PSQ and TRS, as well as the HSQ and SSQ, to assess drug efficacy. The latter questionnaires help to show which *situations* are still problematic, while the Conners scales show which *behaviors* are still so. In addition, parents are given the Side Effects Questionnaire shown in Figure 5.4. Each month, when parents call to obtain another prescription, this questionnaire is reviewed with them to determine whether new side effects have arisen. In addition, at each monthly contact (usually by telephone), a checklist of questions is reviewed with parents in order to assess continued drug efficacy. This checklist is shown in Figure 5.5.

When parents call to complain about ineffective doses that were formerly effective, physicians should use caution in deciding to increase the dose. Often some family crisis or uniquely distressing incident with a child has arisen that may make the child's general behavior seem worse than it is. All parents experience days in which, because of stress, illness, or other factors, their level of tolerance for the child is much lower and may lead them to complain. Such complaints can often be construed as pleas for help from parents. It is not always necessary to increase the dose in such situ-

Child's Name _____ Date _____
Name of Person Completing This Form _____

Instructions:
Please rate each behavior from 0 (absent) to 9 (serious). CIRCLE ONLY ONE NUMBER
BESIDE EACH ITEM. A zero means that you have not seen this behavior in your child during
the past week; and a 9 means that you have noticed it and believe it either to be very serious
or to occur very frequently. Thank you.

Behavior:	ABSENT									SERIOUS
Insomnia or trouble sleeping	0	1	2	3	4	5	6	7	8	9
Nightmares	0	1	2	3	4	5	6	7	8	9
Stares a lot or daydreams	0	1	2	3	4	5	6	7	8	9
Talks less with others	0	1	2	3	4	5	6	7	8	9
Uninterested in others	0	1	2	3	4	5	6	7	8	9
Decreased appetite	0	1	2	3	4	5	6	7	8	9
Irritable	0	1	2	3	4	5	6	7	8	9
Stomachaches	0	1	2	3	4	5	6	7	8	9
Headaches	0	1	2	3	4	5	6	7	8	9
Drowsiness	0	1	2	3	4	5	6	7	8	9
Sad/unhappy	0	1	2	3	4	5	6	7	8	9
Prone to crying	0	1	2	3	4	5	6	7	8	9
Anxious	0	1	2	3	4	5	6	7	8	9
Bites his or her nails	0	1	2	3	4	5	6	7	8	9
Euphoric/unusually happy	0	1	2	3	4	5	6	7	8	9
Dizziness	0	1	2	3	4	5	6	7	8	9

FIGURE 5.4. The Side Effects Questionnaire, to be reviewed monthly with parents of
children taking stimulant drugs.

ations, but it is necessary simply to listen to the parent in a reflective,
supportive, clinical way, and perhaps to refer the parent to someone who can
deal with the precipitating event. If the physician is unable to determine any
familial or occupational stress that has caused such a complaint, then it may
indeed be true that the current dose has become ineffective. Careful questioning of the parent as to the ways in which the child's behavior is different
or worse can be useful in making this decision. Although it is certainly not
true in all cases, mothers of hyperactive children are occasionally likely to
have hysterical personalities associated with overly excitable behavior and
emotions. Thus the crisis that has precipitated the call to the physician may
in fact not be a crisis at all. Clinical judgment and experience are crucial in
handling these parental complaints effectively without unnecessarily increasing the child's medication.

1. What dose have you been regularly giving to this child over the past month?

2. Have you noticed any of the following side effects this month?

   loss of appetite/weight loss   rashes

   insomnia   dizziness

   irritability in late morning   dark circles under eyes
   or late afternoon   fearfulness

   unusual crying   social withdrawal

   tics or nervous habits   drowsiness

   headache/stomachache   anxiety

   sadness

3. If so, please describe how often and when the side effects occurred.

4. Have you spoken with the child's teacher lately? How is the child performing in class?

5. Did your child complain about taking the medication or avoid its use?

6. Does the drug seem to be helping the child as much this month as it did last month? If not, what seems to have changed?

7. When was your child last examined by the doctor? (If more than 1 year, schedule the child for a clinic visit and exam.)

8. Have there been problems in giving the child medication at school?

FIGURE 5.5. A checklist of questions to be reviewed monthly with parents of children taking stimulant drugs.

Approximately every 6 to 8 months that a child is on medication, it is advisable to administer a follow-up clinic examination. During this time, height, weight, blood pressure, and heart rate can be recorded to determine potential side effects. The parents again complete the Conners PSQ, the HSQ, and the Side Effects Questionnaire. Difficulties that continue to plague the child or family can be discussed, and referrals to appropriate professionals can be made when necessary. When parents are called for the appointment by the clinic secretary, they should be encouraged to write down in advance any concerns or questions they may have, so that the clinic visit can be as useful as possible.

Discontinuing Medication

It is less difficult to determine when to discontinue medication than it is to know when to start it. Many physicians recommend that children spend their first few weeks of school each year *off* medication, in order to determine whether their problems from the previous year continue with new teachers. Sometimes, the 3 to 4 months between the ending and the beginning of school result in substantial maturation in the child's behavior, especially as the child approaches puberty; in such cases, medication may no longer be needed. Cantwell has found that as many as 26% of the children can discontinue the medication because of improved self-control after 2 years of medication. This is not to say that the children are cured or have outgrown the problems; only that the problems are not sufficiently severe to warrant the continued use of stimulants. However, a child's reaching puberty is not a reason in itself to stop medication, as is commonly believed. The drugs are just as useful for teenagers as for children. They should be discontinued only when no longer needed, not at some arbitrary age.

Contraindications and Interactions

As stated earlier, children with a history of tics, Tourette syndrome, thought disorder, or psychosis should not be given stimulant medications, for these often exacerbate the symptoms of such disorders. Children with high levels of anxiety are also likely to respond poorly to these drugs. Furthermore, children under 4 years of age are poor responders to medication. There is very little research on drug effects and side effects in this age group. There is some controversy over whether stimulants should be given to children with seizures or epilepsy; doubts about the practice are based on the possibility that the stimulants may lower seizure thresholds. This phenomenon is rarely seen clinically, however, and it can be avoided by a slight increase in the level of anticonvulsants. Since many epileptic children are hyperactive, the stimulants can be useful in their management if the drugs are judiciously prescribed.

The stimulants can alter the actions of other drugs, though such interactions are often not clinically serious or significant. The stimulants may antagonize the effects of hypnotic drugs and may also increase their toxicity in overdosage. In addition, the stimulants have been shown to heighten the activity of antidepressants and monoamine oxidase (MAO) inhibitors. Interestingly, the use of thioridazine in one study was shown to enhance the effects of methylphenidate. The stimulants may also decrease the efficacy of anticonvulsant drugs, although this remains to be empirically demonstrated. In general, the stimulant drugs have few, if any, serious interactions with other drugs.

COMBINED TREATMENT PROGRAMS

One issue frequently raised is that of whether stimulant medication, behavior therapy, or a combination of the two is the best treatment approach to hyperactivity. Some studies using extremely small sample sizes have found that behavior therapy can be as effective in managing classroom misbehavior as stimulant medication can be. Certainly behavioral approaches seem better suited to improving academic achievement, accuracy, and productivity than the stimulant drugs, which, as noted earlier, have few if any effects on these academic areas. With respect to managing hyperactive behavior in general, however, the controversy continues.

In the most extensive study of this issue (1980; see "Suggested Reading"), Rachel Gittelman-Klein and her colleagues studied 61 hyperactive children randomly assigned to one of three possible treatments: Ritalin alone, behavior therapy with a placebo, and behavior therapy with Ritalin. Teacher ratings, direct classroom observations, and global ratings of improvement by parents, teachers, and physicians served as the dependent measures. On the teacher ratings, all treatments produced significant improvements after 8 weeks, but the ratings of the two drug-treated groups were consistently superior to those of the group receiving behavior therapy alone, and were indistinguishable from each other. On the direct classroom observations, only the two groups receiving medication showed any significant improvements in their behavior during treatment, whereas little change in the behavior-therapy-alone group was observed in these measures of disruptive behavior. Again, there was no difference in ratings between the two drug-treated groups. Parents' global ratings found all treatments equally effective; teachers found the combined program the most effective, though both treatments used alone were rated as producing improvements in more than 63% of the children in each group. Psychiatrists rated 100% of the children in the combined group as improved, versus 81% in the drug-only group and 58% in the behavior-therapy-only group.

These results suggest that behavior therapy alone is not as effective as stimulant medication in managing hyperactive and disruptive behavior. On all measures, the combined program of drugs and behavior therapy was the most optimal, although only it received slightly better ratings than medication used alone. Obviously, from a standpoint of cost alone, medication is far more cost-effective than behavior therapy or a combination of these two treatments. These results indicate that, when medication is not sufficient, behavior therapy programs may be added to improve hyperactive behaviors. They do not support the notion that behavior therapy should be the only treatment, or even the first treatment, to be used with hyperactive children.

ALTERNATIVE MEDICATIONS

Other medications have been suggested for use with hyperactive children or have in fact received some study.

Other Stimulants

The possibility that both deanol (Deaner) and caffeine may be useful with hyperactive children has been suggested. Deanol is an organic salt (2-dimethyl amino ethanol) that is believed to operate primarily on cholinergic rather than catecholaminergic pathways in the CNS. The little research that exists does not support its efficacy with hyperactive children.

Caffeine is a xanthine derivative whose use with hyperactive children was the subject of some public attention and support 3 to 5 years ago. At least five or six studies were done to compare its efficacy with that of other stimulants. Some studies found no effects, while those which did noted the improvements to be far inferior to those brought about by the more commonly used stimulants. At present, caffeine is not seriously considered to have much utility with hyperactive children.

Tricyclic Antidepressants

The reader seriously considering the use of these drugs with hyperactive children is referred to the chapter on antidepressants by Judith Rapoport and Edwin Mikkelson in a text edited by Werry (1978; see "Suggested Reading"). The antidepressant most widely studied with hyperactive children is imipramine (Tofranil). The antidepressants are slower-acting medications that have recently been shown to produce behavioral effects similar to those of the stimulants with hyperactive children. An added advantage of this medication with depressed hyperactive children is the mood elevation it produces after several weeks of use. We have found the drug particularly useful with hyperactive children over 10 years of age, in whom depression is usually a significant associated clinical feature.

THE ROLE OF NONMEDICAL PROFESSIONALS IN DRUG TREATMENT

Pediatricians and child psychiatrists obviously play a pivotal role in the drug treatment of hyperactive children. Other professionals can, however, play instrumental roles in such treatment by assisting physicians in monitoring medication effects and by administering psychoeducational therapies to which drugs may serve as adjuncts.

School Psychologists and Educators

At first glance, it may seem to school staff members that there are few if any roles they can play in the drug management of hyperactive children. This attitude is misleading, for the role of the school staff can often prove an important one.

1. School psychologists and educators play an obvious yet critical role in the initial diagnosis of hyperactivity. Families often seek assistance from their pediatricians because of complaints from the school of poor classroom behavior. School personnel are second only to parents in the useful information about hyperactive children with which they can provide physicians, and they are the most important informants when classroom performance is the primary problem. While physicians may query the families for information, they weigh heavily the advice received from school staff in deciding whether or not to medicate such children.

2. The school personnel are also viewed by families as an important source of professional opinion and advice as to whether their children's behavior is deviant and, if so, where they might best seek help. This is especially true if a child is the only offspring of young parents who are naive about normal child behavior and development. Even when a family recognizes the existence of a behavior problem, it may be the advice and urging of the school that finally prompt the parents to seek medication or other assistance.

3. Once drug therapy is implemented, medical staff will again heavily weigh the school personnel's opinion of a child's drug response in determining the proper dose. When physicians do not request this information, it is imperative that school staff members contact them with their observations of the child's reactions. Indeed, the school staff should not automatically assume that physicians prescribing such medication will monitor it adequately. The survey by Solomons mentioned earlier found that 43% of those children on stimulants were not being adequately monitored by physicians. Adequacy was defined merely as contact between family and physician twice within 6 months or three times within 12 months—a minimal monitoring criterion for drugs having considerable abuse potential. In addition, 29% of the families were allowed to "juggle" the dose of medication freely without consulting their physicians. Thus, close monitoring by school staff of a child on stimulants may reveal periods when the child is being overmedicated by the family or when side effects preclude adequate classroom adjustment. Contact with the child's physician under such circumstances is imperative.

4. When the stimulant drug has been properly titrated, school psychologists can greatly assist in identifying residual learning and social skill deficits that will require additional educational programs. As noted above, teachers may be less likely to see these residual problems once children are managed with medication.

5. Finally, school psychologists are in a unique position to implement additional therapies for hyperactive children if drugs should prove ineffective, insufficient, or undesirable to the children, their families, or their teachers. Designing behavior modification or education programs and assisting teachers in their implementation are roles that can be filled most effectively by school psychologists. In addition, school psychologists must see that in-service training programs are developed to instruct other staff members and teachers in the uses and abuses of psychopharmacology in the classroom, as well as in alternatives to medication for children with behavior problems.

Child/Pediatric Psychologists

Like school staff members, child psychologists, especially those trained in pediatric psychology, can play an important role in drug therapy with hyperactive children.

1. Because of child or pediatric psychologists' training in tests and measures, they usually have better knowledge than physicians do of the questionnaires and rating scales best suited to monitoring children's drug responses.

2. In addition, the psychologists are also trained in direct observational methods for recording home or classroom conduct and social interactions. These methods can prove useful not only in monitoring drug responses, but also in suggesting nonmedical methods for modifying deviant behavior.

3. The psychologists' background in psychometric testing is often called upon for the assessment of learning or personality problems that drug management is unlikely to affect. Alternative educational, counseling, or psychotherapeutic methods may be required in addition to medication.

4. Many child psychologists are skilled in training parents in effective child management methods. These methods will be required whether or not drug therapy is used, since the medications are not effective during all the waking hours of children. Parent training has been shown to be as effective as drug therapy and should be considered before drug treatment for many hyperactive children.

5. When parents manifest personal or marital problems that can interfere with effective drug treatment of their children, child psychologists can provide direct counseling to the parents or refer them to other psychologists more skilled in these problems.

This section clearly suggests that the treatment of hyperactive children, even when stimulant drugs are involved, must often be an interdisciplinary matter if broad spectrum programs are to be designed to address the many problems with which hyperactive children present. Drugs alone will not be enough to alter the prognosis of these children.

DISCUSSING DRUG USE WITH PARENTS

One of the most critical aspects of drug treatment with hyperactive children, yet one receiving little or no attention, is the counseling of parents on the drug treatment of their children. Simply providing the parents with a prescription and telling them to call back in a week or two will not do. Physicians need to take time to explain the rationale for drug therapy, to discuss its effects and side effects, and to explain carefully how the drug will be titrated. Often, too, it is important to explain drug response rates, results that the drugs will *not* achieve, and areas in which other therapies will be necessary. Parents often have many misconceptions and concerns about drug treatment that should be addressed by physicians. "Are they addictive? How long will my child need them? How will I know what changes to expect? What will we do if the drug doesn't work? Is my child likely to come to view drugs as an acceptable way of handling problems?" These and other questions frequently plague parents who are faced with a recommendation of drug treatment for their children.

Parents obviously need to be cautioned against adjusting the dose without calling their physicians. In addition, the drugs should be kept in a safe place out of reach of children and adults prone to drug abuse. This is an excellent time to provide the family with the questionnaires they should mail in when the drugs seem to be appropriately titrated. Regardless of the frequency with which physicians must explain medication use to families, it is essential that they remain sensitive to parents' concerns, naive at times as these may seem, and that they not deal too glibly with them if the parents are to become an effective part of the drug management team.

At this point, physicians should take time to discuss the drug treatment with the children themselves. Are the children scared? Do they understand why the drugs are being given and what they will accomplish? Are they willing to take them? What do they think their friends will say when they learn of the treatment? While difficult, these and other issues must be addressed with the children. Often, the parents are left to fumble through or to fabricate explanations as to the purpose of drugs. The children's cooperation with therapy must be enlisted; this requires that appropriate time with physicians who are sensitive to the children's concerns and questions be made an integral part of drug treatment.

ETHICAL AND SOCIAL ISSUES
IN DRUG TREATMENT WITH CHILDREN

It is not the intent of this chapter to engage in lengthy philosophical discussions of ethics and morals in treating deviant behavior in children with drugs. The reader is referred to Cantwell and Carlson (1978) and to Sroufe (1975; see "Suggested Reading") for a more thorough discussion of these issues. Nonetheless, brief mention of the various ethical and social issues is required, as these questions will be put to confront physicians at one time or another by parents, teachers, or the highly vocal antidrug minority, not to mention the local press. How physicians personally choose to resolve these issues will probably contribute more to their decisions about using drugs with children than will any number of research findings on such drugs efficacy and safety. What follows is only a partial listing of the issues worthy of consideration:

1. How ethical is it to treat children with drugs of little-known long-term efficacy because of the intolerance of their parents or teachers?

2. Have drugs simply become too easily available as a method of treatment? In other words, have professionals abdicated their responsibilities to implement less convenient but equally effective nonmedical therapies?

3. Can society afford the apparent double standard of instructing children not to turn to recreational drugs to solve their problems while using similar drugs to solve its own?

4. Are hyperactive children learning to view medicine as the solution to their social problems?

5. What are the implications of the politics of drug therapy? We seem to be more likely to use drugs with children of lower educational and socioeconomic backgrounds, whose parents may be less literate and may also be members of racial minorities.

6. Are the research findings clear enough to warrant medicating 700,000 or more children every year?

7. Should schools and physicians team up as they do to "coerce" parents into using drugs with their children? Are we simply patching up an obsolete educational system?

I believe that drug treatment with some hyperactive children is both necessary and beneficial. Nevertheless, these ethical concerns should not be too far from our thinking as we engage in the modification of children's social conduct through psychopharmacologic means.

CONCLUSION

In summary, stimulant drugs are a highly effective therapy for the management of hyperactive and disruptive behavior. These drugs appear to have their primary effects on attention span and impulse control, perhaps because of their ability to energize inhibitory brain mechanisms. Changes in other behaviors seem to be the result of these improvements in attention and impulsivity. Children who receive stimulants tend to show improvements in their play, social conduct, and compliance to commands and rules; these result in a lessening of supervision, reprimands, commands, censure, and punishment from those adults who must frequently interact with them. Despite these behavioral changes, medication causes little improvement in the academic achievement or performance of hyperactive children, nor is their long-term outcome altered appreciably by drug use during childhood. While these drugs are highly effective in improving the day-to-day management of hyperactive children, other treatments are required if the goals of therapy include the improvement of academic achievement as well as that of long-term social adjustment.

SUGGESTED READING

Barkley, R. A. Predicting the response of hyperkinetic children to stimulant drugs. *Journal of Abnormal Child Psychology*, 1976, *4*, 327–348.

Barkley, R. A. A review of stimulant drug research with hyperactive children. *Journal of Child Psychology and Psychiatry*, 1977, *18*, 137–165.

Barkley, R. A. Using stimulant drugs in the classroom. *School Psychology Digest*, 1979, *8*, 412–425.

Barkley, R. A., & Cunningham, C. E. Do stimulant drugs improve the academic performance of hyperactive children? *Clinical Pediatrics*, 1978, *17*, 85–92.

Barkley, R. A., & Cunningham, C. E. The parent–child interactions of hyperactive children and their modification by stimulant drugs. In R. Knights & D. Bakker (Eds.), *Treatment of hyperactive and learning disordered children*. Baltimore: University Park Press, 1980.

Bradley, C. The behavior of children receiving Benzedrine. *American Journal of Psychiatry*, 1937, *94*, 577–585.

Cantwell, D. P. Drugs and medical intervention. In H. Rie & E. Rie (Eds.), *Handbook of minimal brain dysfunctions*. New York: Wiley, 1980.

Cantwell, D. P. A clinician's guide to the use of stimulant medication for the psychiatric disorders of children. *Developmental and Behavioral Pediatrics*, 1980, *1*, 133–140.

Cantwell, D. P., & Carlson, G. A. Stimulants. In J. Werry (Ed.), *Pediatric psychopharmacology*. New York: Brunner/Mazel, 1978.

Conners, C. K., & Taylor, E. Pemoline, methylphenidate, and placebo in children with minimal brain dysfunction. *Archives of General Psychiatry*, 1980, *37*, 922–932.

Conners, C. K., & Werry, J. S. Pharmacotherapy. In H. Quay & J. S. Werry (Eds.), *Psychopathological disorders of childhood* (2nd ed.). New York: Wiley, 1979.

Gittelman-Klein, R., Abikoff, H., Pollack, E., Klein, D. F., Katz, S., & Mattes, J. A controlled trial of behavior modification and methylphenidate in hyperactive children. In C. Whalen & B. Henker (Eds.), *Hyperactive children: The social ecology of identification and treatment*. New York: Academic Press, 1980.

Golden, G. S. The effect of central nervous system stimulants on Tourette syndrome. *Annals of Neurology*, 1977, *2*, 69–70.

Greenspoon, S., & Singer, S. Amphetamines in the treatment of hyperkinetic children. *Harvard Educational Review*, 1973, *43*, 515–555.

Hastings, J. & Barkley, R. A. A review of psychophysiological research with hyperkinetic children. *Journal of Abnormal Child Psychology*, 1978, *6*, 413–447.

Katz, S., Saraf, K., Gittelman-Klein, R., & Klein, D. F. Clinical pharmacological management of hyperkinetic children. In D. F. Klein & R. Gittelman-Klein (Eds.), *Progress in psychiatric drug treatment* (Vol. 2). New York: Brunner/Mazel, 1976.

Molitch, M., & Eccles, A. K. Effects of benzedrine sulphate on intelligence scores of children. *American Journal of Psychiatry*, 1937, *94*, 587–590.

Rapoport, J. L., Buchsbaum, M. S., Zahn, T. P., Weingarten, H., Ludlow, C., & Mikkelsen, E. Dextroamphetamine: Cognitive and behavioral effects in normal prepubertal boys. *Science*, 1978, *199*, 560–563.

Roche, A. F., Lipman, R. S., Overall, J. E., & Hung, W. The effects of stimulant medication on the growth of hyperkinetic children. *Pediatrics*, 1979, *63*, 847–850.

Safer, R. P., & Allen, D. J. Factors influencing the suppressant effects of two stimulant drugs on the growth of hyperactive children. *Pediatrics*, 1973, *51*, 660–667.

Safer, R. P., & Allen, D. J. *Hyperactive children: Diagnosis and management*. Baltimore: University Park Press, 1976.

Safer, R. P., Allen, D. J., & Barr, E. Depression of growth in hyperactive children on stimulant drugs. *New England Journal of Medicine*, 1972, *287*, 217–220.

Satterfield, J. H., Schell, A. M., & Barb, S. D. Potential risk of prolonged administration of stimulant medication for hyperactive children. *Developmental and Behavioral Pediatrics*, 1980, *1*, 102–107.

Solomons, G. Drug therapy: Initiation and follow-up. *Annals of the New York Academy of Science*, 1973, *205*, 335–344.

Sprague, R., & Sleator, E. Methylphenidate in hyperkinetic children: Differences in dose effects on learning and social behavior. *Science*, 1977, *198*, 1274–1276.

Sroufe, A. Drug treatment of children with behavior problems. In F. Horowitz (Ed.), *Review of child development research* (Vol. 4). Chicago: University of Chicago Press, 1975.

Werry, J.S. (Ed.). *Pediatric psychopharmacology*. New York: Brunner/Mazel, 1978.

Whalen, C. K., Collins B. E., Henker, B., Alkus, S. R., Adams, D., & Stapp, J. Behavior observations of hyperactive children and methylphenidate (Ritalin) effects in systematically structured classroom environment: Now you see them, now you don't. *Journal of Pediatric Psychology*, 1978, *3*, 177–187.

Whalen, C. K., & Henker, B. Psychostimulants and children: A review and analysis. *Psychological Bulletin*, 1976, *83*, 1113–1130.

CHAPTER SIX

PRINCIPLES OF BEHAVIOR THERAPY

Educate your children of self-control, to the habit of holding passion and prejudice and evil tendencies subject to an upright and reasoning will, and you have done much to abolish misery from their future lives and crimes from society.—Daniel Webster

Earlier chapters in this book have demonstrated that hyperactive children display a variety of primary as well as associated problems that warrant intervention. Primary difficulties with attention, impulse control, and rule-governed behavior arise early, are relatively pervasive in nature, and are chronic in their persistence throughout such children's development. Associated problems with aggression, noncompliance, poor peer relations, academic achievement, and emotional expression further complicate the lives of these children and their families. Such children often have increased medical problems, such as frequent upper respiratory infections, colds, and allergies, and increased physical problems, such as enuresis, encopresis, and generally immature physical development.

Besides problems with the children themselves, there is an increased occurrence of psychiatric problems in other family members. Mothers are more likely to be depressed and suffering marital discord. Problems with hysteria, and in some cases alcoholism and minor tranquilizer abuse, are seen. Fathers, if they are in the home setting at all, are more likely to have conduct problems, alcoholism, or depression than are fathers of normal children. The siblings of hyperactive children seem more likely to be at risk for hyperactivity, conduct problems, and learning disabilities than siblings of normal children seem to be.

THE CLINICIAN'S ATTITUDE TOWARD TREATMENT

Such interlocking sets of child and family problems require that therapists modify their approach to therapy in several respects. First, it is obvious that no single professional discipline can hope to treat all of the problems facing hyperactive children and their families. Physicians will be needed to handle

231

the associated physical problems and use of medication, but they are unlikely to have the skills or time to train parents in child management or to consult with schools on classroom misbehavior and learning disabilities. Psychologists may be capable of coping with the latter problems but not with the physical and drug-related issues. Social workers may be better able to work with the child and family problems, but they cannot generally be expected to consult with schools on the assessment and treatment of classroom misbehavior and achievement problems or to handle medical or medication concerns. Clearly, each group of professionals must seek out and be willing to coordinate its activities with those of the other professionals who are needed to manage each child's individual profile of personal and familial problems.

As has been stressed repeatedly in this book, therapists will have to settle for teaching hyperactive children and their families and teachers to cope with rather than to cure the primary difficulties of the children. No treatment has yet achieved any more than short-term improvements in hyperactive symptoms. Even when improvements are seen, they are rarely sufficient to constitute such children as "normal"; their behavior still remains deviant, although it is less distressing. In addition, future problems at home, in the community, or at school are still likely to arise with these children within months or years of seemingly successful intervention efforts. Hence, interventions must be designed to facilitate coping and reduce distress and must be periodically reintroduced throughout the children's development.

A third consideration for clinicians is the need to adopt an attitude toward the families and schools that is supportive, empathetic, and positively constructive. Too often, child clinicians engage in psychological "prosecutions" of parents during evaluation and treatment that are counterproductive and misguided. There is no room for blaming or finding fault with the parents of these children if effective coping is to be taught to them. Often, the parents (especially the mothers) of these children are already heavily guilt-ridden and depressed over their inability to manage the children. Therapist attitudes of blaming or fault-finding will only reinforce these emotional problems further; moreover, they have no empirical support in the current scientific literature. The parents need encouragement that they are not directly at fault for their children's problems but that the ways in which they choose to handle the children can make their problems better or worse. Hence, the parents need to learn new methods of child management but not to do so in the conviction that they have done something wrong.

A fourth issue facing clinicians is that direct treatment of these children outside the social contexts of family and school that does not include significant adults or siblings in the process is doomed to abysmal failure. It is these individuals, not clinicians, who must live with the hyperactive children in their natural environment and who must learn new ways of adapting to the children's problems. The view espoused by Roland Tharp and Ralph Wetzel in the classic text *Behavior Modification in the Natural Environment* (1969; see "Suggested Reading") seems most appropriate here. This approach stresses that the natural agents who normally interact with the children should be trained as the primary therapists, with clinicians serving as trainer-consultants to these individuals. While training may occur in clinics or natural settings and use the children in the process, therapists need to bear in mind that the problems with the children do not normally occur in the presence of the therapists themselves, but with parents and teachers. At some point, these are the people who must be the direct focus of therapeutic strategies if there is to be any shred of hope for generalization of treatment effects or persistence of these effects over time.

A final consideration for clinicians is the need to know behavior modification concepts and principles in working with hyperactive children and their families. Aside from drug therapy, no other form of treatment has demonstrated any reasonable degree of effectiveness in assisting families and teachers to improve hyperkinetic symptoms. Such methods as individual psychotherapy or play therapy have shown no utility in managing the problems of these children. They are expensive, are often long-term in nature, and frequently ignore the needs of parents to learn how to cope with their children's problems in the home. Hyperactive children are often unresponsive to these approaches because of their reduced awareness of their own behavior, its consequences, and its implications for others around them as well as for their own future adjustment. Further, the goals of such therapies are to get children to express and deal with the psychic and emotional conflicts that are ostensibly causing their problems. Such an approach conflicts with the view taken here that hyperactivity is initially a biologically based disorder of temperament and social conduct that is shaped by its familial and social environment, rather than a disorder spawned by psychic conflicts or parents' poor child management methods. Because hyperactive symptoms, like other behaviors, are affected to some degree by their social contexts and consequences, behavior modification methods can result in some improvements in hyperactive children's problems when they are effectively and consistently employed.

The present chapter therefore adopts a behavioral approach to working with hyperactive children and their families; it fully acknowledges that these methods are not likely to result in permanent cures or complete normalization of these children and that drugs may serve as useful adjuncts to these methods, or in some cases as the primary mode of treatment. The approach espoused here is an empirically based one that sets specific behavioral goals and uses methods with some demonstrated utility in the scientific literature. Its focus is the environment of the children, particularly the social contexts of their behavior; in these contexts, the relationship between precipitating events and behavioral consequences is examined and manipulated to produce improved child behavior.

A REVIEW OF BEHAVIORAL PRINCIPLES

It is not my intent here to provide a review of behavioral principles that is sufficiently exhaustive to allow clinicians lacking experience with them to use them effectively. Many excellent texts, some of which are listed at the end of this chapter, will give clinicians a more thorough grounding in these principles. The purpose here is merely to acquaint clinicians with these concepts and principles. The sophisticated reader may wish to go on to the next section.

A behavioral approach focuses on the observable behavior of children, both verbal and motoric or nonverbal, as the target of assessment and therapy. It is based on the empirically supported assumption that those events immediately preceding and following given behaviors have substantial control over the nature and occurrence of these behaviors. The historical aspects of the behavior are given considerably less import than they are in other approaches to child clinical practice. Through alteration of the events in the immediate situation, child behaviors can be dramatically changed, regardless of the historical factors that may have given rise to them.

This approach to child behavior is best illustrated by the model set forth by Fred Kanfer and George Saslow (1969) as the "$S-O-R-K-C$ relationship." Here, the stimuli (S) that immediately precede given behaviors are viewed as having some control over what behaviors occur and when they occur. That is, they serve as cues to children to behave in certain ways. Behaviors that occur in the presence of these cues and that generally do not occur in their absence are said to be under "stimulus control." For instance, when a child throws temper tantrums after commands from the mother but not after commands from the father or teacher, the temper tantrums are under stimulus control by maternal commands. The way in which stimulus control develops will be discussed shortly.

This model also recognizes the importance of organismic (O) factors in determining the occurrence of child behaviors. The developmental status of a child's nervous system, its integrity, and the effects of illness on its current functioning are viewed as contributing to the nature and occurrence of child behaviors. Other states of the organism, such as hunger, thirst, and sexual drives, also contribute to the probability of the occurrence of particular behaviors and are incorporated into this step of the model. The behavioral view therefore gives some acknowledgement to the role of individual differences in biological structures and functions of organisms in determining behavioral expression.

The actual behavior or response (R) of a child can vary in its frequency and topography, depending on both the stimuli and organismic factors that precede it and the events that follow it. Those consequences (K) that occur immediately following a behavior also influence its frequency, intensity, or topography. Events that increase a behavior are said to be "reinforcing," while those that reduce a behavior are labeled as "punishing." Reinforcement and punishment, the processes of increasing and decreasing behavior by controlling the types of events that consequate it, are primary concepts in behavioral treatments. Reinforcement can be both positive and negative. When the introduction of an event increases a behavior, the event is positively reinforcing. Giving a child candy or praise following compliance to commands often increases compliance, and such events are therefore called positive reinforcers. The concept of negative reinforcement has been introduced in Chapter 2; negative reinforcement is believed to play an important role in aggressive and aversive child behaviors. The *removal* of an event following a behavior that increases that behavior is said to be negatively reinforcing. For instance, when a child throws a temper tantrum after the mother repeats a command and the mother withdraws the command, the child is more likely to throw a tantrum the next time the mother gives a command. Here, the repeated commands of the mother are aversive to the child, and their termination following a tantrum reinforces the occurrence of tantrums. In contrast, an event that *reduces* a given child behavior is said to be punishing. Punishment can be the introduction of an aversive event or the removal of a positive one following a behavior. Spanking a child for aggression or removing a privilege would both be considered punishing if they reduced the likelihood of child aggression.

The final stage in this model is that of the *schedules* by which punishment and reinforcement occur following a particular behavior; these are referred to as "contingencies" (C). These schedules or contingencies can be either "continuous" or "intermittent." For example, when a reinforcing event follows every occurrence of a child behavior, the sequence is said to be a continuous schedule of reinforcement. Very few behaviors are continuously reinforced by the environment, with the exception of such events as eating, drinking, the use of certain drugs, and sexual behavior. Behaviors increase very quickly in frequency when they are continuously reinforced, but they do not continue very long once the environment ceases to reinforce them. When a reinforcing event does not follow every occurrence of a behavior but only occurs some of the time, it is called an intermittent reinforcement. Intermittent or partial schedules of consequences, such as reinforcement, seem to take longer to change the frequency of a behavior. However, the behavior is more likely to continue once reinforcement ceases than is a behavior that has been maintained on a continuous schedule. Almost all human behaviors are probably maintained by intermittent schedules of reinforcement or punishment.

A related behavioral principle is the concept of secondary reinforcement or punishment. This occurs when a normally neutral event or stimulus is paired with an already reinforcing one in consequating a child's behavior. After several pairings, the formerly neutral stimulus can also serve as a reinforcer. This is illustrated in the use of poker chips, gold stars, stickers, or "points" as rewards for children's good behavior. These items alone are not usually reinforcing, but they can become so when they are paired with praise and allowed to be exchanged for food, special activities, toys, and other things that already serve as reinforcers. Secondary punishment can also be developed with children by the same method, except that an aversive event is paired with the neutral one. For instance, parents can be instructed to place a small hash mark with an ink pen on a child's wrist for misbehaving in public. Each mark is exchanged for 10 minutes of sitting in a time-out chair when the child gets home. Eventually, the hash mark itself becomes punishing because of its association with the time out procedure.

Stimulus control, mentioned earlier, develops when a behavior is typically consequated (reinforced or punished) in the presence of a stimulus but not in its absence. The stimulus will eventually serve as a cue for a child to behave in a certain way to increase the likelihood of being reinforced or to decrease the occurrence of punishment. When a child throws a tantrum following a maternal command and is reinforced for doing so, the maternal commands are more likely to cue or precipitate tantrums in the future and therefore to gain stimulus control over tantrum behaviors. A stimulus can also serve as a cue for a child to stop a behavior if that behavior has been previously punished in the presence of that stimulus. For instance, when a father verbally threatens to spank a child for continuing to take cookies from a kitchen cupboard and the child gets spanked for continuing to do so, the father's threat will eventually come to serve as a cue for the child to stop taking cookies.

Extinction of a given behavior occurs when the environment no longer provides reinforcement for that behavior; it does not, however, occur all at once. Behaviors that were formerly reinforced but are not reinforced now frequently show a slight *increase* in occurrence when reinforcement is first withdrawn. Eventually, however, they decline until they occur rarely, if ever. This "postextinction burst" in behavior is important to understand; parents must be prepared for it when they are instructed to ignore undesirable behaviors for which their children may previously have received attention. Parents are often surprised to find their efforts at ignoring disruptive behavior resulting in increases in that behavior rather than in decreases.

Frequently, they may stop using the suggested procedure before it has a chance to decrease the children's undesirable behavior.

These and other behavioral principles are more thoroughly discussed in the books listed at the end of this chapter. All of the principles are, in one way or another, incorporated into the specific program for training parents in child management that is described in the next chapter. Some research suggests that hyperactive children may not respond in quite the same way as normal children do to some of these principles. Such differences are discussed with parents as part of the training program. Suffice it to say here that hyperactive children seem less responsive to delays in reinforcement and to intermittent schedules of consequences, and they may be more responsive to punishment than to reinforcement. These findings require more replication before their certainty is accepted, but they are suggestive of problems clinicians might encounter in training parents in the management of hyperactive children.

GENERAL APPROACH TO BEHAVIORAL INTERVENTION

The typical approach to behavioral interventions with behavior problem children involves several steps. First, the parents of such a child, with the assistance of the therapist, must select and define a particular target behavior as the focus of the behavioral interventions. Although it may seem helpful to select the most severe behavior noted by the parents, it is probably better to choose one that is less serious in nature for the initial intervention. The fact that the family will have learned behavioral procedures from the therapist only recently suggests that they should not attempt to implement them immediately with the most difficult child behavior, as their inexperience with the procedures may result in failure. By selecting a less serious, somewhat simpler behavior to modify, the parents are likely to experience initial success; this will keep them motivated to use the behavioral methods with other problems. The selection of a behavior for the initial intervention is therefore based upon the likelihood that the parents will experience problems at first in implementing the procedures with that particular behavior. With parents who seem intelligent, well-motivated, and capable of following through with behavioral principles, it would seem likely that a more serious behavior could be selected for the initial intervention. Once a particular target behavior has been selected for treatment, it is necessary to define the nature of this behavior problem further with the parents. Parents will often state that they are concerned about the child's restlessness, poor impulse control, short attention span, or noncompliance. These are rather general descriptions of behaviors and are not likely to prove amenable to treatment unless the specific behaviors that comprise them can be further defined. For instance, it would be better to design an initial treatment to teach a child to follow the command "Pick up your toys" than it would be to implement an initial program aimed at all noncompliance to all parental commands. Furthermore, more specific delineation of the target behavior makes it more amenable to observation and recording so that fluctuations in its occurrence can be detected.

The second step in a behavioral intervention is to observe and record the occurrence of the target behavior. Parents can be encouraged to keep records on the frequency of a given behavior problem, the time of day that it typically occurs, the factors that seem to precipitate the misbehavior, and especially the consequences that the parents typically provide for the misbehavior. In other words, the therapist should encourage the family to record not only the occurrences of the particular target behavior, but also the cues and consequences surrounding the behavior and the particular setting in which it occurs. In view of the position taken here that hyperactivity is in part a disturbance in social conduct, the social interactions of the child with others are of some importance in the keeping of records. As discussed in Chapters 3 and 4, the records that the parents keep should describe to some extent the interactions surrounding the particular target behavior. In other words, what are the parents and child typically doing just before the behavior problem develops, what is the nature of the child's misbehavior, and what is the parents' reaction to the child's difficulties? How will the child react to the parents' initial response, and how will the parents handle further immediate misbehavior in this situation? All of these factors are relatively simple for many parents to record over a given period of time.

In the third step of this approach, the therapist then reviews the records with the parents in order to analyze the frequency of the behavior's occurrence, the factors apparently precipitating the behavior, its nature, its time of occurrence, and the consequences that the family provides for it. In addition, the timing of the consequences is reviewed for delays and inconsistencies.

The fourth step of a behavioral approach is that of altering the controlling cues for the behavior, the consequences for the behavior, and the timing with which these consequences are delivered. The therapist can then evaluate the changes made in the child's behavior by these alterations through the continued observation and recording of the child's behavior. This continued assessment is the fifth step in the procedures. Finally, in the sixth step, the therapist revises the treatment program on the basis of the success or failure of these initial alterations in the child's environment.

These six steps for behavioral intervention with hyperactive children are best illustrated in the following case history. Tommy was a 6-year-old hyperactive boy who presented numerous behavior problems for his family in the areas of restlessness, noncompliance, short attention span, aggression, poor self-control, and difficulties in classroom behavior and academic achievement. The parents were particularly concerned about this child's failure to listen to them when he was given tasks to do. The therapist assisted the family in isolating a particular target behavior for treatment from the initial complaint of noncompliance. It was decided to focus on Tommy's failure to comply with the command to pick up his toys. Once the behavior was selected, the parents were instructed to keep a written diary of the events that followed every instance in which Tommy was requested to perform this command. This meant recording the particular date and time of day when the command was given; the activity in which Tommy was engaged at the time the command was specified; the way in which Tommy reacted to the command; and the way in which the parents responded to Tommy's behavior, whether or not he complied with the command. If Tommy did not comply, the parents were further to record the nature of their subsequent reactions to him and the final outcome of the interaction.

In a subsequent session, the therapist reviewed these records with the family and discovered that Tommy was indeed responding frequently with temper tantrums to this particular command. The command was given on the average of three to four times each day, and temper tantrums and noncompliance followed approximately 90% of the commands given. The parents frequently followed Tommy's noncompliance by repeating their commands an average of 7 to 10 times. These repetitions eventually culminated in the child's being threatened with punishment if his noncompliance continued further. It was also determined that the parents would frequently leave after the initial command had been given but would later return to find that Tommy had not complied with the command. This would result in their repeating the command to him. The interactions concluded with acquiescence to Tommy's temper tantrums and noncompliance in 65% of the occasions on which the command was given. More specifically, the parents often gave in, and the child was not required to follow through with the command. On approximately 35% of the occasions, Tommy was physically disciplined for his noncompliance. It seemed from the notes kept by the parents that physical disciplining was likely to occur when Tommy misbehaved in the presence of both parents or when company was visiting the family. When this fact was drawn to the parents' attention, they remarked insightfully that this probably occurred because they were afraid to have the other person or persons think that they would not follow through in punishing Tommy when they had threatened to do so. However, they probably acquiesced to the child's temper tantrums in the absence of another adult because it simply wasn't worth the bother to continue confronting Tommy and arguing with him over his noncompliance. In these situations, it was more convenient for the parents to fulfill the requested chore themselves (i.e., to pick up the toys). Further discussion with the parents revealed that Tommy's mother was having more difficulty in getting him to comply with this command than his father was, and that the mother's reaction was one of anger and depression over her greater inability to gain compliance from her child.

In accordance with the fourth step listed above, the therapist made several suggestions to the family as to how to alter their management of this particular problem behavior. The parents were instructed to give Tommy the command "Pick up your toys" only once and to wait 5 seconds. If Tommy had not begun to comply with the first command in 5 seconds, the parents were to warn him in a firm voice that, if he failed to pick up the toys, he would be placed in a chair in a corner of the dining room. If Tommy did not comply with the warning in 5 seconds, he was to be taken to the chair immediately. The parents were also instructed to remain in the room after giving the initial command to determine whether compliance or noncompliance would occur. If Tommy in fact complied with the command, the parents were to provide him with positive attention and praise, indicating specifically that they appreciated his compliance to the command. The parents were instructed to continue recording the occurrence of this target behavior and the circumstances surrounding it, as in the fifth step above.

In a subsequent session, a review of the records kept by the parents indicated that they had in fact implemented the above reinforcement and punishment programs. This had resulted in a 75% decrease in the occurrence of temper tantrums following the command and a commensurate increase in compliance with the command when it was given. However, the records indicated that the family was still having some difficulty in getting Tommy to comply with the command on some occasions. The records indicated that, on these occasions, the parents were not following up Tommy's noncompliance and temper tantrums with the time-out program. The parents reported that this was because these occasions involved their preparing to leave the house for some outing; as a result, they did not have the time to follow up the command with the use of the time-out procedure. The therapist advised the parents that, if they expected Tommy to behave himself during times when the family was preparing to leave the house, they had to follow up his noncompliance with the negative consequences, or he would continue not to comply in those circumstances. The parents agreed to do so. In addition, a review of the records showed that Tommy was not likely to comply with the first command given, but was often waiting for the warning to occur before beginning to pick up the toys. To improve this situation, the therapist suggested that in the subsequent week the parents should give only the initial command; Tommy was to be taken immediately to the time-out chair if compliance did not begin within 10 seconds. When compliance did occur, the family was instructed to continue the use of positive attention and praise. A week later, a review of the records kept by the parents indicated that Tommy was now complying 100% of the time when the parents asked him to pick up his toys.

There is frequently a tendency among therapists to dispense with the record-keeping requirements of this program. Certainly, this chore is cumbersome, requiring additional time from the parents and therapist. Nonetheless, it is imperative that some sort of behavioral records be kept—not simply to help delineate the problem, though this is very important, but also to monitor responses to treatment. Behavior changes in the child during therapy may be quite subtle and may go unnoticed by the parents without the records to reflect them. Furthermore, parents at times tend to draw overly pessimistic conclusions about treatment progress when a particularly distressing negative event occurs with the child. This can be countered by showing the parents the consistent improvement in the child's behavioral records, apart from this one negative event. Without the records, the therapist could be easily deceived into adopting the parents' overly pessimistic view in response to a crisis with the child.

This example illustrates the general steps followed in designing behavioral intervention programs for hyperactive children. The specific methods that can be employed to alter a particular inappropriate behavior are discussed in the next section.

SPECIFIC BEHAVIOR MODIFICATION METHODS

A variety of methods of managing inappropriate child behaviors are discussed in the books listed at the end of this chapter. These methods are too numerous to review here in any great detail, but some mention will be made of the ones more frequently used. These appear to vary along several dimensions. The first dimension is that of the type of target behavior being selected for intervention. The nature of the behavior will often dictate the nature of the intervention to be implemented with a child. A second dimension along which programs seem to vary is that of the individual who is to implement the procedure. Some procedures are implemented by parents, while others may be best implemented by teachers because the misbehaviors in question occur in the classroom. In some cases, a child's siblings or peers may also be trained to implement the behavior management methods. In the case of hyperactive children, it is usually the parents and teachers who implement the behavior modification programs. A third dimension along which programs may vary is that of the types of consequences provided to a child for the occurrence of the target behavior. If an inappropriate behavior is selected for intervention, then some methods of punishment will probably be used upon its occurrence. When the child appears to be deficient in appropriate alternatives to the inappropriate behavior, the behavior modification procedure is likely to employ some system of reinforcement when appropriate alternative behaviors do occur. Many behavior modification programs employ both positive reinforcement and punishment with hyperactive children. This is probably based upon the fact that many of the problems of the hyperactive child involve high-rate, aversive, negative behaviors; the application of positive consequences to the occurrence of the appropriate alternatives is not likely by itself to result in a complete reduction of the inappropriate behavior. In these cases, the addition of a punishment procedure often serves to reduce the inappropriate behavior further while helping to accelerate the occurrence of its more desired alternatives.

Before discussing the types of programs that may be implemented, it is necessary to discuss several types or aspects of behavior that can serve as targets for behavior modification programs. As noted earlier, parents of hyperactive children are likely to single out the child's negative behaviors as the targets for intervention. This is probably the result of the fact that many of these behaviors have a high irritant value for them, are quite obtrusive, and are viewed as primary stumbling blocks to the achievement of a more positive family environment. It is often necessary, however, to point out that the occurrence of high-rate negative behaviors can actually be construed as a deficiency in positive, more actively social behaviors. In this case, the target for intervention would not be the high-rate negative behaviors, but the low-rate appropriate ones. This point is discussed in some detail in Chapter 8. It must be reiterated here, however, that the therapist must continually guard against the temptation to design programs simply for the reduction of inappropriate, negative behaviors, without giving equal if not more time to designing positive programs aimed at increasing the more appropriate, actively social forms of child behavior.

It is also possible to focus on the time period over which a given behavior should occur, instead of focusing on a specific behavior. For instance, it may be that when a child is requested to pick up his toys, he or she initially complies with the command. However, the child's compliance may occupy a considerable period of time, more than is realistically necessary to accomplish the requested chore. The child may often be slower at complying than the family would like or may be dawdling or malingering along the way. Hence, the target of intervention in this particular instance is not the quality or occurrence of compliance, but the duration of compliance. The program selected should be one that assists the child in quickening the pace of compliance to the parents' commands. Such programs are often greatly facilitated by the use of a simple kitchen timing device, such as the one found on a stove or a spring-loaded timer frequently used for baking. The parents can then be taught to specify the length of time the child has for compliance, and then to consequate compliance or noncompliance when the interval has elapsed.

Finally, in selecting a target behavior, the therapist should insure that the behavior is of some social significance in that its alteration is likely to benefit both the child and society. In some cases (e.g., low-rate minor nervous tics), the modification of the behavior simply alleviates parental distress; it may not have any value to the child or the family other than this. In other words, the therapist needs to insure that the behavior selected for intervention is one that is not only disturbing to the parents, but also threatening to the child's adjustment, welfare, and prognosis.

Positive Reinforcement Methods

One of the most important aspects of providing children with positive consequences for their behavior is the fact that such consequences can be used to develop new behaviors or to increase the frequency of those desirable behaviors already occurring in such children's repertoires. By contrast, the most that punishment accomplishes is a reduction in or the elimination of certain inappropriate behaviors. It does not help children to develop new and more appropriate behaviors in place of the inappropriate ones; when used alone, it leaves the children to decide for themselves what behaviors to substitute for the ones just eliminated. In the case of hyperactive children, the behaviors likely to be substituted may well be just as inappropriate as the behaviors that have been eliminated by the punishment. It is therefore necessary to begin any behavior modification program with a hyperactive child with positive reinforcements for desirable alternatives to the inappropriate behaviors that have been targeted.

One of the most frequently employed methods of positive reinforcement is that of giving a child social attention and praise upon the occurrence of desired behaviors. Many studies demonstrate that low-frequency behaviors can be increased when positive attention and praise are given immediately following the occurrence of the behaviors. Other social reinforcers besides praise and attention are physical contact, affection, facial expressions, and other nonverbal gestures of approval. Again, numerous studies show that the occurrence of these reinforcers after a child's display of appropriate behavior frequently increases the occurrence of that behavior.

Therapists must consider several things in the use of social reinforcers with hyperactive children. First, as indicated in Chapter 2, the reinforcement value of the parents' social praise and attention for hyperactive children is likely to be lower than might be the case in other families. In other words, the effect of parental praise on hyperactive children's behavior is less than the effect of such praise on the behavior of normal children. The effect is also less than if the praise is delivered to the children by novel adults. Thus, families with hyperactive children are probably going to require positive reinforcement methods in addition to social attention and praise if they are to change the children's behavior to any significant extent. Furthermore, the relatively low value of parental praise in families with hyperactive children must itself be addressed. A method for improving the value of parental attention is given in the parent training program discussed in Chapter 7.

A second consideration in deciding to use social reinforcement with hyperactive children is the convenience of this method. Praise, physical affection, or merely approving facial expressions are convenient to administer, are rarely disruptive to the behavior being reinforced, are capable of being dispensed in virtually any location, and require little if any training in their use. However, I have found that it is of some benefit to train families of hyperactive children in more effective methods of delivering social attention to their child (again, see Chapter 7). Other advantages of social praise and attention are that they are not expensive to deliver and not subject to the criticism that they are causing children to expect material rewards for the occurrence of any appropriate behavior. Social reinforcers may also be much more likely to result in generalization of the target behavior to other settings because of the already widespread use of these reinforcers across many different situations.

Other reinforcers that can be used with hyperactive children are food and other consumable products. Food is often considered a biological reinforcer because it can be used virtually from the moment of birth to influence child behaviors. Its effect on children is considered to be unlearned, aside from the fact that individuals do show some learned preferences as to the types of foods they consider rewarding. In addition to food, other consumable reinforcers are juices, soda, candy, and gum. A number of studies demonstrate the powerful influence of food and other consumable reinforcers on child behavior.

My typical approach to hyperactive children is *not* to employ food or other consumable reinforcers at the beginning of behavior modification programs. Generally, hyperactive children are responsive to praise as well as to other reinforcers discussed later in this section; these are more convenient to use and less subject to criticism from parents. Parents often believe that using food with children will teach them that food will always be given for the performance of desired activities. In addition, the use of food reinforcers makes treatment programs seem highly similar to methods of training animals to perform tricks, and parents perhaps develop disdain for such programs as a result. Furthermore, the usefulness of food reinforcers depends heavily on the degree to which a child is deprived of or satiated with that particular food. For instance, attempting to use candy to reinforce a child for an appropriate behavior after he or she has already eaten a great deal of candy is not likely to prove especially effective. Many foodstuffs are also perishable, which limits their usefulness in some situations outside the home. If food reinforcers are to be employed, then a variety of foodstuffs should be available so that the child does not become satiated with any particular one. Instead of candy, more nutritive foodstuffs that are more likely to meet with acceptance from the parents can be employed. Such foods as fruits, graham crackers, crackers or bread with peanut butter, certain vegetables, and natural fruit drinks may be more desirable than candies made from refined sugars. In my opinion, food substances as reinforcers should be reserved until other types of reinforcers have proven ineffective for use with a particular hyperactive child.

Another group of reinforcers often used with children is that of intrinsically rewarding or high-rate activities. These may include television, games, and access to playground activities, as well as a virtually limitless number of recreational pursuits. Many studies demonstrate the efficacy of activities such as swimming, play within gymnasiums or playgrounds, games, and television in increasing appropriate child behaviors. Such activities are easily available, may cost little if any money, and are often highly reinforcing to children. On the other hand, they are not always convenient to administer in particular situations, may sometimes in fact require moderate to large amounts of money, and may not prove reinforcing to certain children. Like social praise and attention, they are less likely to fall prey to the criticism that they are encouraging children to want tangible rewards for the occurrence of future desirable behavior. If such activities are to be used as positive reinforcers, however, therapists do have to give some consideration to ethical problems that may arise in their use with behavior modification programs. This is especially true in inpatient or residential-care situations, in which children have basic rights to access to such activities as eating, sleeping, and exercising, not to mention educational activities. Therapists should be wary of using such activities as reinforcers because of the possibility that they will be depriving children of basic legal rights.

One type of reinforcer that has demonstrated great versatility, is convenient to use, and is frequently successful with hyperactive children is a system of secondary reinforcers, such as tokens, points, or other symbols, which represent or can be exchanged for already established reinforcers. These secondary reinforcers acquire their reward value because of their pairing with already pleasurable activities or, more specifically, because of their ability to be exchanged for such activities. Money can be used as a secondary reinforcer, though it is frequently discouraged because it is unlikely to be useful with very young children and is likely to be subject to the criticism noted above of spawning materialism in children. In addition, many families may not find it economically feasible to employ money as a reinforcer. Tokens or points, on the other hand, can be used with young children who do not appreciate the value of money. Furthermore, they do not necessarily have to be exchanged for activities or tangible rewards that cost money. Setting up such systems merely requires that parents or teachers have available poker chips, bingo chips, tokens, or simply pieces of paper with certain point values indicated on them. The parents and children can then discuss the types of activities the children would like to have access to as rewards and the number of tokens or points the children will have to earn in order to have access to those particular privileges. Upon the occurrence of appropriate behaviors by the children, the parents reward the children with one or more points or tokens. After the children have accumulated a specific number of points or tokens, these can then be exchanged for the children's chosen activities. It is often helpful in employing token or point programs with children to have them develop what is known as a reinforcement "menu." This is simply a list of 10 to 15 activities that a child desires and a corresponding list of point values for each activity. Such reinforcement menus avoid the possibility that children may become satiated with some particular activity, thereby depriving it of its effectiveness. Furthermore, if children do not desire a particular activity at any given time, there are others of equal or greater value from which they can choose. A detailed manual for use with families in establishing home token systems has been developed by Edward Christophersen, James Barnard, and Susan Barnard; it is reprinted in Appendix B.

The use of secondary reinforcers has a number of advantages. First, the reinforcers can be conveniently dispensed in practically any situation in which appropriate behavior may occur. Unlike food, they are not perishable, and they can be easily administered to children without disrupting ongoing appropriate behavior. Second, the tokens or points may help to bridge the time delay between the occurrence of an appropriate behavior and the actual availability of a primary reinforcer. For instance, a child being reinforced for appropriate behavior in public settings, such as churches or stores, can be given points or tokens for the appropriate behavior. These can be cashed in for the desired activity when the family returns home. Third, tokens and points can be used to purchase a wide array of other rewards and activities; they thus reduce the likelihood that children will become satiated with any particular one. This helps the tokens to remain more consistently effective across a wide variety of situations and over time. Finally, this type of reinforcer permits various gradations of reinforcement to be given, according to the degree of appropriateness of a particular behavior. For extremely desirable behaviors, more points can be given than for those that, although desirable, are quite trivial, or for those that are positive but not of quite the quality that adults desire.

In spite of their attractiveness, secondary reinforcers do have some limitations. First is the problem of the way in which such programs will be phased out once the desired rates of appropriate behavior have been obtained. Second, such reinforcers may be linked to primary reinforcers that are disruptive to the occurrence of given activities. For instance, employing tokens to purchase food within a classroom situation may lead to all the problems with consumable reinforcers that have already been discussed.

Third, when children accumulate a large number of tokens, they may suspend the occurrence of the appropriate behaviors for a while and yet still have access to all of the reinforcing activities available because of their "savings accounts." Fourth, when large accumulations of tokens occur, they may lessen the value of those points or tokens that may be given in the future. It is sometimes necessary in such token systems to require that the "savings account" be spent at regular intervals to prevent the extreme accumulation of points.

Although not a type of reinforcer, one method of dispensing reinforcement that has proven especially useful with hyperactive children, particularly older children and adolescents, is the system known as "contingency contracting." Contingency contracts are merely written statements of the relationship between desired future behaviors from children and the positive consequences that will accrue to the children when those behaviors occur. Such arrangements are often made in writing and may be signed by all parties to the agreement. An example of a contingency contract is provided in Figure 6.1. For instance, the contract can specify that Johnny will clean up his room every morning before leaving for school. If this in fact occurs, Johnny will earn 10 points each day toward the purchase of a trip to a movie, which in this case will cost 120 points.

The advantages of contingency contracting are that it is convenient to use, often allows the child to take part in the negotiations over the agreement, can involve the specification of any particular type of reinforcer, and often carries with it the influential aura of a legal document. Furthermore, the specific nature of the agreement prevents any argument from developing later, should either party feel that the other has not lived up to the specified agreement. However, these contracts do have some limitations. They have not been widely studied as to their efficacy, or as to which aspects of the contract seem to be the most influential. In addition, they are difficult to use with children who are too young to know how to write. Another problem is that the drafting of such a contract may become a one-sided agreement in which the parents attempt to impose their standards or expectations on a child with little if any input from the child. Finally, the contract may contain a stipulation of delayed reinforcement, which is likely to weaken the effectiveness of this method. Nonetheless, these contracts are quite useful, especially when adolescent hyperactive children are involved and when children can participate in the negotiation of the contracts.

Parents of hyperactive children often complain that they have tried reinforcement methods before and that they have failed to make any appreciable change in their children's behavior. The failure of the parents' use of reinforcement is likely to be the result of several factors. Chief among these is probably failure to employ reinforcers consistently and immediately upon the occurrence of desirable behaviors. Another reason for the failure of

I, _____, agree to do the following:

_____

_____

_____

_____

_____

_____

_____

If I do these things successfully, then I will receive:

_____

_____

_____

If I do not do these things as I promised, then I will lose:

_____

_____

_____

I hereby agree to fullfill this contract to the best of my ability.

SIGNED:

                                    _____
                                    (Signature of child/adolescent)

DATE_____   _____
                                    (Signature of parent)

FIGURE 6.1 A sample contingency contract.

reinforcers may be that the parents have not adequately specified the behaviors they have desired to increase. Instead, they have unsystematically increased their praise to their children for various vaguely specified behaviors and then have complained about the failure of this praise to increase the general behaviors. In addition, the parents may have used reinforcers that they believed to be of some reinforcement value to the children but that in fact were not. Parents often tend to second-guess what may be reinforcing to children and may find that the reinforcer thus chosen is ineffective. Finally, the parents may have given up on the use of a reinforcer before it had a chance to show whether it was in fact effective at increasing a desirable behavior. Many parents, especially those of hyperactive children, may become impatient if behavior change methods fail to show immediate improvements in the children's behavior. Therapists should therefore attempt to explain these reasons for previous failures to the parents before attempting to design new reinforcement procedures.

In some cases, parents may be accurate in pointing out that many of the things they have tried have simply not proven reinforcing to their children. At this point, it may be helpful to have families keep diaries for a week or two on the activities the children engage in when provided with free-play opportunities. These records may reveal certain high-rate activities that can be used to reinforce low-rate desired behaviors as part of a behavior modification program. The use of high-rate activities as reinforcements for low-rate behaviors is known as the "Premack Principle." This principle simply states that when access to high-rate activities is made contingent upon the occurrence of extremely low-rate activities, the low-rate activities will increase in frequency. Hence, access to the high-rate activities serves as a reinforcer for the low-rate activities. An example of this is the often-stated rule that children are not going to be permitted to watch television until their homework is finished. Watching television is an extremely high-rate activity for most children, while finishing homework is often a low-rate activity. Making television watching contingent upon completion of homework frequently increases the completion of homework by these children.

Other methods of determining which reinforcers may be effective for a particular child include formal reinforcer inventories or simply interviews with children as to which activities they would like to work for as part of a behavior management program. In any case, parents should not be discouraged if their initial efforts at reinforcing child behavior are not especially successful. Simply observing the children more closely, talking with them about favored activities or rewards, or recording their activities over a period of several days to several weeks may reveal activities or rewards that can serve as reinforcers in behavior management programs.

A number of variables should be considered in attempts to maximize the effect of positive reinforcers. Obviously, the amount or magnitude of the reinforcers being employed will have some effect on the success of the behavior management program. Within a token system, for instance, 50 tokens are likely to achieve a more dramatic increase in the desired behavior than are 10 tokens awarded for the same behavior. In addition, the time period between the behavior and the actual reinforcement will also affect the efficacy of the reinforcer to some degree. This is frequently a problem for parents who attempt to reward children for appropriate behavior in public places such as stores, restaurants, or churches. Often the parents promise the children a particular reward or reinforcer upon their return home, which may not be for several hours. A delay of several hours, or even several minutes, between the occurrence of the target behavior and the reinforcer will probably result in a diminution in the effectiveness of the reinforcer. The obvious corollary of this is that the more immediate a reinforcer happens to be, the more effective the behavior management program will be in changing a child's behavior.

Certainly the types of reinforcers that are chosen for any particular program will have some influence on the effectiveness of the program. Money or tokens given to a 2-year-old hyperactive child are less likely to be effective than are food reinforcers, physical affection, or social praise. On the other hand, the use of food reinforcers with adolescent hyperactive children is much less likely to be effective than is the use of contingency contracting for intrinsically rewarding activities, such as talking on the telephone, watching television, or going to a movie on the weekend. Hence, the selection of the reinforcer is obviously dependent, in part, on the age of the child in question as well as on the results of the reinforcement survey made during the initial assessment.

Finally, the efficacy of reinforcement procedures hinges partly on their schedule of occurrence. As noted earlier, reinforcers given continuously or upon every occurrence of a desired behavior are likely to increase the behavior more effectively and quickly than reinforcers dispensed on an intermittent basis. As further noted, however, reinforcers given on a continuous basis result in behaviors that are much more likely to disappear when reinforcement is terminated than behaviors reinforced on an intermittent schedule. An apparent solution to this dilemma is to begin a behavior management program with very frequent reinforcement but to gradually reduce the frequency to a more intermittent schedule.

Punishment Methods

The use of punishment methods with children generally involves one of two procedures: the presentation of aversive or unpleasant events following a behavior, or the removal of positive reinforcers upon the occurrence of a behavior. Obviously, both methods are designed to decrease the occurrence of the behaviors that they follow. Probably the most frequently employed punishment method, and certainly the best studied, is that of withdrawing attention from children upon the occurrence of misbehavior. This procedure is in some sense equivalent to an extinction procedure; the ongoing occurrence of positive reinforcement for a misbehavior is now terminated. In other words, instead of paying attention to children for disruptive behavior, parents now choose to ignore the children when misbehavior occurs. As noted earlier, this may result in what is known as a "postextinction burst." That is, the misbehavior may actually increase in frequency immediately after ignoring is introduced as a punishment method. Over time, the behavior will decrease until it becomes rare or nonexistent if parents continue to employ the ignoring procedure. Parents who are not informed of this postextinction burst may conclude that their initial efforts at ignoring are ineffective and may discontinue the procedure before it has had a chance to prove its effectiveness. Although many studies show that ignoring is an effective procedure for decreasing inappropriate child behaviors, several studies show that in some cases it may worsen child misbehavior to quite serious if not dangerous levels. This is likely to occur with children whose misconduct is especially severe or whose repertoire includes self-injurious behavior as a device to gain attention. Once parents decide to withhold attention upon the occurrence of these behaviors, the children may display postextinction bursts that result in increased rates of self-injurious behavior, destructiveness, or actual physical assault against the parents. Therapists must therefore consider the consequences of the initial postextinction burst with a particular target behavior if they are going to recommend that the parents employ an ignoring procedure.

Another form of punishment that involves removing a positive event is termed "response cost." This procedure is most frequently used when secondary reinforcers or token systems are being employed. In this case, when children display an inappropriate target behavior, they must give back tokens or points that were previously earned. Many behavior therapists have expressed the opinion that response cost should always be part of a secondary reinforcement or token system, as it frequently increases the effectiveness of these programs. This would seem to be especially true with hyperactive children; research has shown that the withdrawal of positive events, in a form such as response cost, is more effective at changing such children's behavior than the use of positive reinforcers for more appropriate behaviors.

Another form of punishment procedure that involves the removal of positive events is called "time out from reinforcement." This method has been gaining popularity with families of deviant children; it typically consists of isolating such children upon the occurrence of misbehavior. It is presumed that the method is effective because the children have been removed from access to ongoing positive reinforcement as a result of being isolated. It is obvious that the effectiveness of this technique will depend greatly upon the activities that the children are missing during the period of isolation. Placing a child in time out for the occurrence of misbehavior during a favorite television show is more likely to prove effective at changing that behavior than is placing a child in time out upon the occurrence of misbehavior at bedtime. In the latter case, the child is not missing much, if any, reinforcement, and therefore time-out programs at bedtime are likely to require longer intervals of isolation than such programs during daytime activities are. The use of a highly effective time-out procedure is discussed in Chapter 7 as part of a parent training program for families with hyperactive children.

When time out is to be used, several factors require consideration. First, Therapists must have some idea as to the time limits that will be used. These will frequently vary with the age of a child and the severity of a misbehavior. Nonetheless, these time intervals should be monitored closely to prevent overuse or abuse of this technique. Second, the location of time out is extremely important. Often, having a child place his head down on his desk during class or sit in a chair in a dull part of a house or the classroom is sufficient to prove effective as a time-out procedure. Some highly disruptive children, however, may have to be physically restrained in their time-out chairs to prevent their leaving time-out situations without permission. In rare instances, usually involving incorrigible, abusive, or assaultive patients, small time-out rooms have been utilized. (This is not the same as employing children's bedrooms for time out; time-out rooms are generally small, boring, and undecorated, and they are sometimes locked to prevent escape. In contrast, children's bedrooms are frequently ineffective as time-out locations because of the wide variety of reinforcing activities available, the possibility that the children might escape through windows or doorways, and the fact that parents often permit children to leave their bedrooms before time-out intervals have elapsed.) In my opinion, it is rarely necessary to resort to the use of a time-out room with hyperactive children. Having a child sit on a chair in a relatively dull area such as a hallway or foyer while at home, or having the child stand in a corner of a store or other public location, is quite sufficient in most cases to reduce disruptive behavior. Therapists not experienced with the use of time out should not employ these procedures without the supervision of more experienced therapists.

Several methods of punishment that involve the presentation of an aversive event to a child upon the occurrence of misbehavior have been developed. One obvious method of this sort involves the use of disapproval or reprimands when a child misbehaves. These may include a loud tone of voice, a verbal statement conveying disapproval, and perhaps a threat of future punitive consequences if the child should continue misbehaving. With many families of hyperactive children, this method of punishment has proven quite ineffective at controlling the children's behavior. The procedure can be made more effective by making other forms of punishment contingent upon failure to heed the reprimand. When reprimands are used, they are most effective if direct eye contact is made with the child in question, if the voice of the adult is loud and conveys a firm statement of consequences, and if a particular child rather than a group of children is addressed.

A second method of punishment involving the presentation of aversive events is known as "overcorrection." With this method, the punishment for displaying an inappropriate behavior is the requirement that the child in question perform some work in the situation or display the appropriate alternative behavior to an extreme or frequent degree. For instance, an older child who continues to urinate on the floor next to the toilet instead of into the toilet bowl can be required to scrub the bathroom floor not simply once, but several times in succession, as a penalty for the inappropriate toileting habit. In my opinion, however, the overcorrection procedure has many problems, and it is not often used in my clinic practice. Primary among these is the frequent need to guide children physically through the overcorrection procedure. Often, children who have misbehaved and are being punished are not in entire emotional control over their reactions, and they are likely to resist or fight the overcorrection procedure. Even if they are not out of emotional control, they may refuse to engage in the overcorrection procedure, and confrontations between parents and children may arise as a result. Furthermore, inadvertent abuses of the overcorrection procedure are likely to lead to serious consequences for some children, as abuses of other forms of punishment, such as ignoring, disapproval, or response cost, are not. The overzealous use of physical guidance as part of the overcorrection procedure may lead to actual physical injury to children, or the overzealous application of work as a punishment may have children spending hours engaged in menial labor as punishment for relatively trivial misbehaviors. Finally, the efficacy of the overcorrection procedure remains to be fully demonstrated, particularly with hyperactive children.

Next to ignoring, the punishment method probably most widely employed by parents yet least studied within the scientific literature is the physical disciplining of children. This may involve grabbing children firmly by the back of the neck, spanking them, pulling their ears, or simply grabbing them firmly by the arm. The relative lack of scientific literature on the use of these methods is obviously related to their unethical nature in terms of standards for scientific research. Nonetheless, some studies have examined the presentation of physically aversive events to children upon misbehavior. These have included slapping children on the hand, spanking them, and, in a few cases, administering electric shock to them. These more physically intrusive procedures have obviously been reserved for severely disturbed children whose misbehavior may pose a threat to themselves and to other children. With one exception, it is highly unlikely that such procedures are needed for use with hyperactive children. The exception is the use of mild spanking as a backup punishment procedure to the time-out system. This method is described more thoroughly in Chapter 7, but it simply involves giving a child two mild spanks on the buttocks for leaving a time-out chair without permission. The technique is often not employed, since the time-out procedure is usually sufficient to change the behavior. However, one or two mild spankings may be necessary in order to teach extremely obstreperous children to remain in the time-out location. After that, physical discipline is no longer required, as the time-out program serves as the first line of punishment for any undesirable activity. This infrequent use of physical discipline to back up a time-out procedure certainly seems much more desirable than the type of physical discipline that has probably been taking place with some children prior to treatment. The parents of hyperactive children often confide that they have at times overused physical discipline and have generally found it ineffective in changing the children's behavior. In a small percentage of cases, actual physical abuse of children has occurred when physical disciplining is implemented following high-rate, rapidly escalating negative interactions between parents and children. It seems wise to conclude that, when possible, the use of physical disciplining or other sorts of intrusive procedures should be avoided with hyperactive children.

As with reinforcement procedures, several factors appear to influence the effectiveness of punishment in changing children's behavior. Certainly the intensity of the punishment will have some influence over the efficacy of the procedure. More intense punishment or aversive events, or larger penalties in a response-cost procedure, will probably prove more effective than less intense punishment. Another factor influencing the effectiveness of this procedure is the manner in which aversive consequences are employed. It has been shown that starting out a behavior modification program with mild punishment and then gradually increasing the intensity of the punishment is much less effective than beginning the program with a full-strength or maximum-intensity punishment procedure. The latter procedure prevents the child in question from habituating to the gradual increments in the intensity of punishment.

A third variable to be considered here is the period of time that elapses between the inappropriate behavior and the onset of punishment. As with reinforcement methods, the greater the delay between the behavior being punished and the actual punishing event itself, the less effective the program is likely to be. Punishment, like reinforcement, should therefore follow the occurrence of the misbehavior as immediately as possible. Like timing, the scheduling of behavioral consequences also has some influence over their effectiveness in controlling behavior. Again, as with reinforcement, punishment that follows every occurrence of a particular target misbehavior is likely to prove more effective than punishment doled out on a sparse or intermittent basis. However, the cessation of continuous punishment is likely to lead to a faster recovery of the misbehavior than the discontinuation of punishment given under a more intermittent schedule. It is therefore recommended that when punishment is first introduced, it should be employed on a continuous basis with the particular target behavior; once the behavior has been reduced or suppressed, the punishment should then gradually be shifted to an intermittent schedule.

A further variable to consider is the possibility that a misbehavior may be maintained by some unidentified source of positive reinforcement. If a misbehavior is being reinforced at the same time that a child is being punished for its occurrence, the punishment method is likely to be less effective than it would be if ongoing reinforcement were not occurring for that misbehavior. For example, if a hyperactive child receives peer attention and approval for making loud vocalizations during class, the behavior is less likely to be affected by teacher disapproval or time out at each occurrence of the vocalizations. In contrast, if reinforcement is being provided for an alternative appropriate response at the same time that punishment is being delivered for the inappropriate response, the punishment procedure seems to be much more effective in suppressing the misbehavior. This underlies the observation that use of a response-cost procedure in conjunction with a token system will often make the response-cost system more effective as a form of punishment.

Finally, research has yet to explore the effects of psychopharmacologic drugs on the responsiveness of hyperactive children to reinforcement and punishment procedures. My clinical experience suggests that sedatives and tranquilizers may decrease the responsiveness of some children to either type of consequence, while stimulant medication may enhance the children's response to either consequence. In a number of cases in my clinic practice, hyperactive children taking stimulant medication have required little use either of punishment and time out for inappropriate behavior or of social praise and tokens for desired behavior—less in either case than was required when the children were off medication. This is probably related to the differences in the rates of appropriate and inappropriate behaviors that the use of medication creates. While on medication, children are much less likely to engage in inappropriate behavior and more likely to engage in appropriate behavior; as a result, they require both less punishment and less reinforcement than they do while off medication. In any event, these phenomena require some investigation in future research before these clinical vignettes can be taken as evidence of drug-induced changes to behavioral consequences.

When therapists implement punishment procedures, they should give some consideration to the possible side effects of these procedures. One side effect that may occur is aggression, either toward other children or toward the parents or teachers implementing the punishment. Aggression is most likely to occur when intrusive, intense, or physical forms of aversive stimuli or punishment are utilized. Milder forms of punishment, such as time out, response cost, disapproval, or simple withdrawal of attention, have not generally been shown to produce high rates of aggression. Aside from this consideration, the appearance of aggression in children as a side effect of punishment depends upon the source of punishment, the nature of the punishment, and the children's previous degree of success at terminating punishment through the countercontrolling effects of aggression. Although it was formerly believed that aggressive children have punitive parents and therefore that the punitiveness of the parents must lead to the childhood aggression, this belief is now questioned. More recent research suggests that aggressive children may drive parents to use more punitive management methods in an effort to control the children's misconduct. In any event, aggression may, on occasion, be a side effect of punishment procedures.

In addition to aggression, children may attempt various escape or avoidance procedures in an effort to terminate ongoing punishment or prevent future punishment. In other words, such children are likely to attempt to avoid the agent of punishment in future circumstances or to attempt to try various ways of escaping punishment once it has been implemented. These particular side effects seem to be lessened by any behavior management procedure that uses positive reinforcement methods for alternative appropriate behaviors. Emotional reactions are also likely to increase as a result of punishment. Irritability, crying, anger, and depression are sometimes immediate yet transient effects produced by punishment. When punishment is the sole management used with a child, the child may eventually come to show these emotional reactions simply in the presence of the individual who typically delivers the punishment, even though no punishment is being used at that time.

A further difficulty with punishment is that it appears to produce more immediate effects upon behavior than reinforcement does. As a result, parents may be more likely to turn to punishment in efforts to deal with misconduct than they may be to adopt more positive methods of developing desirable behaviors. Finally, children may learn to imitate overly punitive adults; that is, they may decide that problems with other children are to be solved through punishment of these children. While these side effects of punishment should be taken into consideration when any form of punishment is being utilized, it is quite unlikely that the milder forms of punishment, such as removal of positive reinforcers, result in any long-lasting emotional trauma to children.

Developing New Behaviors

The previously described methods of reinforcement and punishment are typically applied to increase or decrease behaviors already in hyperactive children's repertoires. They are unlikely, however, to influence behaviors that are in fact unknown to such children. Other methods must be taken into consideration in accounting for or in developing new behaviors in children. One such method, mentioned earlier, is the frequent tendency of children to imitate or model the behavior of others. Role models for behavior are ubiquitous in society; they are often observed through television and other visual media or described in literature and audio braodcasting. Obvious and frequent sources of behaviors to be modeled are children's families, particularly their parents. Albert Bandura of Stanford University (1969) has conducted an extensive amount of research on imitative learning in children. His research, and that of others, suggests not only that modeling or imitation is an integral part of the development of new behaviors in normal children, but that it can serve as an effective method of treatment for children with behavioral disorders. It would therefore seem that exposing hyperactive children who are deficient in appropriate social skills to live or videotape models, or even to verbal descriptions of appropriate child behavior, would help to facilitate the development of more actively social forms of conduct. As Bandura has shown, however, even though such children may acquire new behaviors by this method, the actual demonstration of these behaviors in a particular situation depends on the incentives or consequences in that situation for the imitated behavior.

A second method that has been used quite successfully to develop new behaviors in children is that known as the method of successive approximation, or "shaping." This method simply involves positive reinforcement of behaviors in a child's repertoire that have even a modicum of similarity to the terminal response desired. As this response increases, the child may emit responses that are closer to the desired terminal behavior, at which time these become the targets of reinforcement. In other words, the child is taught to perform the desired behavior simply through the application of positive reinforcements to successively closer approximations of it. Although shaping is most frequently applied to the development of new behavior, it can also be used to change the duration of behavior or the time between the occurrence and the initial cue for a behavior. For instance, hyperactive children can be trained to play independently of their parents without interrupting them by successive reinforcement of increasing intervals of time spent away from the parents. Therapists simply instruct the parents to begin with very brief intervals of time with which the children can be successful and to increase the time between reinforcements by small increments until the desired duration of independent play is achieved. Similarly, children can be taught to increase the amount of time by which they delay the display of a particular behavior. For example, if parents wish to teach hyperactive children to sit and wait politely at the dinner table until food is passed to them, they can begin by reinforcing very brief intervals of impulse control under such circumstances. Eventually, they reinforce the children for longer and longer intervals of impulse control in this situation until the children are showing normal delays in responding at mealtimes. Another variant of the shaping technique is the use of physical guidance, often used with handicapped or retarded children. In this case, adults simply move the children's arms, legs, or other body parts through the desired motion in order to demonstrate the desired terminal response. The children are reinforced at a high rate throughout this procedure in order to facilitate acquisition of the response.

One method of learning related to modeling or imitation is known as "vicarious learning." In this form of learning, children observe certain consequences accruing to other persons for displaying a particular type of behavior. Research has shown that under such conditions, the children are likely to change their own behavior to resemble the behavior they have observed as a result of witnessing the consequences of such behavior. For instance, if a child observes that another child displays aggression and is successful in gaining reinforcement through such aggression, the observing child is more likely to increase his or her rate of aggression in that or similar situations. The difference between modeling and vicarious learning lies in the aspects of a behavior that affect the observers in each case. In modeling, children's attention is drawn to a particular behavior in and of itself. In vicarious learning, children are affected by the consequences that they have seen accrue to another individual as a result of a particular behavior. It is quite likely that vicarious learning of consequences is not a primary source of acquiring new behaviors, but an influence on behaviors already in the child's repertoire. Nonetheless, modeling and vicarious learning are often closely related in many situations; as such, both are likely to affect the development of child behaviors.

Teaching Stimulus Control

As discussed at the beginning of this chapter, the term "stimulus control" describes the occurrence of behaviors in the presence of a particular cue or stimulus that do not occur in the absence of that stimulus. Stimulus control is developed when consequences are provided for a particular behavior in the presence of a desired cue or stimulus, while different consequences, or no consequences at all, are provided for the occurrence of that behavior in the absence of that cue. In the vast majority of instances, parents desire their hyperactive children to show greater stimulus control, especially in response to commands and to the passage of time, than the children are likely to be demonstrating. That is, the parents would like to see the children show more compliance to adult commands when these are given, and to have a clearer perception of the amount of time they should take to comply with commands, than they are likely to be showing in most instances. Developing stimulus control, or compliance, under these circumstances simply means providing positive reinforcement to the children when compliance immediately follows a command, while providing punishment to the children for noncompliance in the presence of that command. Eventually, this method of training does help children to develop greater compliance to a particular command. A similar procedure can be used to train children to pay closer attention to the passage of time or to his duration of compliance once a command has been given. Usually, parents start this procedure by bringing out a timing device that the children can observe and specifying the time interval that will be employed for determining the consequences for the children's behavior. It may be that a parent wishes a child to clean up his or her room within a 15-minute period. If so, the timer is set for the 15 minutes and the child is instructed that if the room is clean when the time period has elapsed, positive reinforcement will be forthcoming. However, if the room is not cleaned to the parent's satisfaction when the time period has elapsed, some form of punishment will be administered. Once the child is successfully complying to this time interval, the time interval can be reduced if desired, or the timer can be gradually phased out of the procedure. In both cases, the child's behavior has been brought under stimulus control, either by commands or by the passage of time.

It is also important to note here that most inappropriate behaviors of hyperactive children are to some degree or another under the control of various cues in the environment. Sometimes, when parents attempt to give commands to a formerly fairly well-behaved child, the commands often provoke temper tantrums or negative behavior. Similarly, parents of hyperactive children have often remarked that when they attempt to praise the children for periods of appropriate behavior, the praise seems to prompt them to display high rates of negative behavior. On the surface, such child behaviors seem counterproductive to obtaining reinforcement. The parents however, may have inadvertently taught such children that when they receive parental reinforcement for appropriate behavior, one way of getting the parents to continue their attention is to begin to misbehave. If the children were not to misbehave, the parents would probably cease paying attention to them much sooner. It is therefore one of the goals of therapy to alter the stimulus control properties of parental commands so that they evoke compliant rather than noncompliant or coercive behaviors from children. This can be accomplished by altering the consequences for the behavior that follows the occurrence of parental commands.

Training Children in Self-Control

Probably one of the most rapidly growing areas of research in behavior modification is the application of techniques for training individuals to manage their own behavior. A number of scientists, such as Virginia Douglas, Bonnie Camp, Donald Meichenbaum, Phillip Kendall, and Paul Karoly, have studied the use of these methods with children. This training procedure simply involves teaching children to apply the methods described above for changing other people's behavior to changing their own behavior instead. Skinner (1953; see "Suggested Reading") has defined self-control as the emission of a response by an individual that alters the subsequent probability of another response. For example, setting an alarm clock in the evening before going to bed increases the likelihood of waking up at a certain time the next morning. As discussed in Chapter 1, self-control is a form of behavior that depends primarily upon the use of symbolic stimuli such as language, private events such as physiologic states, or nonsocial stimuli. Individuals bring their behavior under the control of these stimuli, instead of being controlled by circumstances in the immediate situation. It is assumed that by exercising such control, such individuals are likely to avoid short-term and long-term negative consequences while maximizing positive consequences in both the short and long run. Recent research in developmental psychology has also come to suggest that mental images, as well as internal language, may also contribute to some extent to self-control behaviors. That is, an individual can bring behavior under the control of images in the "mind's eye," instead of responding to cues in an immediate situation.

There is very little question that self-control in children develops as a result of both formal and informal training of the children by the community in which they are raised. In addition, an increasing body of literature also suggests that it is the community of individuals surrounding the children that reinforces the children for exhibiting self-control and thus accounts for the maintenance of such behavior. In studies in which this type of environmental supervision and consequation for self-control behaviors has been terminated, self-control behaviors on the part of children tend to diminish.

It is also quite likely that the development of self-control is related to the integrity of particular neurologic substrates in the CNS. This is especially true of that region in the forebrain known as the prefrontal cortex. This is the region of brain that sits immediately behind the forehead and that is more fully developed in man than in any other species of animal. Research on adults and children who have experienced injuries to the prefrontal cortex indicates that such individuals are likely to develop hyperactive-like behavior and to show great difficulty with self-control. In other words, they become very impulsive individuals who tend to have little regard for the future consequences of their behavior for themselves or for others. It is therefore likely that deficiencies in self-control in children can be identified as the result either of poor training of such children within the community, or of poor functional integrity in those neurologic substrates underlying the development of self-control skills, especially in the prefrontal cortex region.

Almost all the research to date on self-control in children has concentrated on the use of language and its ability to control children's behavior. Several studies, however, have demonstrated that training children to fantasize about their behavior and its consequences can produce some changes in the children's behavior. This suggests that symbolic nonverbal stimuli, such as mental images, may also play a role in self-controlled behaviors in humans.

Before discussing specific aspects of self-control, it is worthwhile to review some of the advantages and disadvantages of attempting to train children in this particular method of modifying their behavior. Probably one of the most striking advantages of this technique, at least in theory, is that it seems to address directly one of the major deficiencies in hyperactive children. That is, as noted in Chapter 1, hyperactive children tend to show a great deal of immaturity in the exercising of control over their own behavior. Highly impulsive, inattentive, and prone to risk-taking, these children show little awareness of the consequences of their behavior or its effect on other individuals. Their perception of their future seems quite deficient in comparison with such perception in other children of the same age, and they are likely to show considerable problems in complying to adult commands as well as to rules of social conduct and etiquette. It would therefore seem that training these children to manage their own behavior might assist in remediating one of their primary deficits. Research has shown some promise in this area, but present results suggest that self-control training results in relatively short-term changes in the children's behavior; the changes typically do not endure beyond treatment termination and are not usually generalized beyond the situation in which the procedures have been taught. Nonetheless, the procedure shows sufficient promise to warrant continued research in this area.

Another theoretical advantage of self-control training with hyperactive children may lie in the fact that such children cannot be supervised at all times by other individuals and yet often require some type of control. A frequent complaint of parents and teachers of hyperactive children is that they require more supervision than other children of the same age. Failure to provide such supervision often results in increased behavior problems, mischievous behavior in the absence of other people, and in some cases risk-taking behavior that may in fact physically threaten such children and their well-being. If the children could be trained to observe, evaluate, and control their own behavior, this would eliminate the need for increased adult supervision. Although in theory this seems to be an advantage, current research, as noted above, tends to suggest that children's use of self-control responses is not usually generalized beyond those situations in which the responses have been taught.

A third potential advantage to self-control training is the possibility of actively involving children in the observation and evaluation of their own behavior. This personal input from the children may enhance their motivation to participate in treatment and may therefore increase the likelihood that they will employ the methods after treatment has terminated. Again, although the idea has some appeal, there is little research to substantiate this point.

Yet another possible advantage of self-control training of children is that the children may become better able to control private events (Skinner's term for these is "events within the skin"), such as anxiety, impulsivity, or inappropriate mental images, that may impede such children's ability to attend to external tasks. Furthermore, since the ultimate goal of any behavior modification program is to have individuals exercise control over their own behavior without therapist involvement, self-control training would seem to be the ideal treatment procedure toward which other procedures strive.

Disadvantages of training children in self-control include the fact that the training continues to rely on external consequences provided by others to maintain the children's use of the self-control procedures. It is still the community that must supervise and maintain the children's performance of desired behaviors, even though such supervision may be less direct than it might be in more traditional behavior modification programs. In addition, self-control methods cannot be taught to very young children in whom language has yet to develop, or to older children who show delays in language or mental development, since the training relies very heavily upon language skills. Finally, nearly all the research to date on self-control training has been based on the work of trained therapists with children on an individual or small-group basis. Few, if any, studies have been made in which parents have been trained to carry out the self-control training of their children, although this would seem to be the direction in which research ought to go if any hope of generalization of treatment effects beyond the clinic situation is to occur. The present administration of self-control training by therapists alone seems highly expensive and not particularly cost-effective, given the findings of research on the poor endurance of treatment effects beyond treatment termination.

Skinner has described several methods that individuals seem to employ in controlling their own responses. One of these is the use of self-imposed physical restraint in situations that might provoke impulsive behavior. For example, some people may grab the sides of a chair firmly in order to avoid taking more food than they actually need; others may bite their tongues in order to avoid saying something that might lead to negative consequences for them in the long run. A second technique employed by many individuals is to change the stimulus conditions of which their behavior seems to be a function. This is exemplified in the earlier illustration of setting an alarm clock before retiring at night in order to increase the likelihood of awakening at a particular time the next morning. Individuals who rely on nonsocial stimuli in this manner are said to show more self-control than those who require other individuals to control their own behavior.

A third technique employed by people to manage their own behavior is to manipulate their state of satiation with or deprivation of a particular consumable reinforcer. If some individuals know in advance that they are going to attend a dinner party and yet do not wish to overeat in public, they can drink a great deal of water or other fluids just before leaving for the dinner party in order to reduce their appetites at the dinner table. Conversely, if they are going out to an "all you can eat" buffet dinner, they may wish to abstain from eating for most of the day in order to put themselves in a relatively deprived state when they finally go to the restaurant. This altering of internal physiological states can be used in other ways as well. For example, if individuals know they are going to have to be especially alert on a certain day to conduct a particular task, they may wish to go to bed earlier the evening before so as to ensure that they are well rested. Another method of manipulating internal states may involve the self-administration of drugs and other behavior-modifying substances to change perception, cognition, feelings, emotions, or more basic biological states. For instance, if individuals wish to ensure that they will be alert and capable of studying late into the evening prior to an examination, they may consume large quantities of coffee or take certain stimulant medications in order to increase their state of concentration and arousal. Conversely, the consumption of mild amounts of alcohol prior to engaging in sexual activity may in fact be done to reduce the anxiety individuals may experience during sexual encounters.

A fifth method that Skinner discusses involves the altering of one's own emotional states in order to increase or decrease the likelihood of subsequent behaviors. This can be seen in individuals who attempt to "psych themselves up" just before participating in a particular athletic activity. Similarly, actors who wish to display a particular emotional state during a performance may invoke mental images of events that previously produced the actual emotion in hopes of increasing the occurrence of the emotion in the present circumstance. A sixth method suggested by Skinner for employing self-control is that of simply "doing something else"; this means merely that individuals perform an action that is incompatible with the one they desire not to perform. For example, if they wish to avoid purchasing sweet rolls while walking past a bakery, they may hold their breath in order not to detect the smell of sweet rolls in the air outside the bakery shop. Detecting such a smell is likely to result in a capitulation to the impulse to buy the baked goods.

Most scientists working in this field have typically subdivided self-control into four components: self-monitoring, self-evaluation, self-instruction, and self-consequation. All of the methods described by Skinner involve these components to one extent or another. It is my opinion that all of the four components of self-control require rule-governed behavior in children. The concept of rule-governed behavior has been introduced and discussed in Chapter 1, where it is noted as the basis for compliance to adult commands, for self-control, and eventually for more complex problem-solving skills. The term "rule-governed behavior" simply refers to the ability of children to use language to guide their own behavior instead of responding impulsively to circumstances within a particular situation. As Donald Meichenbaum has frequently suggested (see Meichenbaum, 1978, in "Suggested Reading"), it seems essential to change disturbed children's use of self-speech and eventually their use of internal dialogue if such children are to control their own behavior successfully.

Initially, the training of children in self-control involves teaching them to monitor their own behavior. That is, the children have to be taught to pay close attention to their behavior within particular situations and to note certain details about that behavior. This is quite similar to the first step in the general approach to behavior modification programs introduced earlier in this chapter. In this case, instead of having adults observe and record the children's behavior, the children are taught to do this for their own target behaviors. It is absolutely essential that children learn to observe and record their own behavior before they can be taught to evaluate its consequences or to alter its occurrence.

Once children have been taught this method of self-observation, they can then be taught to pay particular attention to certain characteristics and controlling variables of their behavior in specific situations. That is, they can be taught to focus on particular controlling cues or on the consequences of their behavior in order to assess what may have to be changed in the performance of particular responses. In addition, as part of this self-evaluation, the children may choose the particular behaviors they wish to display in certain situations or may set goals as to the results desired from the performance of particular behaviors.

Once the children have determined the aspects of their behavior, its controlling cues, or its consequences that require changing in order to achieve the desired goals, they can then engage in a series of self-directed commands or instructions that will help them through the particular problem situations. Finally, they must be taught to evaluate the degree of their success or failure in changing their own behavior and achieving the desired goals. This may then culminate in the children's making positive or negative statements to themselves or awarding themselves certain reinforcement or punishment consequences for the degree of success shown in this attempt at self-control.

More specifically, the format for training children in self-control and problem-solving behaviors consists of the following:

1. Training the children to watch, to note, and perhaps to record their behavior in a particular problem situation.

2. Teaching the children to recognize what types of situations are likely to prove especially problematic for them.

3. Teaching the children to inhibit active responding rather than to respond heedlessly and impulsively in particular problem situations.

4. Teaching the children to voice the nature of problem situations and the controlling variables that seem to be getting them into trouble.

5. Helping the children to generate a set of possible responses or solutions to the problem situations.

6. Helping the children to evaluate the short-term and long-term consequences of each response.

7. Assisting the children in active implementation of what seem to be the best of the responses or solutions.

8. Helping the children to evaluate the results of the changes in behavior in relation to the desired goals in each situation.

9. Encouraging the children to engage in self-reward or self-criticism, depending on the success of the program.

It is interesting that the above set of procedures closely parallels the steps involved in a therapist's implementation of a particular behavior modification procedure with the parents of a hyperactive child. In this case, however, children are applying the method to their own behavior instead of having the method applied to them by adults.

One approach to training hyperactive children in self-control has been developed by Virginia Douglas at McGill University. The steps of this program appear in Table 6.1. An interesting facet of this program is its emphasis on explaining the nature of their deficits to children (see Level I of Table 6.1). Although it is laudable in its intent, there is no research to suggest that this sort of explanation in itself results in any change in hyperactive children's self-control. Nonetheless, it seems from a clinical viewpoint to be a necessary first step toward introducing the rationale for the later treatment procedures and toward establishing rapport with the children.

The most common use of self-control training in previous research with children has been in the training of behaviorally disordered or impulsive children in laboratory tasks designed for the assessment of impulsive responding. Some studies have extended this self-control procedure to training children in more academic-like tasks, while only a few have employed the method to train children in responses to social problems. Generally, the children are trained on a one-to-one basis with particular therapists in a laboratory or clinic situation. It is hoped that the children will show some generalization of the treatment effects outside the laboratory or clinic situation, although research on this point has not been especially successful. In spite of the relatively limited application of self-control methods in previous research, I believe that such methods have sufficient promise to warrant their being taught to parents of hyperactive and impulsive children so that the parents may serve as therapists for their own children outside clinical situations. For this reason, one session of the parent training program described in Chapter 7 may actually be used to train parents in the development of self-control behaviors in their children. This session is likely to be implemented

TABLE 6.1. Levels of Training Children in Self-Control

Level I: Helping children understand the nature of their deficits and the ways in which training can help.

1. Providing an explanation of the nature of the children's attentional, inhibitory, and arousal-modulating deficits.

2. Helping the children recognize how these deficits affect their daily functioning and create problems for them.

3. Convincing them that the deficits can be modified and motivating them to share actively in the process.

4. Introducing the children to the basic elements of the cognitive training approach.

Level II: Strengthening the children's motivation and capacity to deal with the problem-solving role.

1. Providing success experiences within the training sessions by the following means:
   Breaking tasks into component parts.
   Presenting tasks in gradually increasing order of difficulty.
   Tailoring teaching material to children's individual capacities.
   Providing systematic reviews of material covered.

2. Arranging success experiences at home and school by doing the following:
   Helping parents and teachers organize demands made on children to coincide with their ability to meet these demands successfully.
   Encouraging parents and teachers to reward genuine attempts at mastery, as well as successes.

3. Teaching the children general rules for approaching tasks, including the following:
   Defining task demands accurately.
   Assessing one's own relevant knowledge and/or the available cues in a situation or problem.
   Considering all possible solutions.
   Evaluating relative effectiveness of solutions considered.
   Checking work carefully.

4. Discouraging passivity and encouraging independent effort by doing the following:
   Addressing children with titles like "Chief Problem Solver."
   Discouraging undue dependence on trainers.
   Discouraging mimicking of trainers' strategies or parroting of instructions; encouraging children to produce their own strategies and to restate instructions in their own words.
   Shifting responsibility for correcting work and administering rewards to children themselves.
   Helping children learn to differentiate between careless errors and errors that reflect genuine problems with understanding.

5. Making children aware of any behaviors and attitudes on their part that interfere with problem solving:
   Drawing their attention to flagging attention or "hyped up" behavior.
   Discouraging excessive talking.
   Reminding them to "work beyond" superficial aspects of a situation or problem.
   Discouraging unreasonably low criteria for success.

TABLE 6.1. (*Continued*)

Level III: Teaching specific problem-solving strategies.

1. Modeling and teaching strategies directed toward improving attention and concentration. These strategies might include the following:
Organized and exhaustive scanning techniques.
Focusing strategies.
Checking for critical factors.
Careful listening for essential information.

2. Teaching strategies and offering management suggestions directed toward increasing inhibitory control and developing organizational skills. This might be accomplished by doing the following:
Teaching the children to sit on their hands until they have thought through possible solutions.
Encouraging parents and teachers to provide special places for keeping important materials and helping the children remember to use them.
Encouraging the use of special notebooks for classroom assignments; keeping notebooks in special place.
Modeling the use of lists for events or assignments to be remembered, necessary materials to be assembled for projects, clothes and books to be laid out for following day.

3. Teaching strategies and offering management suggestions directed toward improved control of the children's level of alertness and arousal. These might include the following:
Labeling of arousal states.
Teaching the children to exhort or calm themselves using verbal self-commands.
Suggesting interesting "breaks" between periods of concentrated work.
Being sensitive to the fact that children may need stimulation to combat boredom.

4. Teaching other specific strategies children have failed to learn:
Rehearsal strategies and mnemonic devices.
Strategies required for particular academic activities (e.g., steps involved in adding fractions or in writing an essay).

Note. Adapted from "Treatment and Training Approaches to Hyperactivity: Establishing Internal or External Control" by V. I. Douglas. In C. Whalen and B. Henker (Eds.), *Hyperactive Children: The Social Ecology of Identification and Treatment.* New York: Academic Press, 1980. Used by permission of the author and publisher.

as part of the standard parent training procedures when the hyperactive child in question is at least 8 years of age or older. It is assumed that older hyperactive children have adequate language development to profit from the self-control and self-instruction training. Whether this is in fact an important factor to consider must await future research on the issue.

ETHICAL CONSIDERATIONS

A number of ethical concerns have been raised by individuals who are critical of the use of behavior modification procedures with children. These will only briefly be mentioned here, but the reader is referred to the works listed at the end of this chapter for a more thorough discussion of these issues. Probably one of the greatest concerns is the fact that behavior modification methods seem to utilize "bribes" for children to behave themselves. Many parents, teachers, and therapists alike show an initial disdain for behavior modification methods; it seems as if adults using them are buying good behavior from children instead of encouraging them to display appropriate behavior for its own sake or for the good of society. The concern and its many aspects seem ill-founded. First, if one considers the dictionary definition of "bribery," one finds the term being applied to the illicit use of rewards, gifts, or favors to pervert the judgment or corrupt the conduct of another individual. According to this definition, individuals are being offered incentives to alter their judgment or behavior in order to display inappropriate, unacceptable, illicit, illegal, or in fact immoral conduct. This can hardly be the case with behavior modification methods, as the behaviors being reinforced or punished are generally selected because of their importance in improving the child's prognosis and adjustment, as well as in increasing the benefits to society. Reinforcing a child for accomplishing his or her homework or cooperating with siblings can hardly be considered a perversion of judgment or a corruption of the child's conduct.

A second complaint about behavior modification methods is that they tend to encourage materialistic thinking in children. That is, children will come to want rewards for any behavior that is even the slightest bit appropriate. In fact, it is believed that such children may eventually attempt to extort positive reinforcement from individuals by threatening to show inappropriate behavior if the reinforcement is not delivered. Although this concern is frequently raised, there is virtually no evidence in the current scientific research to suggest that its occurrence is at all widespread. A related concern is that the children will come to want tangible rewards or edible reinforcers each time they engage in an acceptable behavior. There seem to be two answers to this concern. First, adults need not employ tangible or edible reinforcers with children; instead, high-rate, intrinsically rewarding activities can be used to reward the children for appropriate behavior. Second, research on this issue has yet to demonstrate that a large number of children develop excessive concerns about material rewards after participating in behavior modification programs.

A philosophical rather than an ethical concern about the use of behavior modification methods is the fact that they seem somewhat mechanistic or primitive in the treatment of children. Proponents of this criticism often claim that behavior therapists are not treating "the whole child"—that they are, in fact, ignoring children's emotional, social, and psychodynamic well-being by focusing simply on their behavior and its antecedent and consequent events. A more careful look at the ways in which behavior therapists actually conduct their clinical practice ought to assuage these critics. Behavior therapists do not launch into behavior modification programs without a thorough consideration of children's developmental, medical, social, and academic histories, as well as their current family circumstances and any emotional behaviors with which they may be having difficulty. Psychometric assessments of intellectual, academic, and social maturity are also likely to be implemented. Readers are referred to Chapters 3 and 4 of this text to determine for themselves whether the type of assessment procedure recommended here is as narrow as these critics would contend.

Another consideration for many individuals, particularly for parents of a hyperactive child who also have other children in the family, is the reaction of these other children to the use of behavior modification methods with the target child. The complaint is often that siblings (or classmates) of the child will witness the administration of positive reinforcement to the target child and come to resent that child for the increased rewards he or she is receiving. Their jealousy may also prompt them to discontinue displaying appropriate behavior in the hope that they may divert the application of the positive reinforcement methods to themselves. There seem to be several answers to this concern. First, there is nothing to prevent the application of positive reinforcement methods to a group of children, even though only one child is considered the clinic case. Such group contingency or group reinforcement procedures are discussed in more detail in Chapter 8. Second, there is very little research available to demonstrate that effects of this sort actually do develop in other children as a response to the use of behavior modification procedures with one child. I have found in my clinical experience that parents and teachers are likely to use the behavior modification methods with other children as well as with the target child because of the success of this procedure in altering the behavior of the target child during the treatment program.

SUMMARY

In conclusion, this chapter has reviewed a number of basic behavior modification procedures and has provided a general orientation to the application of these procedures to hyperactive children. The reader is referred to the works listed at the end of this chapter for a more thorough discussion of these methods and their application. At this time, it can be said that behavior modification procedures are one of the two most effective interventions for coping with hyperactive behavior. Certainly, in the improvement of classroom academic achievement, behavior modification approaches are in fact superior to other methods, including stimulant drug management. This point will receive more attention in Chapter 8. Finally, it should be reiterated that these particular treatment methods are intended simply to assist the family in coping with the child's hyperactive behaviors rather than to cure them completely. It is recognized that there will have to be periodic interventions with the hyperactive children throughout their development in order to bring their difficult behaviors within a reasonable degree of control.

SUGGESTED READING

Bandura, A. *Principles of behavior modification.* New York: Holt, Rinehart & Winston, 1969.

Douglas, V. I. Treatment and training approaches to hyperactivity: Establishing internal or external control. In C. Whalen & B. Henker (Eds.), *Hyperactive children: The social ecology of identification and treatment.* New York: Academic Press, 1980.

Franks, C. M., & Wilson, G. T. (Eds.). *Annual review of behavior therapy: Theory and practice* (Vols. 1–7). New York: Brunner/Mazel, 1973–1979.

Goldfried, M. R., & Davison, G. C. *Clinical behavior therapy.* New York: Holt, Rinehart & Winston, 1976.

Goldfried, M. R., & Merbaum, M. *Behavior change through self-control.* New York: Holt, Reinhart & Winston, 1973.

Graziano, A. M. *Behavior therapy with children* (Vols. 1 & 2). Chicago: Aldine, 1971 & 1975.

Kanfer, F. H., & Saslow, G. Behavioral diagnosis. In C. M. Franks (Ed.), *Behavior therapy: Appraisal and status.* New York: McGraw-Hill, 1969.

Kazdin, A. *Behavior modification in applied settings.* Homewood, Ill.: Dorsey, 1975.

Krasner, L., & Ullman, L. P. *Research in behavior modification.* New York: Holt, Rinehart & Winston, 1965.

Lahey, B. B. *Behavior therapy with hyperactive and learning disabled children.* New York: Oxford University Press, 1979.

Leitenberg, H. *Handbook of behavior modification and behavior therapy.* New York: Appleton-Century-Crofts, 1976.

Mahoney, M., & Thoresen, C. *Self-control: Power to the person.* Monterey, Calif.: Brooks/Cole, 1975.

Mash, E. J., & Dalby, J. T. Behavioral interventions for hyperactivity. In R. Trites (Ed.), *Hyperactivity in children: Etiology, measurement, and treatment implications.* Baltimore: University Park Press, 1979.

Meichenbaum, D. Teaching children self-control. In B. Lahey & A. Kazdin (Eds.), *Advances in child clinical psychology* (Vol. 2). New York: Plenum, 1978.

Rimm, D. C., & Masters, J. C. *Behavior therapy: Techniques and empirical findings.* New York: Academic Press, 1974.

Skinner, B. F. *Science and human behavior.* New York: Macmillan, 1953.

Tharp, R. G., & Wetzel, R. J. *Behavior modification in the natural environment.* New York: Academic Press, 1969.

Ulrich, R., Stachnik, T., & Mabry, J. *Control of human behavior* (Vols. 1–3). Glenview, Ill.: Scott, Foresman, 1966, 1970, 1974.

Whaley, D. L., & Malott, R. W. *Elementary principles of behavior.* Englewood Cliffs, N.J.: Prentice-Hall, 1970.

Yates, A. J. *Behavior therapy.* New York: Wiley, 1970.

CHAPTER SEVEN

TRAINING PARENTS TO COPE WITH HYPERACTIVE CHILDREN

Parents who wish to train up their children in the way they should go, must go in the way in which they would have their children go.—*Francis Bacon*

A number of programs for training parents in child management skills have been developed; probably the best known is that of Gerald Patterson and his associates (1975). None of these programs, however, was designed specifically for hyperactive children and their families. Therefore, over the past 5 years, I have designed a program primarily for hyperactive children that borrows partly from other well-established parent training procedures, with additional procedures and modifications added where necessary. Many parent training programs teach parents to focus on and intervene with select child misbehaviors such as occur during dressing, at mealtimes, at bedtime, or in stores or restaurants. Parents design different interventions for each problem area. Such programs are fine for children with only one or two specific behavior problems, but they become quite cumbersome with hyperactive children whose problems extend across multiple situations. This necessitated the design of a program whose methods were relatively simple, could be applied across many problem situations, and would address the core problems or symptoms of hyperactive children.

My numerous research endeavors relating to social behavior and our vast clinical experience with these children, as well as over 1000 interviews with their parents, suggests to me that the major problems for which these children are referred are their noncompliance and poor self-control. This is supported as well by findings that the parent rating scales of hyperactivity described in previous chapters correlate more highly with measures of child noncompliance than with measures of activity or attention (with which they show few, if any, significant correlations in most studies). It therefore seems that chronic and pervasive noncompliance underlies most parental complaints about hyperactive children. Obviously, methods aimed at improving child compliance to adult commands have to be a necessary component of any parent training program that is to be effective in teaching parents to cope with hyperactivity. This focus on compliance also simplifies the methods that parents have to learn and is applicable in almost every situation in which the children manifest problems. In fact, many of the problems of hyperactive children could be reinterpreted as problems with noncompliance to commands, to rules implicit in the setting, or to rules of social etiquette or conduct. As noted in Chapter 1, noncompliance and poor self-control are both problems in rule-governed behavior. Hence, our program involves training in those methods that foster the development of rule-governed behavior in children.

One already established program that seems to meet these needs is that originally designed by Constance Hanf at the University of Oregon Medical School and widely researched by Rex Forehand and his associates at the University of Georgia. The first stage of this two-stage program focuses primarily on increasing parental attention toward compliance, independent play, and other desirable child behaviors, while decreasing attention to inappropriate behaviors. The second stage involves teaching parents the use of time out from reinforcement (isolation to a chair) as a punishment for noncompliance. The apparent simplicity of this program is quite deceptive. As is not the case in many other programs, the parents are actually trained in their manner of paying attention to child behaviors in order to enhance the reinforcement value of the attention to the children. Training in the disciplinary stage of the program also includes instruction in the style with which commands, warnings, and eventual time outs are given. The program is highly effective at improving child compliance and the overall relationship between parents and children, as demonstrated in Hanf's initial papers and in a series of articles by Forehand and his associates (see Hanf, 1969, and Forehand, Sturgis, McMahn, Aguar, Green, Wells, & Breiner, 1979, in "Suggested Reading").

The initial Hanf program has been modified to include training sessions on hyperactivity and parent–child interactions as well as on managing public behavior and increasing appropriate independent play (i.e., teaching children not to bother parents when they are busy). Depending on the needs of individual children, later sessions are devoted to problems other than noncompliance, such as enuresis, encopresis, and social skills training. The initial core program remains the same, and noncompliance remains the initial focus of intervention, since dealing with noncompliance is felt to be a prerequisite to dealing with other problem areas. For example, it is extremely difficult to use a program for enuresis or encopresis with a belligerent, noncompliant child until the child learns to comply with requests. Furthermore, current research suggests that when treatment focuses solely on child compliance, positive changes in other deviant behaviors occur without treatment being designed expressly for them.

PRACTICAL CONSIDERATIONS

Before discussing the program in detail, it is important to consider the various pragmatic issues involved in training parents in child management. For one thing, therapists need to review training procedures to ensure that the methods to be taught are relatively simple, are easy to learn, and fall well within the educational level of most parents. Information is presented in units arranged in a hierarchy so that each unit builds on the last and no unit is so complex or detailed as to discourage the parents. Clinicians should give some consideration to the amount of homework that is feasible for the average parent to accomplish between sessions. In deciding this matter, clinicians should also consider the amount of behavioral record keeping parents should do between sessions to assess children's progress, the behaviors that should be recorded, and the recording method that should be used.

Another general consideration is the screening of families so that only those who are likely to profit from and participate in the training are provided these services. Recent research as well as clinical experience has suggested several important family characteristics that contribute to success or failure in such programs. Chief among these seems to be serious marital discord that is not simply the result of disagreement between parents over child management. The latter is often a problem that is resolved during training as both parents adopt the child management style taught in the program. Marital problems stemming from other sources, however, often result in poor attendance at the sessions and ineffective parental compliance with the recommended procedures. One parent may often actively sabotage the other's efforts at applying the program, so that failure in training is inevitable. In other cases, the marital discord creates so much confusion and tension in the home that systematic and consistent use of the procedures is all but impossible. The Locke–Wallace Marital-Adjustment Test used in the assessment of families can often help to screen out such families. When discord is great, clinicians would be better off referring the parents for marriage (or divorce) counseling first and then attempting child management training only when the conflicts are resolved.

Another factor that may complicate effective training is parental educational level. Parent training methods such as those taught in this program require substantial verbal exchange between therapists and parents, some note taking by the parents, and some reading of parent handouts. Poorly educated or illiterate parents will probably require more intense modeling of the methods and perhaps direct observation and shaping of their child management efforts if therapy is to prove effective.

The severity of a child's problems at referral can also impede effective parent training. In a few cases in which a child is completely unmanageable, temporary placement in a residential treatment facility may be necessary to gain greater control over child behaviors. In other cases, placing children on stimulant medication is necessary to permit parents to practice their newly acquired skills on more manageable children. In short, child management training is not useful to and should not be provided to all families with hyperactive children, regardless of their circumstances. Clinicians' time is more useful spent in working with those families most likely to benefit from therapy.

An additional practical consideration is that of whether both parents should be required to attend the training sessions: if not, the question of which one should must be resolved. Some clinicians require both parents (if present in the household) to attend, and therapy is not offered to them if either refuses. Others believe that the presence of only one parent is necessary for effective change to occur in child behaviors, and that this parent can communicate the information to the one not able to attend the sessions. Some research suggests that the presence of only one parent is necessary to achieve the desired effects from training. Most often it is a child's mother who will attend the sessions because of her husband's inconvenient work schedule, the greater time she spends with the child, or the fact that she may be experiencing more problems with the child than her husband. However, I have found that if late afternoon appointments are scheduled, a majority of fathers will attend the training sessions.

A fourth issue of practical import is that of whether training should be conducted on an individual basis with each family or in a group parent training format. This decision will be partially dictated by clinicians' case loads and experience in conducting group forms of therapy. Each method has its advantages, and current research suggests that both are equally effective. This might automatically suggest a group parent training approach because of its greater cost-effectiveness and utilization of clinicians' time. Group formats, however, do not permit clinicians as much time to tailor the program to each family's circumstances and problems; nevertheless, group approaches provide opportunities for commiseration and cameraderie among parents that may produce intangible yet positive effects during training. A few of our completed parent groups have continued to meet outside the clinic and without therapists on a monthly basis as parent support and information groups—something that would not have happened in an individual training format. Clinicians experienced in both approaches will probably use both, depending on the circumstances involved in the families whom they see.

Probably one of the greatest problems with any form of treatment is the extent to which parents comply with the suggested methods. This can occur either as failure to appear consistently for appointments or as failure to implement the suggested methods or homework assignments outside the sessions. Obviously, such problems must be discussed with parents candidly, if not sternly, with great emphasis being placed on the need for parental compliance if the methods are to work. In many cases, discussion as to what has precluded satisfactory compliance to the methods unveils other family problems not obvious during evaluations or earlier treatment sessions. The course of training is temporarily suspended at this point to address and treat, when possible, the problems that have hindered compliance. If this is not possible, treatment may be suspended until these other issues are resolved, perhaps by referral of the parents to other professionals for marriage or individual therapy. In some cases, simply seeing that therapists are quite serious about assignments results in some improvement in compliance. In other cases, families' schedules of activities may have to be recorded and altered if these preclude compliance. Some therapists have used "breakage fees"—deposits of money left by parents with the therapists at the beginning of treatment. Incidents of broken appointments or failure to complete assignments result in deductions from the deposit so that less money is returned to the families in question at the end of therapy. Some clinicians have even mailed the defaulted money to the parents' most hated political or charitable organization by prior arrangement with the parents. Patterson (1976) has found that most parents are not averse to this procedure. Other clinicians have made progress in therapy contingent on compliance to assignments, so that advancing to the next step in training requires that all prior assignments be done. Whichever method therapists choose, it is essential that the issue of treatment compliance receive some attention.

A final consideration in training is that of whether it is best conducted in the clinic or at home. To many clinicians, in-home treatment is a luxury that reduces the number of clients with whom they are able to work because of transportation time and that increases the expense to families to whom additional fees must be rendered for that time. There is little if any research addressing itself to this issue in parent training. At this point, however, there is no reason to assume that training in the home yields any particular benefits that are not offset by the additional expense and inconvenience.

STYLISTIC CONSIDERATIONS

It is a well-known fact to most clinicians that treatment efforts can succeed or fail merely on the basis of the manner or style in which they are presented to a family. A large part of treatment efficacy has long been known to be the "placebo" or nonspecific factors associated with clinicians, their characteristics, and their confidence in and enthusiasm for the methods they are attempting to teach. The specific treatment procedures, while obviously important, are of little effectiveness if clinicians cannot convincingly persuade parents of the procedures' importance and efficacy. These remarks and those that follow may seem obvious to skilled clinicians, but they are rarely stated in scientific papers on treatment outcome research and are often overlooked by even experienced clinicians. Granted, there are varying preferences among clinicians on these issues of style. The points presented here are obviously ones that I favor and have found to work well in previous treatment cases. The reader should therefore view them as the suggestions they are, rather than as an inflexible set of rules to be applied to every case, regardless of their utility.

I have found a generally Socratic style of conveying concepts and behavioral principles to parents to be most helpful. This seems to help parents consider themselves an important part of the process of engineering programs for their children instead of fools or simpletons who must receive direct lecturing. Clinicians using such a style question the parents and led them to the "correct" conclusion, concept, or method in such a manner that the parents feel they have achieved the solution on their own. It is felt that this method leaves a more lasting impression of the material with the parents and perhaps helps to maintain their motivation in treatment. Moreover, it avoids the implication of any directive styles of teaching that the parents are ignorant of child management principles—a myth that will be quickly dis-spelled by only a few cases of parent training. While parents may not be able to use professional terminology to describe these principles, they are often accurate in describing the actual processes involved. Certainly, there will be times where a more directive style will be necessary, particularly in describing homework assignments or discussing little known or subtle principles of behavior. When pressed for time, clinicians may elect to engage in directive lecturing in order to cover large amounts of material, but this is generally detrimental to parents' long-term acquisition of that material.

A corollary of this Socratic style is that professional jargon is to be avoided where possible. Efforts to teach parents the terminology of behavioral psychology hardly guarantee that they have understood the underlying principles sufficiently to insure their use of the principles outside of therapy. Employing such jargon as "contingencies of reinforcement," "extinction," and "stimulus control" unnecessarily restricts the educational or intellectual range of parents to whom these methods can be taught. They are also likely to be viewed as dry, boring, or unintelligible by most parents who lack college educations, and this certainly affects such parents' compliance to therapy and motivation. There is also no empirical evidence to show that using such jargon enhances treatment efficacy. In the absence of these data, I feel that behavioral jargon is more of a hindrance than a help to teaching effective child management. It is left to readers to decide whether they, as parents, would prefer to hear that they should provide social secondary reinforcers on an intermittent schedule upon the occurrence of compliant responses to verbal stimuli, or that they should periodically praise their children's compliance to commands immediately after it occurs.

A Socratic method of teaching parents also seems to avoid a problem that is probably quite common in therapy—parental dependence on the therapist. When clinicians alone design behavioral programs and then hand them to parents for use, the parents may fail to gain the problem-solving skills needed for dealing with present or future child behavior problems. Week after week, such parents come to therapy to lay additional problems at the feet of the great behavioral engineers, without ever understanding the basic principles used by the therapists to design these programs. Such dependence will be hard to discontinue as treatment termination nears. While the problem has not received wide study, many clinicians would agree that parents who understand the principles and concepts that serve as the basis for a management method are more likely to use it than those who have been shown only the method. A recent study addressing just this issue demonstrated that the children of parents who were taught general behavioral principles were more likely to continue to have improved behavior after treatment termination than were the children of parents taught only concrete, highly specific methods.

Many behavioral therapists have noted that the principles they are attempting to convey to parents for use with their children are quite similar to those that they use in training the parents themselves. This obviously means that ample praise and appreciation are shown to parents upon their participation in therapeutic discussions, accomplishment of behavioral record keeping, and implementation of suggested treatment methods. Disapproval and withdrawal of reinforcers (such as breakage fees), as noted earlier, are often contingent on parental noncompliance to the suggested methods.

During each session, it is imperative that clinicians periodically stop the discussion of new material and pause to assess the parents' understanding of what has been presented. In addition, therapists should invite the parents' opinions as to how they believe the method under discussion will fit into their particular schedule and how it may be used with children in particular. This often reveals factors that would have hampered or precluded compliance to the method and suggests that it may have to be modified to form a "best fit" with a particular family. Similar mistakes are often made by physicians in prescribing drugs that must be taken chronically in several daily doses without taking the schedules or life styles of patients into consideration. For example, it may be theoretically useful to have a child take Ritalin at 7:30 A.M., 10:30 A.M., and 2:00 P.M. because of its rapid "wash-out" period for that child. Such a schedule, however, is unlikely to be adhered to consistently, if at all, if the child's class schedule at school or schedule of weekend activities does not coincide with the dose schedule. The greater the discrepancy between treatment schedules and family life styles is, the less compliance to the schedules there will be. While this may be obvious to the reader, it is often overlooked in clinic situations when time is at a premium and case loads are large.

A similar caution applies to leaping into new material at the beginning of a therapy session without first reviewing what has transpired in the life of a family since the last session or determining how well the homework assignment has succeeded. Inexperienced clinicians who overlook such obvious stylistic precautions will often have their errors forcefully brought to their attention later in the session by a variety of client reactions. One may be apparent boredom or inattention to what clinicians are saying because of preoccupation with the as yet unacknowledged problem. Other clients may more assertively interrupt to present the complication, such as the fact that a spouse has deserted the home, a serious medical problem in a parent or a child has been discovered, or the method assigned for homework has resulted in serious misfortune for a parent or a child. I recall a case where a parent interrupted my discussion of a new treatment method for her child halfway through a session to say that she had learned she had cancer of the kidneys since the last session occurred. Such revelations often dictate that the course of therapy be altered or set aside until these new issues are addressed.

In discussing the behavioral methods, clinicians should take care to invite the parents to modify or embellish them if they see where such changes would aid the individualizing of the program to their children. Here it may be the clinicians' turn to learn a new thing or two from the clearly greater experience parents have with their particular children. This is nicely illustrated by a case in which parents were being taught to use time out in public settings, such as stores, in which a time out chair or corner was not available. In this case, the therapist explained that using a small black notebook to record the child's misbehavior might help. For every entry in the book, the child would have to spend 10 minutes in a time-out chair upon his return home. In the next session, the parents explained that they had tried this method but added a quite novel twist to it. They had taken a Polaroid picture of the time-out chair at home and placed it in the black "bad behavior book." When the child misbehaved in a store, they handed him the photo and reminded him that this was where he would wind up at home if his misbehavior continued. I have found this embellishment to be of such practical value that it is now described to each new set of parents we train. As noted earlier, parents are rarely ignorant of effective behavioral methods or principles and can serve as satisfactory "cotherapists" at some points in a therapy aimed at improving their children's behavior. I have found it of great help to make out the need for such parent–therapist collaboration clear at the outset of therapy. This serves a secondary function of letting the parents know that clinicians do not necessarily have all of the solutions to their children's problems. While the clinicians may be experts about general behavioral principles and technology, the parents are the obvious experts about their particular children, their habits, their temperaments, and their reaction patterns. Acting as if the parents know nothing about child behavior principles is both patronizing and professionally naive. Without the integration of information from both sets of "experts," therapy is much less likely to succeed.

It almost goes without saying that interspersed throughout therapy should be periodic expressions of compassion for parents' or families' current conditions, as well as acknowledgements that the methods being discussed are easy to read but not so easy to put into effect. Reminders as to the importance of homework being accomplished and methods being practiced should also be periodically given. Often it can be helpful to draw analogies between learning child management skills and acquiring new skills with musical instruments or recreational sports. Parents are usually quick to give therapists total credit for any success at improving their children's behavior. It should be made obvious to them that the success is partly if not solely due to their use of the behavioral method, since no tool left on the shelf miraculously fixes a problem.

GENERAL CONCEPTS IN CHILD MANAGEMENT

The program to be discussed below contains a number of key general concepts that are repeatedly stressed throughout parent training, regardless of the particular method being presented in each session. The first of these to be introduced to parents is the notion of immediacy of consequences for a child's behavior, be they positive or punitive. It is repeatedly emphasized that parents need to provide consequences for a child immediately after the behavior of interest occurs, instead of waiting several minutes or hours to confront the problem or appreciate the desired behavior. Because of hectic life styles, most parents delay dealing with behaviors, especially positive or appropriate ones. They are often much quicker to attend to undesirable or especially intrusive behaviors, but, even with these, they often wait until after the fourth or fifth repetition (or more!) of a command before consequating their children's noncompliance. The need to stress immediacy of behavioral consequences for children is evident, particularly since hyperactive children have greater than normal problems in responding to delayed consequences.

Parents are also taught that consequences, especially verbal or social ones, should be quite specific. Both praise and criticism should refer specifically to the behavior that is at issue, instead of being vague, general, or nebulous references to the children themselves, their general behavior, or their personal integrity. Similarly, with punishment, the consequence should be tailored to fit the "crime" and not based upon the parents' level of impatience or frustration over this or prior episodes of misbehavior.

A hallmark of virtually all behavioral approaches to parent training is an emphasis on the consistency of parental management. This refers to consistency across settings, over time, and between parents. Consistency "across settings" simply means that if a behavior is to be punished or rewarded in one setting, it almost always should be handled that way in other settings as well. This is contrary to the common practice among many parents of handling child behaviors one way at home, while in a different way (if at all) in public situations such as trips to stores or visits to others. The implicit message to the children is often clear: misbehave in public and you will succeed, but misbehave at home and you will be less likely to do so. Consistency "over time" merely means that what is good or bad child behavior today should probably be judged as such tomorrow, and that a behavior should be handled in the same way no matter what time it occurs. Punishing a child today for "raiding" the refrigerator because a parent has a headache, while ignoring or actually assisting a visit to the refrigerator at a future time, is a ludicrous yet common practice in some homes. Similarly, if a behavior is rewarded today, it should be rewarded in the future and certainly should not be subjected to punishment later. Consistency between parents in the rules they establish for a child and in the consequences they provide is an obvious yet essential principle in parent training. Quite frequently, mothers of hyperactive children tend to manage their problems very differently than their fathers do; this often leads to conflicts not only in the development of a consistent set of rules for the children, but in the marital relationship as well.

Patterson (1976) has shown that parents of children who are seriously behaviorally deviant have a tendency to resort to punitive methods of management rather than to reinforcement, even after completing parent training sessions in which both methods have been taught. This may be the result of the fact that punishment seems to produce a more immediate improvement in negative parent–child interactions because it brings about an immediate cessation in coercive or intrusive behaviors. In any case, throughout training, parents should be given periodic reminders to use positive methods before negative ones. That is, when parents are concerned about a negative child behavior, they should first define the more social or desirable behavior that they wish their child to display in place of the negative one. Having done so, they should then formulate positive reinforcement systems or incentives to increase that behavior. Only then should punishment methods be employed to reduce the negative behavior. Especially at those times in training when disciplinary methods are being taught, therapists need to present this caution periodically.

It has become quite evident that many of the parents who we treat spend a tremendous amount of effort in reacting to child misbehavior when it occurs, yet very little in analyzing and anticipating those situations in which the children are likely to create problems. If such parents were to do so, they might discover methods which, if implemented, might tend to reduce the occurrence of misbehavior. Perhaps this apparent lack of forethought or anticipation is merely the result of being so overwhelmed with incorrigible behavior that it is difficult to "take the offensive" and try to anticipate and ward off future problems in a particular setting. Another intriguing possibility, however, is that many, though not all, parents of hyperactive children have as many problems with impulse control for their age as their children do. As a result, they may resort to management strategies of dubious long-term effectiveness as an impulsive reaction to misbehavior. For whatever reason it exists, this lack of anticipation and preparation is a repeated focus of parent training sessions.

Reciprocity, a concept that is strongly emphasized in Chapter 2, is also reviewed with some frequency throughout training. Without belaboring the point, it is stressed with parents that their behavior toward their children is in part a function of their children's actions toward them. Further, the ways in which they choose to manage the children will in part determine the children's subsequent responses to them. Although seemingly trite or superfluous, this principle is often lost to parents and therapists alike if the therapists become immersed in the specifics of a particular child's behavior and the training of his or her parents.

It has been noted frequently in this book that therapists must adopt an attitude of coping with and not curing hyperactive behaviors. Although these behaviors may be manipulated and reduced to a great extent, no therapy yet available has shown a "normalization" of all of the problems with which these children present. It is of equal importance that this attitude also be instilled in the parents of hyperactive children. In my opinion, this new attitude will often help parents who tend to drift from one therapist to another, always seeking the "quick fix" or elusive cure for their hyperactive children while never being satisfied with those services that are delivered, even if these are helpful. By a rough estimate, it seems that the majority of the families I treat have been through the services of at least four or five different professionals before reaching my clinic; often they have been told that the children are likely to outgrow their problems or that the problems are the parents' fault. By the time I see them, they are frequently receptive to the truth about their children's problems and the need to acquire coping skills. This point is so vital to an adaptive approach to living with hyperactive children that it requires repeated emphasis during parent training.

In summary, several general principles deserve periodic emphasis throughout the parent training program. Immediacy and specificity of consequences, as well as consistency across settings, over time, and between parents, should be stressed. Having parents establish incentives for desirable behavior *before* implementing punishment is also a key concept. The importance of anticipating and preparing for problem situations in the near future must be reiterated throughout training, as must the reciprocity of effects in parent–child relations. And, finally, parents are encouraged wherever possible to view hyperactivity as a developmental disorder to be coped with and diminished where possible, but not as a disorder likely to be cured. In years of conducting parent training programs for hyperactive children, I have not been disappointed at the positive reception these concepts have received from most of our parents. The shift in the perspective and expectations of parents that occurs with the adoption of these concepts is often half the battle in reducing distress in parent–child relations with hyperactive children.

OVERVIEW OF THE COURSE OF TRAINING

In order to provide a broad framework within which the details of the program described below can be presented, it is valuable to review the general sequence of training sessions used in this particular program. To my knowledge, it is the only such program based on a theory of the deficits of hyperactive children as well as on the ever-burgeoning literature on parent–child interactions in deviant children. It will be recalled from Chapter 1 that hyperactive children display problems not only in attention, but also in rule-governed behavior. These two deficits may obviously interact to compound each other, but neither is necessarily subordinate to the other. Both are primary deficiencies. The difficulties with rule-governed behavior translate into ones of noncompliance, poor self-control, and deficient problem-solving skills (especially in social areas) for hyperactive children or adolescents. To look at the situation from a developmental perspective, children learn compliance to external commands and rules before internalizing these commands and rules for use in self-directed speech or self-instruction. This phase is referred to as self-control; when adequately developed, it serves as a basis for the later development of self-questioning and problem-solving strategies— critical components of self-awareness, reflection, and anticipation of future behavioral consequences. It is probably no coincidence that hyperactive children have been found to have deficits at all three levels of rule-governed behavior in comparison with normal peers. Such a theory, however, serves as only part of the reason for so structuring the program. Other reasons will be noted as the details of each session are presented.

The first session of the program serves as a general orientation to hyperactivity, its nature, its prognosis, and its etiologies. Practical suggestions for altering families' homes to make them safer are also provided. The second session proceeds to a discussion of parent–child interactions, reciprocity, and factors outside the interactions that might affect them; the principles discussed in Chapter 2 are presented here. Session III presents a highly specific approach to developing and enhancing parental attention for use with children's play. In Session IV, parental attention and other reinforcers are extended to children's compliance and independent play (insofar as these are occurring). The fifth session sees the introduction of time out and other disciplinary methods for use with in-home child noncompliance. In Session VI, the use of disciplinary methods is closely analyzed and then extended further with in-home noncompliance. The seventh session presents the modification and use of reinforcement and disciplinary programs in public situations, such as stores or restaurants. The core sequence concludes with a review session and directions for developing parental problem-solving skills for future child behavior problems. A "booster" session a month after the last regular session completes the sequence, although other sessions can be added for dealing with such associated problems as enuresis, encopresis, or learning disabilities.

While the sequence parallels the previously discussed theory of the development of rule-governed behavior, it is hardly intended to be an inflexible course of events for every family. Circumstances of parental noncompliance, or parental psychiatric or marital problems, can at times sidetrack the sequence while these more critical problems are addressed. Nor is this sequence intended to cure or remediate developmental deficits in rule-governed behavior simply because it focuses on a developmental sequence in acquiring that behavior. The problems of hyperactive children may well prove to be neurophysiologic in nature and not likely to be cured simply by backtracking and retraining such children in a seemingly developmental course. Improvements in behavior may occur, but these are not likely to result in a permanent normalization of child behaviors. It is ludicrous to assume, as some in the area of developmental disabilities have, that developmental disorders can be corrected by regressing children to an earlier stage of development and re-emphasizing through exercise a normal course of development. It remains to be shown that impaired, immature, or dysfunctioning neurophysiologic systems automatically right themselves through such methods. In contrast, it is equally simplistic to attempt to train children in more advanced developmental skills when they lack the prerequisite abilities from an earlier developmental period. This would seem to be the situation in trying to train 3- and 4-year-olds in self-instruction and self-control when they are severely noncompliant to the instructions of others and when it is now recognized that internalized self-speech probably does not develop until somewhat later years. In short, the present program is guided by current theories of development, but hardly viewed as curative in nature simply because of this fact.

Sequence of Activities within Each Session

As will be made clear below, a common course of events occurs within each parent training session. Except for the first session, each session opens with a review of events that may have transpired within a family since the last session that might influence the course of therapy or a particular child's problems. A review of homework then occurs, and problems that may have arisen with the homework or parental reactions to doing it are discussed. New material, concepts, and principles of that session are then introduced and tied in conceptually with the previous sessions' material. Parents practice this new set of methods, when possible, in front of their therapist so that corrective feedback can be rendered. A discussion as to how the new method will fit in with this individual family's home circumstances then takes place. Homework is assigned, and the session is concluded. Ample praise, positive feedback, and encouragement are provided throughout each session for the parents' compliance to the instructions and homework.

SESSION I: A REVIEW OF HYPERACTIVITY

The activities occurring in the first session of parent training are relatively straightforward. Initially there is a review to determine how family status or a child's major problems may have changed since the evaluation. It is quite useful to have the family again complete the HSQ (see Figure 3.10) to aid in redefining current problem areas. In addition, the questionnaire can serve as a pretreatment baseline that can be compared against the results obtained when it is administered later in or at the termination of therapy. Its role in the fifth session in selecting deviant target behaviors will be discussed in that section of this chapter. The therapist then explains the sequence of sessions and the general purpose of the training program. A breakage fee may then be establised if the therapist so desires.

Using a series of slides especially prepared for this purpose, the clinician reviews with the parents in general terms what is known about hyperactive children. (Slides for use in this session and the next are available for a fee from myself or from the publisher.) If the use of slides is not feasible, then obviously a verbal discussion must suffice. Nonetheless, I have found the visual aids to be quite helpful in making this session both interesting and informative. Most parents have very little information available to them about the disorder, and much of what is available in lay periodicals is often inaccurate. Parents, more than anyone, need to have an understanding of this disorder if they are to learn to cope not only with their children but with the myriad of professionals likely to be consulted throughout the children's development. This knowledge base helps parents to distinguish fact from fad as they read about hyperactivity in lay publications and receive information from well-meaning but often intrusive relatives. The visual presentation of slides or the discussion begins with an overview of the definition of this disorder as set forth in Chapter 1 of this book. Parents are often quite curious as to how diagnoses of hyperactivity are made, especially if this has not been covered with them in the feedback session following the evaluation. Besides the primary symptoms, the most common associated problems— aggression, poor peer relations, achievement problems, accident proneness, and so on—are also discussed. The day-to-day and cross-situational variability of the hyperactive children's problems are emphasized, so that parents can understand that a child can be diagnosed as hyperactive and yet can still behave relatively well in certain situations. This is followed by a presentation of prevalence rates, with emphasis on the disproportionate occurrence of hyperactivity among males and in lower socioeconomic circumstances. Time is then spent reviewing those factors that show promise as early predictors of hyperactivity in children, as well as the developmental course likely to be observed with these children. Facts about adolescent and adult outcome as gleaned from the follow-up literature are then reviewed, as are those factors that seem to predict outcome. This leads into a review of the possible etiologies of hyperactivity as they are now understood.

At this point, questions from the parents are solicited and are often found to be numerous. This provides an opportunity for them to discuss the ways in which this information contradicts many of the myths and misconceptions they may have about hyperactivity. This is also an excellent time to introduce the concept of hyperactivity as a developmental disorder for which there is no real cure. The view of coping, not curing, is presented as part of this discussion, and parents are invited to share their feelings about this often radical shift in perspective. Many parents find this view refreshingly honest, though somewhat discouraging; on the one hand, they acknowledge their hopes that their children could be "normalized," while, on the other, they admit their recognition of the now pervasive problems with the children and their growing suspicion that the problems would be relatively chronic ones. Therapists can greatly assist such parents in coming to this somewhat discouraging yet realistic adjustment by placing hyperactivity in perspective with more serious developmental disorders, such as autism, mental retardation, cerebral palsy, and epilepsy. The parents learn that their children are certainly likely to have a better prognosis than children in most of these other groups, and that there is no reason to give up hope that the children might one day make a satisfactory or better adjustment to life. Therapists should emphasize the ability of certain treatments to result in substantial symptomatic relief of the children's problems, provided the parents are willing to work at learning more effective management methods. The phrase "take it one day at a time" seems as apropos to this group of parents as it does to individuals who follow the guidelines of Alcoholics Anonymous. In the years of conducting this training program, it never ceases to amaze me how easily parents accept this perspective on hyperactivity; in most cases, it seems to agree with their own dimly formulated intuition about their children's problems. The heightened motivation of parents to work at coping and achieving a "best fit" relationship with their children can be striking when the parents come to feel they have found a professional who truly understands the disorder and the distress they have been living with these many months or years.

The slide presentation or the discussion then proceeds anew with a brief review of the most commonly used treatments for hyperactivity. Greater time is often given to the stimulant drugs than to other treatments, as many of the children may at one point or another be tried on them. Again, the many misconceptions that parents have are often disspelled by this discussion, as they come to achieve an understanding of the drugs as good as, if not better than, their physician's. The major effects and side effects, as well as the ways in which the drugs are prescribed, receive brief discussion. Many parents are quite curious as to why and how these drugs may work. Behavior modification, self-control, and dietary approaches also receive brief attention. The goal of this part of the presentation is not to train the parents in the use of any of these therapies, only to acquaint them briefly with the remedies that have been tried with hyperactive children and the relative success rates of each.

In short, the first part of this session is a review of Chapter 1 of this book with the parents, as well as a brief discussion of possible treatment alternatives. While this part of treatment is hardly designed to result in any behavior changes in children or in direct changes in parent management skills, its indirect influence on parent–child relations is often sizable. This is seen not only in increased parental motivation and rapport with the therapist, but also in more relevant changes in the expectations parents have for their children themselves, their behavior, and their future. As noted in Chapter 2, parental expectations of child behaviors and parents' views of the precipitants or causes of such behaviors in any given situation partly determine the parents' reactions to their children. If they feel that the children can control their behavior but are misbehaving to irritate others or merely to gain attention, parents will respond quite differently than they will if they feel that the children's misbehavior is not entirely within their control or designed expressly to irritate them. Simply absolving parents of blame for their children's problems often results in their newfound motivation to try to adapt to the children's problems, which they formerly attributed to their own failure as parents. This issue is raised again and dealt with in more detail in the discussion of the second session.

Once the slide presentation (if given) is completed, the therapist discusses the practical implications of this information on hyperactivity. One obvious conclusion is that children and families are likely to require periodic professional assistance throughout the children's development, regardless of how successful the initial intervention might be. Parents are also directed to provide their children with increased activities during leisure time to avoid or reduce the likelihood of the children's getting into trouble as a result of their impulsivity and lack of direction or self-supervision. Particularly during the summer months, parents are encouraged to enroll their children in as many structured, supervised activities (e.g., Scout groups, swimming lessons, YMCA activities) as possible, including summer school for those children whose academic achievement has been marginal during the regular school year. If this latter program is not feasible, then parents should devote time regularly to a review of academic subjects with these children in order to prevent them from losing skills over the summer months.

Another practical implication to be reviewed is the need for families of hyperactive children to "childproof" their home. Toxins, medicines, or other substances usually accessible in cupboards and closets should be removed and locked in a secure place. Accidental poisonings are more frequent with these children, for they are likely to climb up to or ferret out the usual places in which parents may tend to hide such poisons as cleaning fluids, combustible liquids, or yard care products. Other items likely to be dangerous in the hands of overly curious, impulsive hyperactive children, such as power tools and workbench supplies, should also be secured. Dangerous stairwells, second-floor windows without screens, and storm doors that appear deceptively open at first glance should all be secured, blocked, or marked in order to prevent accidental injuries. Each year several hyperactive children are admitted to Milwaukee Children's Hospital for traumatic injuries sustained from falls down stairwells or out of unscreened windows above the first-floor level, or from crashes through unmarked glass doorways. Obviously, if the children are to be outdoors, then greater supervision of their play may be required even where fenced-in yards are available. Again, several children each year are admitted to our hospital for injuries resulting from running into streets, playing behind parked cars in driveways, falling off low roofs or fences, or attempting high-risk stunts while playing with other children.

Besides decreasing the possible risks for injuries to these children about the home, families should pay close attention to protecting property and valuables as well. Such items as jewelry, large sums of money, valuable electrical appliances and tools, and other cherished items should be kept out of reach or secured to prevent their damage. This is true even when parents feel they can protect their property merely by closer supervision, since hyperactive children are more prone to night waking and unsupervised wandering. I am aware of one family who had to watch their young hyperactive child's behavior so closely that they had their newly built home specifically designed to reduce likely problems; they even had one-way mirrors installed in the child's bedroom and other rooms to facilitate closer supervision. While extreme, this case clearly illustrates the need of families to "childproof" their homes for their hyperactive children more closely than parents might consider doing for normal children.

It is also wise advice to families at this point in training to enlist the aid of neighbors, relatives, and friends in watching the children more closely while they are away from home. Explaining the nature of the children's problems and the parents' concern for the children's welfare to these people can help with the children's safe adjustment within their community. Parents should take care in selecting babysitters to stay with these children while they go out, as inexperienced sitters are likely to have as difficult a time with the children as the parents or teachers but are much less likely to know how to cope with the children safely. Once sitters are chosen, it is worthwhile to have them arrive well ahead of scheduled outings to review management methods and precautions in handling the children.

One concern raised by many parents in the initial stages of training is that of how to discuss the issue of hyperactivity with relatives, particularly grandparents. Having relatives read certain articles on hyperactivity can help to alleviate the pressure they may be placing on parents about these children. Grandparents are often likely either to deny the children's problems or to go to the opposite extreme by refusing to permit the children into their home, obviously on the basis of their prior experiences with these children. In either case, the parents are likely to be blamed for the children's problems or to be accused of being overly sensitive or intolerant of what relatives may perceive as normal child exuberance. Both Chapter 1 of this book and Chapter 2 of *Hyperactivity* by Dorothea Ross and Sheila Ross (1976; see "Suggested Reading") provide excellent resource material for parents and relatives wishing to have more information on the nature of the children's disorder. If all else fails, a separate session with the parents and with critical or skeptical relatives, if they are willing, can be used to review this material and perhaps to reduce the stress associated with such problems on the parents.

The homework assigned during this first session may consist simply of implementing the suggested "childproofing" of the home or of further reading on the subject. Often parents may request that this information on hyperactivity be conveyed to the children's teachers by telephone, correspondence, or a visit to the school. Here, too, pressure being placed on families by teachers naive about the nature and etiologies of hyperactivity can be alleviated or reduced by the simple act of communicating information to them.

SESSION II: A REVIEW OF PARENT-CHILD INTERACTIONS

At the beginning of this session, the therapist should review with the parents the incidents that may have transpired since the previous session. Again, this is to determine whether or not there have been important changes in the life style or activities of the family that may influence the continuation of therapy. In addition, the therapist may wish to inquire whether the family has any questions about the material covered during the last presentation. Often, so much information is presented on hyperactivity during the first session that many families are unable to digest all of the information until they have more time at home in which to consider it. Such further consideration may lead to many questions about hyperactivity or about a particular child. Once these issues have been covered, the new material in this session can be presented. Basically, this session is devoted to a review of the principles and concepts on parent-child interactions introduced in Chapter 2 of this book, especially as these apply to families with deviant children. These principles and concepts are presented in a simplified form so that they may be easily understood by a lay audience. It is often quite helpful for the therapist to utilize slides or blackboard drawings to illustrate the points to be made in this chapter. In order to facilitate such a presentation, the slides that I typically use in this session are presented as figures throughout this section of the chapter. The reader is encouraged to have these illustrations developed into slides or more useful drawings to aid in the presentation of this information to individual families or to parent training groups.

A number of issues relating to parent-child interactions are covered within this session. It is helpful to review with the family the fact that many people, scientists and parents alike, continue to view parent-child interactions as a one-way street in terms of the influence that each person has on the other. That is, they continue to view adults as the most powerful influence within these interactions. Children are often viewed as passive recipients of the influences of the parents; as a result, the final outcome of the children's socialization and personality growth is attributed primarily to the manner in which they were treated by their parents. As Richard Bell (1977) pointed out, scientists in child development research have followed this sort of unidirectional viewpoint of parent-child interactions for well over 50 years. This view is illustrated by much of the research that took place on childhood aggression during that time period. Many correlational studies were under-taken with aggressive children to determine what family factors seemed to be associated with the aggression. Research in this area repeatedly demonstrated that aggressive children tended to have more punitive, more negative, and generally less affectionate parents than nonaggressive children did. Despite the fact that these findings are purely correlational and do not indicate in any way which variables have a causal influence here, researchers and clinicians alike were quick to draw conclusions from these data. Probably the most frequent conclusion drawn was that aggressive children are so because of the punitive styles of their parents. That is, greater than normal rates of parental punishment toward a child were viewed as the cause of the children's aggression. This was explained on the basis that the children may become quite frustrated in response to the punishment and attempt to act out their frustration aggressively outside the home. Some scientists believed that the children were simply imitating the punitiveness of their parents in expressing aggressive behavior toward peers and toward other members of their families. In either case, the parents were viewed as the primary causal agents in the development of the children's aggression. Bell has now pointed out that it is just as likely that aggressive children create punitive parents. That is, the original data, being purely correlational, would support either viewpoint. Bell has gone on to explain that children may become aggressive for many reasons besides the possibility that they may be imitating their own parents' punitiveness or expressing frustration. Chronically aggressive children, with whom families must interact over considerable periods of time, may actually come to influence their parents to develop progressively more punitive styles of managing their behavior in order to exercise some control over it. From this vantage point, the parental management style is viewed as a reaction to the children's characteristics and behavior, rather than as the cause of them. Many parents of hyperactive children are able to identify quite closely with this example when they reflect upon the develop-ment of their own style of managing their children over the years.

The unidirectional viewpoint of parent–child interactions is illustrated in Figure 7.1. The figure depicts the approach taken not only in the research on childhood aggression noted above, but also in other areas of scientific literature, such as autism or child abuse. In all of these areas, previous research has laid heavy stress on the role of parents in developing these particular problems. The therapist can then point out how a more accurate view would be to take a child's characteristics and particular behaviors within a situation into consideration in determining both the parent and child behaviors and interactions.

Having demonstrated that many scientists tend to have this unidirec-tional viewpoint of parent–child interactions, it is also helpful to go on and point out that many child clinicians, or professionals working with children,

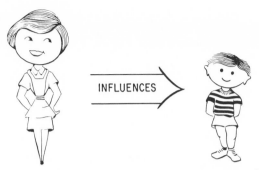

FIGURE 7.1. The typical yet erroneous unidirectional view of the effects of parents on children.

tend to think along similar lines, whether they do so consciously or not. In many cases, it is quite obvious that when parents take their children to child guidance centers for evaluation and treatment, the evaluations consist primarily of reviewing the manner in which the parents have raised the children and are attempting to deal with the children in current contexts. Explicit or implicit in such evaluations is an effort to find what the parents may have done wrong or failed to do in raising these children that could account for the children's current difficulties. The result of this approach to evaluation and treatment is to blame parents for their children's difficulties. Again, many parents of hyperactive children can identify with this particular issue because of their own experiences with pediatricians, child psychiatrists and psychologists, social workers, teachers, and other professionals with whom they may have come into contact in the course of seeking treatment for the children. A number of the parents will probably report particular occasions on which they were in fact explicitly blamed for their children's difficulties. Inviting parents at this point in the session to speak about their experiences with previous professionals who may have taken this approach is often helpful not only in providing the family with an opportunity for catharsis over frustrations experienced with prior evaluations and treatment, but also in increasing their rapport with the current therapist. It is at this point in therapy that many families will remark that this is the first time they have found a therapist who genuinely seems to understand their predicament.

Not only do many professionals who work with children seem to have this unidirectional view of parent–child interactions, but many parents do as well. Long before such parents may have come into contact with professionals, they too have often reflected upon and found fault with the manner in which they have attempted to raise and manage their children. Mothers especially will often remark about their frequent comparisons of their own management strategies with those of friends and neighbors whose children are behaving quite normally. These sorts of comparisons often lead such mothers to experience feelings of guilt, inadequacy, incompetency, low self-esteem, and depression, because they believe that their inability to manage their children is their own fault. Again, helping these families to discuss these feelings and particular incidences in their past can often improve rapport and aid in the adoption of the different view of parent–child interactions to be presented below. In summary, it is the purpose of this particular discussion on unidirectional viewpoints of child development to teach parents that this view is an erroneous explanation of their children's current predicament and the way in which it may have come about. As noted in Chapters 1 and 2, there is absolutely no evidence to suggest that poor child management practices are the primary cause of hyperactivity in children.

The therapist should then go on to point out the more accurate view-point that ought to be taken in understanding parent–child interactions and relationships. The current view, illustrated in Figure 7.2, is that of a bidirectional or reciprocal approach to parent–child interactions. In this view, both parents and children influence interactions and their outcomes to an equal degree. In some instances, parents may actually have more influence over the outcome of the interaction, but in others it may be the children who are the principal determinants of the ways in which the interactions evolve. At this point, it is helpful to discuss with parents the fact that the influence of children will be heavily stressed in the discussion during this session, but that they should remember that both parents and children are influential in any given interactions. Greater emphasis is being given to children's influences because of the relative neglect of this influence both in terms of previous research and clinical practice, as well as in terms of the way families may have previously viewed the development of the children's problems.

FIGURE 7.2. A more appropriate bidirectional view of the effects of parents and children on each other. Interactions are viewed as reciprocal.

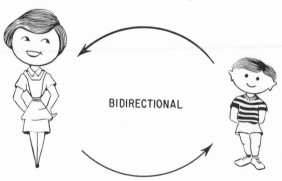

The discussion should then progress to the manner in which parental expectations about child behaviors may help to determine how a parent reacts to a particular behavior of a child. As discussed in Chapter 2, parents seem to have thresholds or expectations for children's behavior within any given situation. These thresholds deal with the appropriateness of the children's behavior in its quality, quantity, or intensity. Parents seem to have an "upper limit threshold," or a set of expectations as to the amount or excessiveness of a behavior that they are willing to tolerate before they will react to change that behavior. Similarly, parents also seem to have a "lower limit threshold," or a set of expectations as to how little of a behavior they will tolerate before acting to increase that behavior. It is helpful at this point to explain to parents that, although this is a highly simplified view of parent–child interactions, it does seem to account for a large percentage of the different types of interactions parents may have with their children. Figure 7.3, or a slide or illustration like it, is then shown to the parents to illustrate the upper limit control behaviors that parents tend to exhibit when confronted with excessive child behaviors. It can be seen that when children emit inappropriate or excessive levels of behavior, parents are likely to respond with controlling behaviors that are probably designed to reduce the children's behavior to more acceptable levels or limits. It is explained to the parents that these upper limit controls often consist at first of efforts at ignoring the children, followed by a series of restrictive commands designed to get the children to stop doing what they are doing, which may then proceed to heated threats against the children if they persist in the behavior. These may then be followed by parental disciplining of the children, either through physical punishment or through deprivation of privileges. Such

FIGURE 7.3. Effect of excessive child behaviors on parents: the elicitation of parental upper limit control responses.

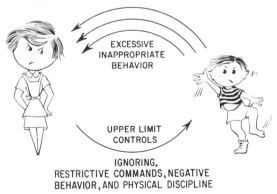

EXCESSIVE
INAPPROPRIATE
BEHAVIOR

UPPER LIMIT
CONTROLS

IGNORING,
RESTRICTIVE COMMANDS, NEGATIVE
BEHAVIOR, AND PHYSICAL DISCIPLINE

behaviors on the part of normal parents are often successful in diminishing temporarily excessive or inappropriate behaviors in normal children.

The parents are then told that when children's behavior falls within the appropriate thresholds or expectations for child behaviors in a given situation, parents are likely to respond with equilibrium behaviors. As noted in Chapter 2, these equilibrium behaviors often consist of generally positive and facilitating remarks and interactions toward the children, perhaps emitted in an effort to keep the children behaving in the manner that they are now behaving. This situation is illustrated in Figure 7.4. The therapist explains to the parents that this is how parents of normal children tend to respond when the children emit appropriate behavior.

The clinician then proceeds to a discussion of the manner in which parents are likely to react to children who are not emitting a sufficient amount of behavior to meet the parents' expectations for that situation. This is best illustrated with examples of shy, withdrawn, retarded, or language-delayed children, who are often found to emit lower than expected levels of behavior. In such cases, it is demonstrated that parents are likely to respond with what are known as lower limit control behaviors. These behaviors are shown in Figure 7.5. As with upper limit control behaviors on the part of parents, these lower limit controls are probably shown by most normal parents during transient situations in which their children may show occasional shyness or fail to demonstrate sufficient behavior to meet parental expectations. Such behaviors on the part of the parents probably exist and continue to be used because of their frequent success in increasing desirable child behaviors.

FIGURE 7.4. Effect of appropriate child behaviors on parents: the elicitation of parental equilibrium control responses.

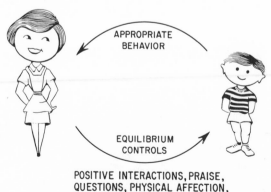

APPROPRIATE
BEHAVIOR

EQUILIBRIUM
CONTROLS

POSITIVE INTERACTIONS, PRAISE,
QUESTIONS, PHYSICAL AFFECTION,
AND FACILITATING BEHAVIOR

At this point in the sequence of Session II, some discussion as to whether the parents agree with or understand the principles just presented is helpful. It is often beneficial to have parents think of examples that illustrate each of the three types of parent–child interactions with their own children. It should also be reiterated that in these examples, the parents are reacting to what the children are doing, not simply causing the children's particular behavioral problems.

The flow of the discussion can now shift to a consideration of factors outside a particular interaction with a child that may influence the way in which that interaction evolves and the outcome it eventually takes. It is first helpful to explain those general factors that seem to influence how any parent may interact with any child. These are listed in Figure 7.6. It should be explained to the parents that these factors, although they may have some indirect influence on the way in which a parent treats a particular child, are outside the influence of the child. That is, in most cases, the child's interaction with or reactions to a parent have no effect on the existence of these factors within the family or within the life of a particular parent. For instance, a parent who has diabetes and is excessively preoccupied with the effects of the disease on his or her life may react differently to a child because of this preoccupation than a parent of normal health might. Here it can be seen that the parent's preoccupation with his or her health may influence the way in which the child is treated, and yet the child has no control over the health status of the parent. It is for this reason that one of the homework

FIGURE 7.5. Effect of infrequent or inadequate child behaviors on parents: the elicitation of parental lower limit control responses.

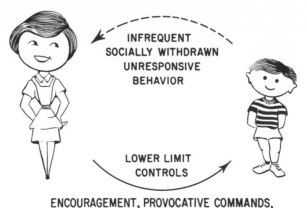

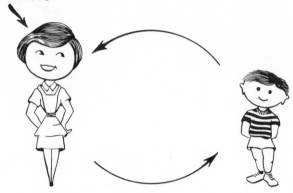

PHYSICAL CONSTITUTION / HEALTH
GENERAL TEMPERAMENT
EMOTIONAL STATE
EXPERIENCE WITH CHILDREN
INTELLIGENCE / EDUCATION
EXPECTATIONS
ENVIRONMENTAL STRESS
PSYCHIATRIC PROBLEMS
SETTING FACTORS

FIGURE 7.6. Variables that affect parental responses to children yet are outside the particular interactions between parents and children.

assignments for this session calls for the family to take some time to reflect upon extra interactional or intrafamilial stressors that may affect the way in which a child is treated to an unfair or inappropriate degree. The homework assignment consists not only of taking stock of these stressors, but also of proposing some solutions for the ones that can be changed. In any case, each of the particular factors listed in Figure 7.6 can be discussed with the family and, if the parent training is not being done on a group basis, they can be illustrated with particular examples from this family. Parents are often quick to understand how acute stress events, such as an argument with a spouse, can carry over into the subsequent treatment of a child. It is somewhat more difficult for them to understand that more insidious stressors, such as a progressive decrease in a parent's social interaction outside the family or a slow increase in financial problems, can also carry over into the treatment of a child.

Following this discussion, the therapist can then demonstrate that there are just as many factors influencing the child and the manner in which he or she treats a parent that are generally outside the direct influence of the parent. These factors are listed in Figure 7.7. The therapist can illustrate this principle with a particular example: for instance, the manner in which a child

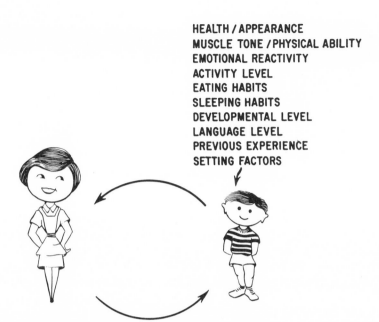

HEALTH / APPEARANCE
MUSCLE TONE / PHYSICAL ABILITY
EMOTIONAL REACTIVITY
ACTIVITY LEVEL
EATING HABITS
SLEEPING HABITS
DEVELOPMENTAL LEVEL
LANGUAGE LEVEL
PREVIOUS EXPERIENCE
SETTING FACTORS

FIGURE 7.7. Variables that affect child responses to parents yet are outside the particular interactions between children and parents.

may have been treated by friends at school that day might carry over into the way in which that child reacts to his or her parents upon returning home from school. Obviously, the parents have no control over what may have happened to the child at school, yet they will be influenced by these events because of their effects on the child's disposition and behavior. Unlike parents, children are unlikely or unable to take stock of those particular factors that may be influencing their behavior or to attempt to change them. It is therefore necessary that, before parents react to a particular child's behavior, they consider the factors that may be influencing this behavior. Parents often do this when interacting with children who are physically ill or fatigued. For instance, a parent may often remark that a particular child is irritable or cranky because he or she has recently missed an afternoon nap; the parent thus takes this into consideration in reacting to the child's irritability. On the other hand, if the parent is not able to identify the stressors that may be influencing the child's behavior, they are likely to hold the child accountable for the irritability, which in this case may be outside the control of the child. It can be seen at this point that the purpose of the last two figures (Figures 7.6 and 7.7) is to try to make parents more aware and considerate of the extrainteractional factors that may be influencing both themselves and their children in parent–child interactions. In doing so, parents may become more tolerant of particular child behaviors, or may in fact be able to change the manner in which they treat the children simply by removing these stressors from the family situation. To borrow a term from Bell's work, it is the effort of the therapist at this point to create "thinking parents" rather than to allow the parents to go on responding impulsively to their children's behavior, as they may have been doing previously.

Although the therapist up to this point has been stressing the simplicity of this theory or viewpoint of parent–child interactions, it is actually more complex than it may seem. This can be demonstrated by showing the parents a diagram similar to Figure 7.8, in which all previous diagrams have been collapsed into one to show all of the forces that come into play when parents and children engage in particular interactive sequences with each other. Obviously, parents may feel overwhelmed by this particular figure, and so the therapist should not spend time in dwelling upon separate aspects of the diagram, as these have actually been covered in previous illustrations. It is, however, quite helpful to show the parents how this model may apply to the particular circumstances involving many hyperactive children. This sequence of events is shown in Figure 7.9, in which those temperament and dispositional factors known to occur more commonly in hyperactive children are

FIGURE 7.8. Figures 7.1 through 7.7 collapsed to show complexity of parent–child interactions.

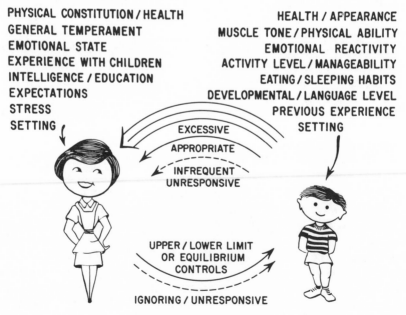

PHYSICAL CONSTITUTION / HEALTH
GENERAL TEMPERAMENT
EMOTIONAL STATE
EXPERIENCE WITH CHILDREN
INTELLIGENCE / EDUCATION
EXPECTATIONS
STRESS
SETTING

HEALTH / APPEARANCE
MUSCLE TONE / PHYSICAL ABILITY
EMOTIONAL REACTIVITY
ACTIVITY LEVEL / MANAGEABILITY
EATING / SLEEPING HABITS
DEVELOPMENTAL / LANGUAGE LEVEL
PREVIOUS EXPERIENCE
SETTING

EXCESSIVE
APPROPRIATE
INFREQUENT
UNRESPONSIVE

UPPER / LOWER LIMIT
OR EQUILIBRIUM
CONTROLS

IGNORING / UNRESPONSIVE

listed on the children's side of the diagram. The parents are likely to understand now how it is that such child characteristics can come directly or indirectly to influence the ways in which children may interact with parents. These temperamental or behavioral characteristics lead to excessive child behaviors in terms of either quality, quantity, or intensity within a particular situation. This figure shows that normal parents who are under no excessive degree of stress are likely to respond to these excessive child behaviors with the upper limit controls discussed above.

However, if a particular family is under certain stresses that are likely to be found in the families of hyperactive children, interactions may proceed a bit differently. This point is demonstrated in Figure 7.10, in which the most frequent family characteristics and possible stress events in families of hyperactive children are shown on the parents' side of the diagram. These particular stress events can lead the parents to overreact to the children's excessive behavior so greatly that intensely negative interactions may ensue. In fact, it seems to be precisely these combinations of characteristics that may result in potentially abusive situations with the children.

If time permits, the therapist may wish to take this opportunity to draw a schematic diagram such as that shown in Figure 7.8 or 7.10, involving those stressors in the particular family that is now in therapy. This can be done by having the parents list the stress events they identify as affecting themselves and potentially indirectly affecting the manner in which they treat the child in question. The parents' attention can then be focused upon what sorts of characteristics of their child may influence the child's reactions

FIGURE 7.9 Effects of hyperactive behaviors on normal parents.

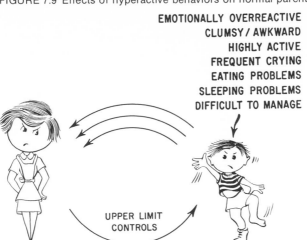

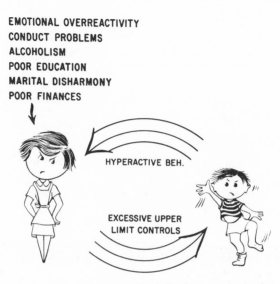

EMOTIONAL OVERREACTIVITY
CONDUCT PROBLEMS
ALCOHOLISM
POOR EDUCATION
MARITAL DISHARMONY
POOR FINANCES

HYPERACTIVE BEH.

EXCESSIVE UPPER
LIMIT CONTROLS

FIGURE 7.10. Effects of hyperactive behaviors on stressed parents.

to them in particular interactions. This individualizing of the model of parent–child interactions presented here often leads to substantial insight on the part of most parents into the reasons why they interact with their children the way they do in many cases. It may also reveal particular stress points in a family that have not been revealed during the initial evaluation because of the family's belief that these factors may not be important to the clinician trying to understand the child's problems. Having been exposed to this model of interactions, the parents may now come to view these factors as influential in the child's behavior and as important for the therapist to know about.

Several additional important issues raised in Chapter 2 also require some discussion with the family. The first involves the manner in which families are likely to move through a hierarchy in attempting to manage chronic child misbehavior. The second pertains to those characteristics that previous research has shown to be more common in the families of deviant children. The hierarchy of parental behaviors is listed in Figure 7.11. The therapist should discuss with the parents the fact that no parent–child interaction remains in a static condition for very long. Each individual in the interaction is attempting to find more successful ways of dealing with the other individual. Those reactions that do not seem to influence the other person in the desired direction are often extinguished, and other behaviors in the hierarchy may take their place. Figure 7.11 indicates that many parents initially respond to difficult child behavior by attempting to ignore it.

```
┌─────────────────────────────────────┐
│                                      │
│   IGNORING                           │
│                                      │
│   RESTRICTIVE COMMANDS               │
│                                      │
│   NEGATIVE AFFECT AND COMMANDS       │
│                                      │
│   PHYSICAL DISCIPLINE                │
│                                      │
│   ACQUIESCENCE                       │
│                                      │
│   LEARNED HELPLESSNESS               │
│                                      │
└─────────────────────────────────────┘
```

FIGURE 7.11. Hierarchy of parent control responses.

Eventually, when the parents learn that this management strategy is of little utility, they may then move on to employing restrictive commands with their children. At this phase in the evolution of the negative parent–child interactions, the parents are likely to be emitting high rates of commands toward the children in rapid-fire succession and often to be repeating many commands. Eventually, the parents move through progressively more punitive phases of child management as previous phases fail to affect the child's behavior. Over several months to several years, families may find themselves near the lower end of this particular figure, vacillating between the use of physical discipline or acquiescence toward the child. Acquiescence, as explained in Chapter 2, occurs when a parent presents a child with a particular task or command but simply fails to enforce the command when confronted with child noncompliance thereby acquiescing to the noncompliance. In my opinion, some parents may reach an end stage of adaptation to severely deviant behavior that is known as "learned helplessness." This concept must be explained to the parents in some detail, as they are unlikely to understand it when it is initially presented. Basically, the concept simply means that when individuals find all of their normally adaptive behaviors to be non-adaptive or nonfunctional in a particular situation, they tend to give up coping with the situation and to accept whatever consequences accrue to them. Individuals at this stage of evolution in parent–child interactions are often significantly depressed, evidencing low self-esteem and feelings of incompetency, and showing very little reaction toward even the most obvious, obnoxious, and intrusive child behaviors. Such parents tend to take whatever abuse their children may dole out to them, and they typically show no reaction whatsoever to these behaviors when they occur.

It is important to explain to the family that most parents of normal children would rarely progress through this entire hierarchy of parent reactions because the children would have responded to earlier methods of management. Normal parents and children interact within a reciprocal system in which each participant is responsive to the other's interactions, resulting in a high rate of appropriate and facilitating interactions between them. When the children's behavior gets out of hand, the parents, like the thermostat in a house, react by attempting to reduce the "heat" of the children's behavior. Such parental reactions are often successful, and thus parents rarely progress to other methods of management as long as those they are using are successful. In families with hyperactive children, the parental reactions normally occurring are not successful at reducing the children's behavior, because many of the children's difficulties are the result of inborn or intrinsic temperamental or behavioral dispositions over which the families have little control. The attention span problems, impulsivity, restlessness, and irregular habits of these children are not likely to respond to typical forms of parental management. Hence, normal reactions of parents are not likely to reduce these behaviors to any great degree, and these parents will therefore progress through the hierarchy farther than parents of normal children will. In short, the typical mechanisms that operate to govern parent–child interactions in families with normal children break down in dealings with hyperactive children because of their lesser responsiveness to these normal management methods. This point helps parents to understand how it is that their families and in particular their interactions with their children may have evolved to their current state; and it also helps to absolve them of feelings of complete responsibility for the current family situation.

This discussion on parent–child interactions concludes with the presentation of a list of attributes generally found in the interactions of parents with deviant children. This list of common characteristics is shown in Figure 7.12; it should be reviewed briefly by the therapist with this particular family. Most of these items are self-explanatory and will not receive any attention here. Several of them, however, require some discussion. One of these is that, as Patterson (1976) has shown, the reward value of the parents' praise in families with deviant children is often reduced in its influence over these children. That is, the children do not seem to respond as well to the praise of the parents as they might to the praise of strangers with whom they have had few negative interactions. This indicates that treatment must first address the reduced reward value of parental attention before parents can be told simply to go home and pay positive attention to desirable child behaviors. Such

PARENTS PROVIDE GREATER POSITIVE REINFORCEMENT TO DEVIANT
CHILD BEHAVIORS

PARENTS PROVIDE LESS POSITIVE REINFORCEMENT TO PROSOCIAL
CHILD BEHAVIORS

PARENTS ARE MORE LIKELY TO PUNISH PROSOCIAL CHILD BEHAVIOR

THE REWARD VALUE OF PARENTAL ATTENTION/REINFORCEMENT IS
REDUCED OVER TIME FOR A DEVIANT CHILD

PARENT-CHILD INTERACTIONS ESCALATE RAPIDLY TO NEGATIVE
INTERACTIONS BECAUSE OF MUTUALLY COERCIVE BEHAVIORS

PARENTS MONITOR AND ATTEND TO FEWER NEGATIVE CHILD BEHAVIORS
OVER TIME

PARENTS EXPRESS FEELINGS OF DEPRESSION, LOW SELF-ESTEEM,
AND INCOMPETENCY AS A PARENT

PROBLEMATIC INTERACTIONS BETWEEN PARENTS OR BETWEEN A
PARENT & INITIALLY NON-DEVIANT SIBLING ARE MORE
LIKELY TO DEVELOP OVER TIME

TYPICAL FORMS OF PARENTAL PUNISHMENT ARE NOT AS
EFFECTIVE IN DEVIANT PARENT-CHILD INTERACTIONS

AFTER TRAINING, PARENTAL PUNISHMENT METHODS ARE MORE
LIKELY TO PERSIST THAN PARENTAL REINFORCEMENT METHODS
(PROBABLY DUE TO NEGATIVE REINFORCEMENT)

AS EXPECTED, THE PROGNOSIS FOR DEVIANT PARENT-CHILD
INTERACTIONS IN FAMILIES WITH ONLY ONE PARENT,
ECONOMIC HARDSHIPS, MARITAL DIFFICULTIES, PARENTAL
PSYCHIATRIC PROBLEMS, AND POOR PARENTAL EDUCATION
IS SUBSTANTIALLY WORSE THAN FOR FAMILIES WITHOUT
THESE FACTORS

FIGURE 7.12. A list of typical attributes of the interactions of parents and deviant children.

attention is likely to have less influence on these children because of this diminished reward value. It is the purpose of Session III in parent training to address this particular problem.

The second item in Figure 7.12 that may require clarification for parents is the one dealing with the operation of negative reinforcement in producing rapid escalations of mutually negative interactions. The therapist should review Chapter 2 again in order to understand fully how negative reinforcement may explain the development of high rate, coercive parent–child interactions. As noted in Chapter 2, it is often the person who can demonstrate intense, high-rate, and aversive behavior the most quickly who will eventually win out in a particular interaction. That a parent management style of this sort may be somewhat successful in the short run is outweighed by the obviously great detrimental influences it will have over the long run in parent–child relations.

To summarize up to this point, it is the goal of this particular session to get parents to view parent–child interactions as reciprocal systems in which both parents and children have an important influence on the outcome of the interactions. In particular, the role of children is stressed in order to get families to recognize how important the children's behavior is in determining the parents' own reactions to the children in a particular circumstance, as well as in determining overall family status over time. In addition, another goal of this session is to get parents to acknowledge, attend to, and perhaps address and correct those intrafamilial and extrafamilial stress factors that may indirectly be influencing how the parents and children interact with each other. Finally, an indirect goal of this session is to get parents to realize that they are not entirely responsible for the predicament in which their family finds itself and that they cannot take complete blame or responsibility for all of their children's deviant behaviors. This point alone often results in a new motivation for parents to learn new management skills that may help them cope with their children's hyperactive behaviors.

The therapist should then take time to discuss the homework that will be assigned for the next week. The first part of the homework assignment involves having a family review those stresses that may be placed on it by the factors listed in Figure 7.6. This can be done by utilizing the family problems inventory that is set forth in Figure 7.13. The parents are instructed to take the form home and complete it at some time during the week when they have a moment to sit down and reflect upon the family's current circumstances. As noted earlier, this questionnaire often brings out family problems that have not been made apparent during the initial interview because of the parents' lack of awareness that such problems might affect their child's behavior. Now that they understand the importance of these intrafamilial and extrafamilial stress events, they are more likely to divulge their nature to

EVALUATING FAMILY PROBLEMS

Some time during the next week, take a moment to sit down and complete this questionnaire. You have been shown that many problems occurring in your life can influence your reactions to your child's behavior. We think it is important that you evaluate your family life to see whether such problems exist, and, if so, what you are doing about them.

In the space provided below each problem area, write down the types of problems you may be having in this area. Then write down what it is you are trying to do about the problem to solve it. Don't be afraid to say you are not doing anything at this time to solve a problem. We simply want to know what types of problems you are having now. Please be as honest as you can, as this information is very important to our helping you with your child.

PROBLEM AREAS   PROPOSED SOLUTIONS
Health problems:

Marital problems:

Financial problems:

Occupational/job problems:

Problems with relatives/in-laws:

Problems with friends:

Problems with other children in the family:

Personal or emotional problems:

Other problems (religion, sex, drug or alcohol abuse, etc.):

Thank you for taking the time to complete this. It will be kept confidential and will not be released to anyone.

FIGURE 7.13. A family problems inventory for parents to complete as part of their homework after Session II.

the clinician. In addition to simply describing the stress events, the parents are asked on the questionnaire to consider possible solutions or ways of coping with the stresses that may reduce their influence on the family.

The second part of the homework assignment involves having the parents begin to record certain child misbehavior. It is my opinion that this is best accomplished by having the family keep a diary that focuses on one or two particularly troublesome types of child noncompliance. For instance, if the child has difficulty getting dressed in the morning before school or going to bed at night when requested to do so, the family may be asked to begin recording the nature of these situations each day. In doing so, the family should be instructed to record the actions they are asking the child to perform, the dates and times at which the command is being given, the nature of the child's reactions, and the ways in which the parents attempt to manage the situation. In addition, some remarks by the parents as to the eventual results of the interactions are also helpful. Note that this diary of interactions is very similar to the more extensive interview on parent–child interactions that the clinician has used in the evaluation phase. If the parents keep such a diary, the clinician will be better able to understand the nature of the interactions the parents and child are having in problematic situations. Further, the diary will help to determine whether or not future sessions of the program are having some positive influence on these noncompliant behaviors. It is my impression that the diary is of greater benefit to the clinician in treatment planning and in monitoring treatment effectiveness than is a simple frequency count of parental commands or child compliance occurring during any particular problem situation. Such frequency counts hardly convey the nature of the social interactions or their context as well as the diary seems to do. Of course, clinicians should follow the method that they are more comfortable with and that provides them with the greatest amount of useful information.

SESSION III: DEVELOPING PARENTAL ATTENDING SKILLS

Like the previous session, this session begins with a review of the family's status since the last appointment, as well as a review of the homework assignments given during the previous session. First, it is helpful to review the family problems inventory assigned for homework. As noted above, this questionnaire can often reveal certain family problems that were formerly unknown to the therapist, in spite of what the therapist may have believed to have been a very thorough evaluation. Some suggestions can be made to the family at this time as to how they might approach solving some of the family stress events raised in the questionnaire. It is stated earlier in this chapter that when severe marital difficulties are revealed, it is perhaps best to have

PAYING ATTENTION TO YOUR CHILD'S GOOD PLAY BEHAVIOR

The first stage of this program involves learning how to pay attention to your child's desirable behavior when it happens during play time. To learn this, it is first necessary to practice the skills of what we call "paying attention." Later, we will show you how to use these skills when your child complies with your commands. Paying attention to ongoing desirable play behaviors involves the following:

1. Find a time when your child is playing something he or she enjoys and that is appropriate. This can be a time when the child normally plays alone, or a special time that you set aside each day. In either case, you are to spend at least 15 to 20 minutes each day in this type of play. The child is to select what he or she wishes to play with, and you are to give no help in this decision. This is essential. In addition, no other children should be involved in this "special play time," just you and this particular child.

2. *Relax!* Casually approach your child, watch the play activities for a few minutes, and then sit down next to the child if he or she is playing at a table or on the ground.

3. Watch, mentally note, or tailgate the child's activities for a few moments to get some idea of what he or she is doing.

4. Begin occasionally to describe to the child what he or she is doing. You might try to do this as a sportscaster at a baseball game would do it—simply describe the action. Another way of thinking of this style of talking to your child is to pretend there is a blind person in the room with you and your child and you must describe to that person what your child is doing. In either case, you simply narrate your child's activities and no more.

5. ASK NO QUESTIONS AND GIVE NO COMMANDS! During this play time, you should avoid asking any questions. You will find this to be very difficult, since most parents interact with their children primarily through questions. Questions are, however, intrusive and commanding and will only serve to provoke confrontations during this play time; avoid them. Also, use no commands. You are not to direct your child's activity at all unless it becomes extremely inappropriate.

6. Occasionally, provide your child with positive, *genuine* feedback. This is not necessarily praise, but a positive statement about what you like that the child is doing: for instance, "I like it when you and I play quietly together." Your comments can be either about what your child is doing that you like, or about what your child is not doing that would be inappropriate: for instance, "I enjoy it when you don't throw the toys around the room."

7. If your child begins to misbehave, simply turn away from him or her and attend to something else in the room. If the misbehavior continues or escalates, then leave the play area immediately. Come back and play with your child later when he or she is behaving more appropriately. If another child tries to become involved (and many siblings do when they see you paying attention to another child), direct them not to play but tell them that you will spend some "special time" with them alone later. If both parents are living at home, then one can take the other children away from the play area while the other plays with the problem child.

8. *Each* parent should spend at least 15 to 20 minutes with the child each day.

9. If the child becomes extremely disruptive or abusive during play, then discipline the child the way that you normally would. We will show you later how to discipline the child effectively during such times.

THIS PROGRAM IS EASY TO READ! IT IS NOT SO EASY TO DO!

FIGURE 7.14. Parent handout on spending "special time" with a hyperactive child, to be introduced during Session III.

the family address the marital difficulties in therapy before proceeding with any further training in child management. Should this be the case, the therapist may wish to stop training at this point and refer the family to a more experienced marriage counselor, with the stipulation that the family return for the remainder of management training once the marital issues have been resolved. If the child management training is to continue, the therapist should then review the record-keeping assignment given to the family for the previous week. It may be necessary to refine the manner in which the parents are keeping records on the one or two noncompliant behaviors selected for recording purposes. Again, this diary may reveal certain things to the therapist that have not been formerly revealed in the initial evaluation. The therapist should always praise the parents for completion of the homework assignments.

The clinician should then introduce the goals of the present session, primary among which is to improve the attending skills of the parents—that is, the manner in which they pay attention to appropriate child behaviors. The need to improve the parents' skills in reward, praise, or attending is based upon the observation made earlier in this chapter that the reward value for hyperactive children of parents' praise is often less than it is for normal children, probably because of the chronic history of aversive interactions between the parents and children. The third session has shown itself to be quite useful in reversing this particular problem. In addition, it will also train the family in new methods of attending to the child's behavior when the child is compliant with adult commands. A second purpose of this session is to improve the relations between the parents and their child through the use of nondirective play so that the child may learn that the parents are still interested in him or her, despite the fact that the child may have behaved badly earlier in the day. In other words, the play behaviors to be discussed in this session are designed to get parents and children interacting more positively with each other on a more frequent basis than is typically seen in families up to this point. This is done in order to reverse the common trend in families of hyperactive children of disengagement between the parents and the children over time. That is, the parents tend to interact less and less with the children because of the frequent confrontations over the children's noncompliant behavior. This disengagement often extends into recreational or leisure interactions as well. By playing together in the manner described in this session, parents and children can often come to find renewed interest and pleasure in interacting with each other on a positive basis. While this goal may seem overly optimistic to the parents at this point in training, it is often noted at the end of one week of play that parents in fact find their children more desirable persons with whom to interact.

The material to be introduced to the parents in this session is provided in a printed handout, a copy of which is shown in Figure 7.14. It is worth reviewing in some detail the way in which this handout should be introduced and explained to the family. As the handout indicates, this session is designed to train the parents in using new methods of paying attention to child behaviors during play. The handout instructs parents to select a time when their children are playing in an activity that the children normally enjoy and that is appropriate. Parents are then to approach the children and begin a period of 15 to 20 minutes of playing with the children in the manner discussed further in the handout. Parents are encouraged to label this as "special time" with the children so that the children may come to view it as a reward or sign of affection. During this play period, the children are to choose whatever they wish to do, provided the activity falls within a broad range of appropriate behavior. It is essential that the children select the activity so that they come to believe that their parents are interested in what they want to do and not interested simply in taking charge of the play and redirecting it to something that the parents desire to do.

As suggested in the second step of the handout, it is critical that the parents learn to relax during this time, and that the parents have absolutely nothing on their minds other than learning to attend to what the children are doing. For this reason, parents should not attempt to play with the children immediately prior to going out on an errand or performing some other activity, as it is likely that the parents' minds would be preoccupied by the other activities and that the quality of attention the children would receive would be quite shallow and probably ineffective. Thus, it is the sole purpose of this play period that parents attend to what the children are doing.

During the playtime, the parents should watch, mentally note, and follow the children's various activities for a few moments before beginning to narrate what the children are doing. This narrative description of the children's activities should occur occasionally throughout the play period. By doing so, the children will begin to develop the idea that the parents are quite interested in what they do, regardless of how trivial it may seem at the time. In addition, the narration of the children's activities necessarily prevents the parents from engaging in asking questions or giving commands in order to redirect the children's play. As indicated in the fifth point on the parents' handout, the parents should avoid the use of commands and questions during this playtime. One method that I have found quite effective in training parents to adopt this style of paying attention is to have the parents consider what it would be like to be a sportscaster at a particular baseball or football game. In essence, the parents' goal should be to describe the children's actions, and not to direct them or take control of them. Depending upon the way in which the parents choose to narrate and the degree to which this narration is embellished by emotional cues of interest and excitement, this style of paying attention can be highly effective at reinforcing the children for appropriate play behaviors.

As mentioned above, it is essential that the parents limit their questions and eliminate any commands that may be given during this time. Commands are obviously designed to take control over an activity, and such control is to be inhibited during the children's playtime. As I have often explained to the parents I have trained, there is virtually nothing that parents need to teach children during this 15 to 20 minutes of special playtime that could not be taught at some other time of the day. Even if the children's play is not up to the standards expected by the parents, the parents should avoid taking charge of the play and trying to teach the children different ways of playing. Questions, like commands, are quite intrusive upon children's play; they necessitate that the children redirect their thinking and their activities toward the parents in order to answer them. Again, this is to be avoided during this special playtime.

Throughout the playtime, the parents should intersperse various comments of positive, genuine feedback. As noted in the parent handout, this feedback is not necessarily glowing praise for what the children are doing. Instead, it is simply a statement that reflects the parents' interest in what the children are doing and perhaps the parents' enjoyment of being with the children. A list of various positive statements and actions that parents can use during playtime is provided in Figure 7.15. We provide this handout to parents so that they do not come to use only one or two phrases of positive feedback predominantly during this special time. It is further explained to the parents that it is possible not only to give the children feedback for the desirable things they are doing at this time, but also to praise the children for the things they are not doing. For instance, the parents can say, "I really like it when you play quietly and don't run around the room." This way, the parents not only specifically attend to what the children are doing appropriately, but also are able to mention the child behaviors they find unacceptable during play.

Many parents ask at this point how they should behave during the special playtime if their children begin to get seriously disruptive. It is my belief that the parents' best reaction at this point is to simply turn away from the children. After several episodes of misbehavior in which the parents redirect their attention elsewhere and ignore the children, it is likely that the misbehavior will decline. If, on the other hand, the children's misbehavior escalates in response to the ignoring, as in the postextinction burst described earlier, then the parents should leave the room. At this point, the parents can simply say that they will return when the children wish to play in a more acceptable manner. Of course, there may be instances in which the children's behavior becomes so unacceptable that discipline may be necessary. If this is the case, the parents are instructed to handle the disciplining in a manner similar to the way in which they have been handling it previously. No effort should be made at this point to introduce the time-out procedure to be used

SUGGESTIONS FOR GIVING POSITIVE FEEDBACK TO A CHILD

PHYSICAL:

Hug	Smile
Pat on head or shoulder	Kiss
Affectionate rubbing of hair	"Thumbs up" sign
Arm around child's shoulder	Wink

VERBAL:

"I like it when you _____."

"It's nice when you _____."

"You sure are a big boy [girl] for _____."

"Thanks for _____."

"That was terrific when you _____."

"Great!"

"Nice going!"

"Good job!"

"Super!"

"Fantastic!"

"My, you sure act grown up when you _____."

"Wow!"

"Beautiful!"

"Wait until I tell Mom [Dad] how nice you were when you _____."

"What a nice thing to do for me by _____."

"You did that all by yourself when you _____ and I didn't have to remind you."

"I am really impressed by the way you _____."

"I know I don't say this as often as I should, but I really like it when you _____."

"Won't _____ be happy when he [she] hears how well you _____."

"Just for behaving so well, you and I will _____."

"I am very proud of you when you _____."

"It makes me very happy to see you _____."

"I always enjoy it when you _____."

NOTES:
1. Always be immediate with your praise to a child—DON'T WAIT!
2. Always be specific with your praise. Tell the child what you liked that he or she did well.
3. Never use "back-handed" compliments, such as "It's about time you did such a nice job cleaning your room," or "This is nice—so why can't you do this more often?"

FIGURE 7.15. Parent handout on possible positive statements and actions for use during "special time" with a child, to be provided during Session III.

later, as this obviously is providing the parents with too many activities to engage in with the children as part of the homework assignment.

It requires mentioning to parents at this point in training that the special time is to be conducted alone with the hyperactive children and with no other siblings. In addition, the play should involve only one parent at a time. This allows a child to learn that both parents are interested in his or her play activities on an individual basis. In addition, the children do not have to share the special time with siblings, whose characteristics and behaviors may be at this point more desirable than those of the hyperactive children and hence may attract more positive attention from the parents than the hyperactive children may. When siblings are in the home, they can be told by the parents that they will also receive some special time later in the day. For now, the parents should be discouraged at permitting siblings to become involved in a hyperactive child's special time period.

Once the therapist has explained these procedures to the parents, they should be permitted to discuss any questions or problems they may have about implementing the procedure. Typically, at this point, several different parental reactions are observed. One of these is that the parents feel that the procedure is extremely simple and will be quite easy to implement in the family's home activities. When parents appear too glib about the procedure, they should be reminded about the statement typed in bold capital letters at the bottom of the parent handout dealing with the playtime (Figure 7.14). As this statement indicates, this program may seem quite easy when parents are reading it, but it becomes quite a different matter as they try to implement the procedure. Parents should be told that one of the most common mistakes made by other parents who have previously been through the program is that they have extreme difficulty in limiting their questions and eliminating all commands during the playtime. Parents are so accustomed to taking control over children's play, teaching the children, or just generally supervising their hyperactive children's behavior that it becomes second nature to them to constantly direct and redirect the children's activities. In addition, many parents find that one of the few vehicles they have of interacting with these children is to question them about what they are doing, how they may have learned to do what they are doing, or about some other trivial aspect of the children's play behavior. Parents seem to be at a loss for other ways of initiating interactions with the children besides using questions. They should be warned about this problem, and the therapist can provide suggestions as to how to translate impending questions into statements or interesting narration of the children's activities. Again, as with commands, there is virtually no question that a parent could ask during this playtime that could not be asked at some other time. It is my custom at this point to ask parents how they might feel if, upon their return home from a quite arduous day's work, a spouse or another adult began to "interrogate" them in the same way that they interrogate their children during play. Most parents find this situation easy to identify with; they often remark that such treatment by another person would be quite aversive and would hardly be what they would consider quality attention. Children's reactions to repeated questions and commands during playtime are probably quite similar to those adults would have if treated in a similar fashion.

A second concern of many parents is that the special time does not seem to be directly connected to the problems with their children's behavior that have brought them to the clinic. This is a particularly frequent reaction of many fathers of hyperactive children. They will often remark that they brought their children here because they do not listen and do not seem to follow through with what they are asked to do. How, they ask, is playing with the children in this manner going to address the problems of noncompliance? At this point, the therapist can respond with the fact that appropriate disciplinary procedures aimed at reducing the children's inappropriate behavior will be taught in a subsequent session. At this time, it is not the goal of this program to teach families to rule the children's noncompliance by fear, but instead to teach positive ways of attending to the children in order to increase their appropriate behaviors. In addition, it is explained that a positive relationship with these children needs to be reestablished before parents are trained in an effective disciplinary method. This is to avoid having the children receive disciplining for inappropriate behavior at home while failing to receive any form of positive attention for appropriate play and compliance. A third rationale for this part of the program is that at this particular time the quality of most parents' attention to these children and hence the reward value of this attention to the children are probably not especially high. Thus, the parents need to learn more effective ways of attending to the children so that they may use this attention in the next session to reinforce child compliance. Simply to tell a family to go home and praise a child for appropriate behavior does not necessarily mean that the parents will know the best ways of paying attention to child compliance or that the attention they use has any effect on the child's behavior. By following through with the assigned special time periods with this child, the parents will often find by the end of the first week that the child views them in a much more positive light and finds their attention and praise significantly more rewarding. This can be illustrated by the fact that at the end of the 20-minute special time period, children often request that their parents remain in order to play for a more extended time period. Parents, however, should attempt to avoid doing so in order for the special time to remain just that. In any case, parents should be encouraged to be patient with the therapist and to direct their efforts at learning the more positive ways of attending to their children's behavior.

A third, though less frequent, reaction of many parents to this particular session is that if they spend special time with the children and praise them for what may seem trivial play behaviors, the children will come to expect praise for almost everything they do. There are several ways a therapist can handle this particular parental reaction. The first is to point out to the parents that this has not happened with any children who have previously been trained in this program. Secondly, it is helpful to explore with the parents the basis for this attitude toward child behaviors. Obviously, the parents are being paid by their employers for their work, which is in a sense a way of reinforcing them for their performance at their jobs. In addition, the parents have expectations of each other that each will appreciate, at least on a periodic basis, what the other is doing to support the family. I have often pointed out to parents the fact that many marriages have difficulty because of a lack in precisely the activities we are trying to teach them to use with their children—appreciation of positive behaviors. Further, the parents can be directed to experiment with this particular method of paying attention to other children and adults whom they may encounter, simply to see how effective it is at encouraging desirable behaviors in others. Of course, the method of paying attention would have to be upgraded to more adult levels of praise and genuine feedback. The discussion on this issue should simply center around the fact that all of us, adults or children alike, have a particular need for and desire to obtain the attention of other individuals. Hyperactive children in this case are no different and are deserving of periodic positive praise and feedback for their positive activities.

Once the parental reactions to this aspect of the program have been discussed, it is instructive for the therapist to model the type of attending behaviors that a parent should use with a child. If the child in question is available, the therapist can do this simply by providing the child with play materials and demonstrating the attending technique directly with the child. Should the child not be available in this particular session, the therapist can have one of the parents role-play the part of a child playing with toys while the therapist demonstrates the attending methods. In some instances, when a videotape machine and monitor are available, it can be of further benefit to show the parents a videotape of the therapist demonstrating the play technique with another child. By whatever method one chooses, it is often helpful to demonstrate the technique to the family, as even after a thorough explanation they may still be doubtful as to precisely how to implement the technique.

Following this modeling demonstration, the parents should be encouraged to practice the skills themselves. Again, if the child is available, the parents can be encouraged to implement the methods in the clinic situation with the child directly. If not, then the therapist or the other spouse can assume the part of the child while the other parent attempts to practice the play techniques. In either case, I find that the practice is essential and should be used when possible. This permits the therapist an opportunity to comment upon and assist in shaping better parental attending skills. In proceeding with both the therapist modeling and parental practice aspects of this session, it can be of great benefit if a clinic playroom is available in which there is a one-way mirror between the playroom and an adjacent observation room. When such a playroom is equipped with a two-way intercom system as well as a "bug in the ear" teletransmitter device, the child in question can be involved directly in both the modeling and parental practice parts of this program. In this case, the therapist enters the playroom with the child, while the parents remain in the observation room listening to the style and observing the technique by which the therapist attends to the child's play behaviors. After a sufficient modeling time, one of the parents can then be sent into the playroom to practice the skills with the child. If the "bug in the ear" device is available, this can be used with the parent in the playroom to comment upon and shape that parent's attending skills without the child being aware that such comments are being made. Granted, both the playroom and the communications devices may be luxuries to many child clinicians. However, when these are available, they can aid substantially in the training of the parents in these and subsequent management techniques.

Following the parental practice period, the therapist can review with the parents their feelings about the progress of the practice session. Many parents respond that they did not believe that the technique was quite so difficult as it now appears to be. Secondly, if the technique has been demonstrated with the child, the parents are often amazed to see how responsive the child can be to the parents' attention even after years of negative interactions within the home. At this point, the therapist should discuss with the parents the times of day that would be most appropriate for each to implement these "special time" homework assignments, as well as any problems they anticipate with siblings or with their daily activity schedules. Care should be taken to explain to the parents that they should not expect substantial improvements in a child's problem behaviors simply as a result of implementing this play method over the next week. The child's negative behaviors are quite engrained in the family's style of interactions and will take some time to diminish. What the parents can expect, however, is that the child will come to view the parents in a somewhat different, more rewarding light as a result of the use of the attending skills at home. This may not occur for some families, but the vast majority often report such changes in the child's behavior toward the parents as a result of only a week of implementing the attending skills.

Finally, the session is concluded with a discussion of the homework assignments for the subsequent week. First, the parents should be encouraged to continue making notes on the one or two noncompliant behaviors they have been recording in the diary since the previous session. Second, the parents are requested to use the 15 to 20 minutes of special time with the child each day, and to try to implement the method at least 5 days during the subsequent week. Finally, the parents are asked to record a second set of observations in their notebook. These observations pertain to the date and time of day that the play sessions were implemented, the child's reaction to the special time sessions, and any particular problems the parent observes during the special time period. By assigning this as homework, the therapist is quite likely increasing the probability that the parents will in fact implement the procedure. How well and how frequently they implement the procedure can be reviewed in the subsequent session while reviewing the diary.

SESSION IV: PAYING ATTENTION TO COMPLIANCE AND INDEPENDENT PLAY

At the beginning of this session, as in previous sessions, the therapist should review the homework assignments with the parents. Initially, this involves reviewing the diary being kept for the one or two noncompliant behaviors assigned during Session II. At this point, the parents will have collected approximately 2 weeks' worth of information on these behaviors. This should help the therapist to discern a trend in the child's misbehavior and in the nature of the interactions the family is having with the child. In a few instances, these noncompliant behaviors may begin to improve as a result of the previous homework on paying attention to the child's play. In most cases, however, there is little improvement in the noncompliant behavior. This, of course, is expected and should have been explained to the parents at the end of the last session. Following the review of noncompliant behaviors, the therapist should review the records kept on the "special time" that the parents were to have spent with the child at least 5 days during the previous week. While reviewing the records, the therapist can inquire as to the parents' opinions on the general results of the special time sessions and the child's reactions to these play periods in particular. In many cases, parents will report that their children's behavior at first was one of unexpected surprise and perhaps dismay that the parents was spending this much time with them. Some children often respond to the initial periods of special time with suspicion, somewhat similar to an adult's reaction if sent a gift when there is no particular occasion for the gift. Eventually, most children come to realize that the attention is being given to them without any ulterior motive or hidden agenda being involved. In a few cases, parents report that the play sessions went satisfactorily, but that they were a little uncomfortable with the fact that the children rarely acknowledged their presence or their periodic feedback. The therapist should respond to this concern by pointing out that such children may have understood the praise but may not have verbally acknowledged the fact that it was given. These parents should be instructed that children rarely openly acknowledge positive feedback and praise from others, and that its true impact must actually be judged by whether or not it increases the behavior upon which it is contingent—in this case, the children's play.

Once the records have been reviewed, the parents are instructed that they should continue spending as much special time as possible with the child; at least 20 minutes per day for at least 5 days out of each week should be allotted for it. No further instructions will be given on the special time, and the parents will only be periodically asked whether they are still spending such time with the child in future sessions. The point to be made here is that the special time should become a part of the family's activities or life style, instead of simply being terminated after a week of involvement.

The purpose of the present session is to train the family in extending their use of positive attention from the child's play behavior to the child's compliance and independent play. That is, the parents are going to be taught how to use the attending skills taught in the previous session to reward the child's appropriate compliance. In addition, they will also be taught how to use the attending skills to keep the child from bothering them at times when they must direct their attention to other activities, such as talking on the telephone. It is explained to the parents at this point that the use of their attention, which has probably increased in value to the child since the previous session, to reinforce child compliance should result in an increase in the child's compliant behaviors. Few parents have difficulty with this particular session because it is such a logical extension of the previous one.

Before reviewing the handouts to be used with this session, it is important that the therapist spend a few moments discussing with the parents the nature in which commands should be given to children in order to insure greater compliance. First, the commands that are given should be brief, clearly and pleasantly worded, and not stated as favors or questions. The latter style of giving commands to children often results in noncompliance because the commands are not firmly stated and because they allow the children to answer "no" to the question or the favor being asked. While command–questions and command–favors may be used successfully with normal children, they should be avoided in the initial stages of this program with hyperactive children, as these children are highly unlikely to respond to them. Secondly, parents should avoid giving multiple-part or complex commands to children. This, of course, depends quite heavily on the children's age and understanding of the task being requested. Nonetheless, it is a common problem with parents of hyperactive children that their commands are often multiple or repetitive in nature and at times more complex than the children are capable of comprehending. In order to ensure that the commands are in fact understood, it is often helpful to ask such children to repeat what they have been asked to do before they attempt to accomplish the assigned task. This not only insures that they understand the command, but also reinforces their memory of the command, which should result in somewhat better compliance. Third, once a command has been given, parents should allow adequate time for the children to comply before following up the command with others. Parents of hyperactive children often make the mistake of providing them with a chain of commands that they cannot possibly comply with in a short period of time. Finally, parents should insure that they have the children's complete attention when giving them commands, and that they are not attempting to compete with other, more attractive stimuli within the room. The best way of achieving the former is to make direct eye contact with the children while giving the commands. The latter can be achieved by insuring that such distracting stimuli as the television set, a stereo or radio, electronic games or toys, or other highly appealing distractors are turned off or removed before attempting to give the children commands. Following these simple rules of providing commands to children can often result in improved compliance without any positive or negative consequences being provided to the children.

There are two handouts provided in this session, and the therapist should review these with the parents. The first handout, set forth in Figure 7.16, is a relatively straightforward series of instructions on ways for the parents to provide positive attention to a child immediately following compliance with commands. A few points deserve additional emphasis. For one thing, parents are instructed in the third step that when they have given a command they should remain in the area in which the command is to be accomplished in order to monitor the child's compliance and provide contingent praise and positive feedback for compliance. In the fourth step of this handout, parents are also instructed that, should a child comply with a household rule without being told to do so, this calls for exceptional attention and praise from the parents. Such attention should increase the likelihood that the child will internalize the household rules without necessarily having them repeated each time the parents desire him or her to comply.

Despite the fact that parents have shown increased attention to their children during the previous week, some deviant children may still be quite unresponsive to social praise alone. Parents of such children need to be reminded of this so that they do not expect inordinate increases in their compliance during the coming week, simply because they are providing increased attention to them. For these children, it may be helpful to supplement the praise and positive feedback with other sorts of reinforcement. The easiest system to implement for further reinforcement of child behaviors is a token or point system. As explained in Chapter 6, this simply involves awarding the children a certain number of tokens (e.g., poker chips, bingo chips, play

---

PAYING ATTENTION TO YOUR CHILD'S COMPLIANCE

Although you first learned the method of "paying attention" to your child when "special time" was introduced, you can now begin to extend it to periods when the child is complying with commands you have given him or her. When you give a command, it is necessary that the child receive immediate feedback or praise for initiating compliance. Don't just walk away from your child when he or she is doing something as directed. Spend a few moments letting the child know you appreciate the compliance.

1. As soon as you have given a command and your child begins to comply, then provide the child with feedback, in statements like these:

"I like it when you do as I asked."

"It's nice that you do what I say."

"Thanks for doing what I asked."

"Good boy [girl] for _____ as Mom [Dad] asked you to do."

Other possible statements of positive feedback are given in the handout on "Suggestions for Giving Positive Feedback to a Child."

2. Again, you can use the same methods you used during play. When your child is complying, simply watch, tailgate the compliance, narrate or describe the compliance to the child, and provide periodic feedback for the compliance.

3. Once you have attended to the child, you may leave for a few moments. Be sure to return to the child when he or she is still complying to periodically reward the continued compliance. Use statements like these as feedback:

"You sure are a big boy [girl] for doing that without Mom's [Dad's] help."

"I really like it when you do as I asked without my having to remind you. Thanks."

4. If you find that your child has done a chore or followed a household rule without having to be told to do so, that is the time to praise and pay exceptional attention to the child. This will help your child to internalize household rules and to want to obey and remember them.

FIGURE 7.16. Parent handout on ways of providing positive reinforcement for child compliance, to be introduced during Session IV.

money) or a certain number of points indicated on a sheet of paper for compliance and desirable behavior. The tokens or points can then be exchanged by the children for household privileges, extra activities out of the home, the purchase of desirable toys or objects, or (in some cases) money. Through the process of this exchange, the tokens or points come to be of considerable value to the children and will frequently serve to increase compliance when used to reward its occurrence. The therapist can also instruct parents to establish a "reinforcement menu" that can provide these children with a list of activities and the number of points or tokens required for access to those activities. The parents can sit down with the children at some point during the coming week and have the children assist them in establishing the privileges and activities and in negotiating the point values for each. For instance, it may be that the children will have to earn 20 points for every hour of television that they watch, 30 points for staying up past their usual bedtime on a weekend evening, or 200 points to attend a movie for the coming weekend. In any case, the tokens or points can be given to the children along with the positive praise and attention from the parents when compliance occurs to parental commands. Further instructions for setting up a home token system have been discussed in Chapter 6 and are also given in Appendix B.

Besides the use of secondary reinforcers such as tokens or points, the use of a simple kitchen timer can often improve children's compliance to parental commands. Kitchen timers are especially helpful when the command or task the children have been given will require an extended time to accomplish, such as picking up toys, cleaning a room, preparing for bed, completing homework assignments, or performing other chores around the home. In such cases, a time limit becomes part of the command. For example, parents can indicate to their children that they should get dressed for school and that they will be permitted 10 minutes to do so. The children are also instructed that the timer has been set for the 10 minutes and that when the bell rings signaling the end of the 10-minute period, the children should be dressed and ready for school. If so, then positive parental praise, positive feedback, and perhaps the use of tokens or points can be used to reinforce the compliance. At this time, should noncompliance occur, the parents are instructed simply to handle it as they have typically been doing, and that in the next session they will be instructed in the use of a different disciplinary procedure. For now, the parents' focus should be on compliance when it occurs rather than on noncompliance and ways of dealing with it.

The therapist should then proceed to a discussion of the second handout, set forth in Figure 7.17, which provides the parents with a set of instructions on the way to reward their child for not bothering them when they are busy. This essentially involves reinforcing the child for increasingly longer periods of independent play, that is, activities that are independent of the parents' involvement. This procedure is quite helpful in training children not to interrupt their parents when they are talking on the telephone, trying to prepare a meal, trying to speak with other people (such as visitors to the home), trying to watch television, or simply trying to accomplish any usual activity within the home that requires the parents' total attention. The procedure involves having parents utilize the attending technique they learned during the "special time" play period to reinforce the children for progressively larger amounts of independent play. In addition, the tokens or points discussed above can be used to increase the children's independent behavior. In essence, the technique discussed in Figure 7.17 is merely a variation of the shaping principle noted in Chapter 6. This principle involves starting with a

---

PAYING ATTENTION TO A CHILD WHEN THE CHILD IS NOT BOTHERING YOU

Many parents of children with behavior problems complain that they are unable to do things, such as talk on the telephone or make dinner, because the child is always interrupting them or misbehaving. The following steps are designed to help you teach your child to behave appropriately when you are busy and can't be around very much to attend to the child. As with any good behavior by your child, you must pay attention to him or her for showing the desirable behavior if you expect him or her to do it again.

1. Take a moment from what you are doing and see if your child is behaving appropriately. If not, then do NOT pay attention to the child at this time. If the child is behaving well, then take just 15 to 20 seconds from what you are doing and go to where he or she is playing. If you are on the telephone, then tell the other person to hold on for just a moment. You would ask the caller to hold on if you had to deal with your child's misbehavior, so you can do it just as easily for your child's good behavior.

2. Go to the child and briefly provide him or her with positive feedback and attention FOR NOT BOTHERING YOU. For instance, you can say:

"I really like it when you don't interrupt me while I'm _____ . Thanks."

"Mom [Dad] really likes it when you play quietly while I am _____ ."

"You're such a big boy [girl] for letting me _____ and not disturbing me."

3. Then return to your activity. At first, you should stop what you are doing every few minutes to go praise your child for leaving you alone.

4. Gradually, you can begin to lengthen the time between your visits to the child. For instance, you may be praising the child every 3 or 4 minutes when you begin this program. The next day, you can begin to praise the child every 6 or 7 minutes. On the next day after that, you can praise the child every 10 minutes. By increasing the time between visits to the child very slowly, you can shape the child so that he or she can behave quietly while you are busy for as long as 30 to 45 minutes.

5. If you have more than one child who bothers you while you are busy, then find the one who is not bothering you and pay attention to that one while you ignore the others. This clearly shows the other children what kind of behavior it will take from them to get your attention—good behavior.

FIGURE 7.17. Parent handout on ways of reinforcing a child for independent play, to be provided during Session IV.

behavior that is already within an individual's repertoire and then reinforcing progressively closer approximations to the desired behavior until the desired behavior is achieved. In this instance, parents will be shaping the amount of time their children are capable of spending away from the parents in desirable play activities without interrupting or bothering them.

Figure 7.17 instructs parents who are busily involved in some activity to take some time away from that activity, perhaps no more than 15 to 20 seconds, to locate the children and determine what they are doing. If they are playing appropriately and have not been interrupting what the parents have been doing, the parents should praise the children or provide them with positive feedback for not bothering the parents. Possible praises are listed within the handout, as well as in Figure 7.15. At this point, the parents do not remain with the children, but return to the activity in which they were previously involved. After a few minutes have passed, the parents again leave the activity and seek out the children; if the children have been behaving appropriately and not bothering the parents since their last visit, the parents again reward the children with social praise and positive feedback. Once more, the positive feedback should involve a clear statement of the parents appreciation for the fact that the children have not interrupted them. The parents then return back to the activity in which they were previously engaged. Eventually, the parents increase the amount of time between visits so that the child will be able to play for a number of minutes without interrupting the parents. The parents provide positive feedback and perhaps tokens or points as reinforcers for the increasing amounts of independent play. Although this technique involves such frequent visits to the children at first that the parents are unlikely to be able to devote their sole attention to the activity in which they are interested, over several days of using the technique they will be capable of shaping the children so that they will play for 30 to 45 minutes or longer without bothering the parents and without requiring frequent reinforcement for their behavior. Figure 7.17 also indicates that if there is more than one child in a family, the parents should seek out the child who is behaving appropriately during this time and reward that child. The other children are likely to observe this and to learn that it is the child's appropriate behavior that results in increased parental attention and rewards. They will, it is hoped, eventually imitate the appropriate behavior. In any case, the main point of this particular series of instructions is that parents should be rewarding children for independent play activities and not providing the children with attention for interrupting what the parents have been doing.

I have found it very helpful to teach this technique through the use of an example. One of the best examples is that of training children not to bother their parents when the parents are talking on the telephone. As previous chapters have shown, hyperactive children often present with quite serious noncompliance and behavior management problems when their parents are trying to speak on the telephone. Parents are told that this technique can be used in order to teach their children not to engage in such behavior while they are on the phone. This is done by initially instructing the children to play in a certain area or to engage in a certain desired activity at the moment that the phone is heard to ring. The children are instructed to remain in that area and not bother the parents while they are on the telephone. If the children comply, the parents praise them for initially doing what was asked, and then the parents turn to answer the phone. Moments after answering the phone, the parents tell the caller in question simply to hold on for a moment and then seek out the children, praising them briefly for not bothering the parents while they are on the phone. The parents then return to the telephone to continue the conversation. Within a few minutes, the parents interrupt the phone call again to seek out the children, again praising them for not being bothersome. Over time, the parents increase the amount of time between visits to the children. Depending on the length of the telephone call, it may be possible to teach these children to play for 5 or perhaps 10 minutes without parental attention during the very first phone call. If not, then in subsequent phone calls, the parents can begin to increase the amount of time between visits to the children.

Initially, parents may respond to this method by saying that this may often result in their being rude to individuals calling them at home. On the contrary, it is quite likely that at present the parents are already interrupting their phone calls frequently in order to cope with the undesirable child behaviors that occur during that time. All this particular method is doing is shifting parents' attention from the undesirable interruptive behaviors of their children to the more desirable ones of independent play. It is explained to the parents that they probably would have gotten off the telephone to attend to negative behaviors, so it is certainly no greater effort for them to shift their attention to getting off the phone to reinforce more positive, independent play activities. The parents should be told further that if they are going to use the telephone situation for practicing this technique during the coming week, it is helpful to have relatives or friends place telephone calls to the home for the sole purpose of teaching the children this particular procedure. That is, when the friends or relatives call, they will be doing so with the understanding that the parents will interrupt the phone calls quite frequently to reinforce the children's independent play. This can often eliminate parental concern over being rude to callers while at the same time begin to shape the children's independent play activities so that when legitimate calls come, the children are already well along in learning to play for long periods of time without interrupting the parents' activity.

Parents often have several reactions to the application of this method. First, many parents operate under the philosophy of "let sleeping dogs lie." This translates simply to not paying attention to their children when they are behaving quietly and appropriately, for fear that the parental attention will only spark new occurrences of undesirable child behavior. In fact, such parents will often say that they have tried to reward their children previously for appropriate independent play, only to find that their rewards triggered new episodes of aversive or hyperactive behaviors. It is explained to these parents that when the independent play of their children is not rewarded, there is no reason to expect that it will recur with any greater frequency. In fact, it is likely to diminish over time because of the lack of reinforcement for its occurrence. Furthermore, it is explained to these parents that the children are probably misbehaving when the parents attend to them because the children have learned that this is one method of keeping the parents in the room for greater lengths of time. If the children were to continue playing appropriately, the parents would simply leave the room again. Thus, these children have learned that when the parents come by to praise them, the best way of getting the parents to stay longer is to begin to act disruptive or to misbehave. The technique taught in this session, by contrast, is simply to reward the children for independent play and to ignore them or to leave the room when misbehavior occurs. A second reaction of parents is that they will not be able to accomplish the activities they desire to perform if they often have to interrupt what they are doing to praise their children for not bothering them. While this may be true initially, after several days it is quite possible to teach a child to play for increasingly longer amounts of time without disturbing a parent. The eventual result is that the child can play alone for the entire time that the parent is involved with another activity without receiving praise from the parent. The parent simply has to invest in frequent visits to the child at first in order to achieve the desired behavior from the child later on.

If the child is available for this session, the therapist should then model the desired behavior with the child. As noted earlier, if a clinic playroom is available with a one-way observation mirror, the desired parental behaviors can be modeled by playing with the child in the clinic playroom while the parents observe from the adjacent observation room. Whether such a play-room is available or not, the method can still be demonstrated in front of the parents with the child as target of the technique. In this case, the therapist can begin playing with the child and then after a few minutes tell the child to remain with the play activity while the therapist reads a magazine at the other side of the room. After going to the opposite side of the room for a few moments and reading the magazine, the therapist can then return to the child and praise him or her for not being bothersome and for playing quietly. The therapist can then return to the other side of the room and continue reading the magazine. At this point, the therapist can begin increasing the time between visits to the child. This will demonstrate to the family how easy it is to get the child to play and not to bother them simply by making the visits to the child less and less frequent. Once this has been demonstrated to the parents, the parents can be asked to practice the method directly with the child. Following the parental practice under the supervision of the therapist, the therapist should discuss with the parents their feelings about and reactions to using the technique, as well as any possible problems with using the method in the home during the subsequent week.

At the close of this session, as in previous sessions, the homework is assigned. The homework for this session involves having the parents continue to keep a record of the one or two noncompliant behaviors selected in the second session. The second facet of the homework assignment may involve having the parents continue to record the "special time" periods they spend with the child. This is often done if there have been problems with the use of special time in the home the previous week. If no problems have been encountered, the parents are told that they no longer need to record the occurrence of the special playtime in the diary, but that they should continue using the method with the child in any case. Finally, the homework to be assigned should involve the parents' selection of one or two activities in which the child would normally interrupt or bother them and to attempt to use the method described above to reinforce independent play. Related to this, of course, is the instruction to the parents that they should now begin to provide positive feedback to the child for compliance to commands when it occurs. This can be aided by having the family select one or two commands that they know the child is likely to comply with during the subsequent week and by asking them to focus on paying particular attention to these compliant behaviors. If necessary, the parents can be requested to use the diary to record these behaviors and the reinforcement with which the child is provided. Whether or not this is assigned, the parents should be asked to record in the diary their efforts at teaching the child to engage in increasing amounts of independent play and not to bother them. In summary, the parents will be requested to record at least two different activities. The first is the continued recording of the noncompliant behaviors selected in Session II. The second is the recording of their efforts to shape the child's independent play during times when the parents wish not to be bothered. The other record-keeping activities may be assigned at the discretion of the therapist.

SESSION V: USING TIME OUT AND RESPONSE COST FOR NONCOMPLIANCE

This session begins, again, with a review of the records that have been kept by the parents over the previous week. This should begin with an examination of those one or two noncompliant behaviors that the parents have been recording for the previous weeks. Again, trends in the data may become obvious by this point, or it may be that there has been a reduction in the noncompliance as a result of the previous two sessions of positive management strategies. In most cases, however, there will be little change in these difficult behaviors, but the parents can be reassured that the current session will be designed to address these inappropriate behaviors. Next, the therapist reviews the records dealing with the parents' efforts at developing greater independent play by the child during times when the parents are busy with other activities. Time should be spent in discussing the parents' use of the procedures, any problems that arose in attempting the shaping procedure, and the extent to which the parents were successful at developing greater independent play. The parents are then instructed to continue using the shaping procedure during the subsequent week for other situations in which the child would normally be interruptive.

It is the purpose of the present session to assist the family in developing a more effective style of disciplining the child for noncompliance and other inappropriate behaviors. In doing so, it is essential that the therapist prepare the family for several things that will take place during the coming homework assignment. First, the parents should be prepared for the fact that this will probably be the most difficult week of the program for them. In many cases when the time-out procedure recommended below is implemented, children may throw temper tantrums lasting as long as an hour to an hour and a half, which may prove quite aversive to their families. During these tantrums, the parents of these children may feel as if they should give in to them in order to terminate this coercive type of behavior. Although this parental response would certainly be effective at stopping such children from crying and becoming disruptive, it would merely serve to teach them that such behavior is an effective means of coping with any discipline that the parents wish to administer. Thus, once the time-out program is implemented for a particular child behavior, these parents must see it through to its final conclusion without acquiescing to the children. The increase in aversive behaviors by these children, as well as in temper tantrums, is probably the result of the fact that the children's aversive behaviors have developed by the principle of negative reinforcement discussed in Chapter 2. That is, the children have learned that when the parents invoke a command (an aversive event for the children), they can effectively terminate this aversive event by emitting aversive or negative behaviors of their own, such as temper tantrums, crying, screaming, or destructiveness. As a result, their behavior has been negatively reinforced by the parents' withdrawing the command or acquiescing to the children's coercion. When the parents attempt to implement a command or subsequently to back it up with a time-out program, the children will attempt to emit coercive behaviors that are as intense as or more intense than those they have found successful in the past. The parents should be told to expect this high-rate aversiveness from their own child when they attempt to implement the time-out program.

A second factor that the parents must be prepared for is that of using discipline consistently for the child's noncompliance, even when it may be inconvenient for them to do so. The parents up to this point have probably been quite inconsistent in the manner in which they have handled the child's negative behaviors. Inconsistency is often found between the parents; that is, each parent treats the child differently. In addition, the behavior of each parent over time may also be inconsistent. That is, a parent may on some occasions have attempted to discipline the child for noncompliance but on other occasions may have acquiesced to the child's refusal to do the command. Both types of inconsistency have probably contributed to some extent to the ineffectiveness with which the parents have managed the child. Part of this parental inconsistency may reflect resistance or ambivalence on at least one parent's part toward any kind of discipline for the child because of a belief that it will harm the child or result in psychological maladjustment. The therapist needs to discuss the issue of discipline with the family to determine whether such a belief is part of either parent's philosophy of child rearing. If so, it will have to be dealt with before any effort at training the parents in specific methods of punishment can occur. By not doing so, the therapist runs the risk of having such parental inconsistency weaken the new methods in which the parents are to be trained.

The therapist should then introduce the parent handout shown in Figure 7.18. It is worth discussing this handout in some detail because of its importance to the overall program and to the diminution of noncompliant behaviors in the child. As it is introduced to the parents, the therapist explains that from this point forward, when the parents give a command to the child, they should be willing to back it up with consequences for noncompliance. No longer are the parents to issue commands that they cannot enforce because of time pressures, family activities, or simple inconvenience. Under such circumstances, it is explained, the parents would be better off if they issued no commands at all. Giving commands under circumstances in which they cannot be followed up with consequences for compliance or noncompliance merely teaches the child that the parents' word is not especially meaningful. As the handout indicates, repeated commands are to be avoided, since most hyperactive children will take advantage of such repetitions to continue with their noncompliance.

When a command is to be given by a parent to a child, the parent should view the sequence of activities as occurring in three stages. I often use the analogy of a traffic signal or stop light to describe these three stages. The first stage involves giving the initial command pleasantly but in a firm tone of voice, and not phrasing it as a question or as a favor. The command should be stated directly and simply, and eye contact should be made with the child as the command is being given. As noted earlier, distractors in the situation, such as radios or televisions, should be turned off in order to capture the child's full attention when the command is being given. This phase of the procedure is equivalent to the green light on the traffic signal. In other words, the interaction with the child is pleasant and straightforward at this point. The parent then silently counts to 5, at which point a warning is issued if compliance has not begun. It should be noted at this point that the

USING TIME OUT FOR CHILD NONCOMPLIANCE OR MISBEHAVIOR

It is important that you never give a command that you are not willing to back up with consequences. Doing so only teaches your child that you do not mean what you say. When your child complies, he or she should be praised and attended to for it. Similarly, when the child does not comply, he or she should be disciplined immediately. As a parent, you should *not* repeat your command more than once before providing consequences for noncompliance.

1. Always give your first command to a child in a firm but pleasant voice. Do not yell it at the child, but also do not ask it as a favor. Make it a simple, direct statement as to what you expect. Do not give complex two- or three-part commands if your child is younger than 8 years of age.

2. After you have given the command, count silently to 5. Do not count out loud, as the child will eventually come to rely on this counting in learning when to comply with a command.

3. If the child has not made a move to comply within these 5 seconds, you should *make direct eye contact* with the child, *raise your voice* to a much louder intensity, *adopt a firmer stance,* and say:

"If you don't _____,
then you are going to sit in that chair [point to where the chair is]!"

This warning should be given in a firm voice, with sharp, firm gestures of the hands and arms to illustrate the warning.

4. Having given this warning, count silently to 5 again.

5. If the child still does not make a move to comply within these 5 seconds, then take him or her firmly by the wrist and say:

"You did not do as you were told, so you will have to sit in the chair!"

This should be said loudly and firmly to the child. The child should then be taken firmly by the wrist and taken to the chair. If the child promises to comply now, do not listen, but take him or her to the chair. The time for compliance was at the first command, not now. If the child falls to the floor kicking and screaming, then drag him or her by the wrist to the chair. In either case, the child goes directly to the chair at your pace. He or she does not get to go to the bathroom, to get a drink of water, or anything else—THE CHILD GOES DIRECTLY TO THE CHAIR.

6. Place the child firmly in the chair and say sternly: "Now you stay there until *I* say you can get up!"

7. At this point, only 10 seconds have elapsed since you gave the first command, so you should not be emotionally upset at all. When you raise your voice during the preceding warnings, it is done for dramatic effect to let the child know you mean business. Leave the child in the chair until he or she is quiet and until it has been long enough to be unpleasant. We will come back to this point in a moment. You may tell the child that he or she is not getting out of the chair until he or she is quiet, but do not say this more than once. DO NOT ARGUE WITH THE CHILD while the child is in the chair. This only encourages further disruptive behavior.

8. DO NOT GO OVER TO THE CHAIR AGAIN UNTIL THE CHILD IS QUIET. If the child is kicking, screaming, yelling, etc., stay away from the chair. When the child is quiet, you may go to him or her and say firmly:

"Are you ready to do what I asked you?"

FIGURE 7.18. (*Continued*)

If the child says "yes," then he or she may leave the chair and go straight to the area where he or she must comply. If the child says "no," then say, "Fine, you stay there until I tell you to get up!"

9. Once the child has complied with the initial command, then say in a neutral voice, "I like it when you do what I asked." This is not to be praise, and you should not apologize to the child for having disciplined him or her.

10. It is important after the child has complied that you watch the child for the next desirable behavior he or she displays. At this point, you should go to the child and give him or her some positive feedback for behaving appropriately. This serves several purposes. First, it prevents you from carrying a grudge over what your child did earlier. Second, and more importantly, it teaches your child that you are not angry and are willing to praise him or her for good behavior. From this, the child learns that it is his or her behavior that gets him or her punishment or praise; therefore, his or her choice of behavior is also a choice of consequences—praise or punishment. This also always keeps the program in balance so that you are never punishing a child more than you are praising that child.

11. If your child gets off the chair before you say it is time, then give the child this warning only once in his or her life:

"If you get off that chair again, I am going to spank you!"

This is to be said very loudly, using firm gestures and clapping the hands loudly in front of the child when the word "spank" is said (for dramatic effect). Direct eye contact is also important here.

12. The child is considered to be off the chair when both buttocks have left the flat surface of the chair. If the child gets off the chair again after the warning, he or she is spanked. In spanking the child, the parent sits in the time-out chair, pulls the child's pants down, places the child over the knee, and spanks the child firmly and quickly twice on the buttocks. The child then has his or her pants pulled up and is placed back in the chair. Once again, you should tell the child, "Now you stay there until I tell you to get up!" The child is not spanked hard, just firmly and swiftly, but is spanked every time he or she gets off the chair. Generally, most children do not get off the chair after the warning about the spanking, and of those who do, most require only one or two spankings before they remain on the chair. After this, there is rarely a problem with the child remaining on the chair whenever he or she is sent there.

WHERE SHOULD THE CHAIR BE?

Choose a rather dull corner of the dining room, foyer, hallway, or other area, and place the chair far enough from the wall so that the child cannot kick the wall while sitting. The child should be facing the wall when seated.

DO NOT USE A BATHROOM, LIVING ROOM, OR CLOSET! We also believe that sending a child to his or her room is not as effective as using a chair since the child has many things to play with in this room. For parents who prefer not to spank their children, however, sending them to the room may be the only alternative to using the chair. However, you will still have to decide what you will do if a child repeatedly leaves his or her room without permission. For that reason, we prefer to use the chair.

Place the chair so that the child is not able to reach anything while sitting in the chair. There should be nothing to play with, and the child should not be able to see a television while seated.

FIGURE 7.18. *(Continued)*

The chair should be in a place where it can be seen from other places in the home, so that the parent can continue doing other activities while watching the child.

If the child begins moving and rocking the chair without getting out of it, then warn him or her that moving the chair around will also result in his or her getting spanked. Other than this, you should not talk to the child while he or she is sitting on the chair. No one else in the family should talk to the child while he or she is on the chair either.

HOW LONG SHOULD THE CHILD STAY IN THE CHAIR?

The child remains in the chair until he or she meets two criteria: he or she is quiet, and it has been long enough to be unpleasant. This last time period will vary with the age of the child. Young children (those under 4 years of age) require only a few minutes. Children between 5 and 8 years may require 10 to 15 minutes. Those over 8 years may require 20 to 30 minutes. The child's perception of time changes as he or she gets older, so it takes longer before an older child feels unpleasant sitting in the chair. In any case, the child does not leave the chair until he or she is quiet, even if this extends to an hour or more. Eventually, the child will learn to be quiet immediately upon being sent to the chair, and he or she may only need to stay there 15 minutes or so.

On the first visit to the chair, the child may have to stay longer because he or she may be fussing and throwing a temper tantrum to try to get out of the punishment. Once the child learns that this will not rescue him or her from the chair, he or she will become quiet immediately upon going to the chair at later times.

The child is not permitted to leave the chair to go to the bathroom or to get a drink of water. In addition, if the child is sent to the chair during mealtime, he or she misses the meal. In other words, the child is to miss whatever is happening in the house while he or she is sitting on the chair. This is what makes the chair so effective. If your child misses a meal, he or she may have a snack later that day if a snack is customary. However, do not prepare a special meal for the child simply because he or she missed one.

If the chair is used for bedtime problems, then its use must be altered somewhat from the above. The therapist will explain these circumstances to you.

FIGURE 7.18. Parent handout on the use of time out, to be introduced during Session V.

parent is not encouraged to count out loud, as many parents seem to do. This merely teaches the child to comply with numbers rather than with the initial command, and also gives the child some idea of how soon it will be before consequences occur. In our program, we would rather have the child attending to the command instead of taking advantage of a counting system.

The warning, like the yellow warning light on the traffic signal, is clearly different from the initial command. The parent is instructed to make direct eye contact with the child again, to raise the voice to a much louder level of intensity, to adopt a firmer posture and stance, to point a finger at the child, and to present the child with the warning, "If you don't do as I say, then you are going to sit in that chair [parent points to the time-out chair]." The parent should adopt firm and sharp gestures during the warning to convey to the child that the parent is very perturbed with the child's continued noncompliance.

After the warning has been given, the parent again silently counts to 5; at this point, if the child has not begun to comply with the initial request, the child is taken immediately to the chair and told along the way, "You did not do as you were told to do, so you will have to sit in the chair!" This should be stated firmly in a loud, intense voice, and should again be backed up with firm gestures. In addition, once the child is placed in the chair, the parent should look at the child and state, "Now you stay there until I say you can get up!" At this point, the sequence of activities has taken no more than 10 seconds, and the command has only been repeated once. It is hard to see how any parent could become so emotionally upset during this brief encounter with the child as to be out of control and unable to discipline the child if necessary. That is one of the benefits of this particular program. Although the parent may be speaking loudly and intensely to the child, the discipline is being carried forth in a businesslike manner. There is no actual risk of the parent losing control with the child, as the parent might have done if he or she had repeated the command 7 to 10 times to the child before finally deciding to take action against the child's noncompliance.

When the child is taken to the chair following noncompliance to the warning, this can be seen as the red light in the traffic signal analogy. In essence, the interaction over the noncompliance stops with the child's being placed in time out. When the child is taken to the time-out chair, this should be done swiftly, regardless of the resistance the child presents. In no instance should the time out be eliminated simply because the child is resisting being placed in the chair. At this point, many children will engage in temper tantrums, kicking, or screaming, while others may offer to comply with the original command now that they see that their parents mean what they have said. Parents should be cautioned not to give in to either of these ploys. The "bargaining" children should have complied with the command when the initial command was given, not now that discipline is actually being carried through. To succumb to the ploy of these children is to reinforce them for their initial noncompliance. In the other instance, with children who are kicking, screaming, and physically resisting time out, to succumb to this type of gross coercive behavior would also be to reinforce its future occurrence. Parents should therefore be prepared for either of these cases to occur and should be forewarned that in no case are children to be excused from time out once they have violated the warning.

An important consideration is that of how long a child should remain in the chair after being placed there. Although many other professionals have offered suggestions on this matter, there actually is no simple answer to this question. First, it must be appreciated by therapists and parents alike that a child's subjective experience of time varies with age. Very young children, of 3 or 4 years of age, may feel that a 5-minute time-out period is extremely long and arduous for them, while 8- or 9-year-old children would not have the same experience with the same 5-minute interval. The time-out criteria must therefore be based upon the particular child, the child's age, and, most importantly, the amount of time it takes for the child to view the time-out interval as having been unpleasant. We therefore impose two criteria that must be met before the child can be permitted to leave the chair. The first is that the child must be quiet before the parent returns to interact with him or her. If the child takes an hour or more to stop screaming and throwing temper tantrums, then this is how long the child will have to stay in the chair for this particular incident. Over several visits to the chair for particular episodes of noncompliance, the child will eventually learn that he or she will be allowed out of the chair much more quickly for quieting down sooner. At this point, the child will often quiet down within a matter of seconds after being placed in the chair. It is obvious then that a second criterion must be implemented in order for the time-out program to remain effective. This second criterion is simply that the child must remain in the chair long enough to feel that doing so is unpleasant. The unpleasantness is judged by the parent in terms of the child's attitude, demeanor, and general facial expression while seated in the chair. Most parents know their children well enough to know when they are not enjoying a particular activity. As noted earlier, for a 3- to 5-year-old child, it may be that 5 or 10 minutes in the chair is sufficient to make the experience unpleasant. On the other hand, for an 8- to 10-year-old child, it may be that 20 minutes in the time-out chair is the sufficient interval of time. Although it may seem to the therapist that this allows a great deal of leeway and flexibility for parental judgment, possibly opening up the opportunity for abuse of the procedure, there has not been a single occasion during the past 7 years in which this program has been implemented that a parent has abused the time-out interval. This is true partly because the parents are keeping records on the use of time out that can be verified during the subsequent session and corrected if need be, and partly because most parents do seem to have an excellent grasp of the time interval that their children require in order to experience subjectively the unpleasantness associated with being seated in the chair. In short, then, the child remains in the chair both until he or she is quiet and until it has been long enough to be an unpleasant experience for that child.

While the child is seated on the chair, there is to be no arguing between the parent and the child and no interaction with the child, other than perhaps a statement at first that the parent will not come back until the child is quiet. Although it is in fairness that the child is given this statement of the connection between the parent's coming back and the child's being quiet, I have rarely found this statement alone to decrease the amount of time that the child is being noisy and disruptive in the chair. When the child is quiet, and when it has been long enough for the child to have experienced unpleasantness at being seated in the chair, then the parent is to go over to the child and ask if the child is ready to do what was originally asked. If the child responds with "yes," he or she is to go immediately to the area of noncompliance and comply with the initial command. If the child's misbehavior was something that cannot now be corrected—for example, swearing at someone or hitting a sibling—then the child simply needs to promise not to do this behavior again. If the child makes such a promise, he or she is allowed out of the chair. If the child still refuses to comply with the command, the parent simply responds by saying "Fine, you stay there until I tell you to get up!" The child is then allowed to sit in the chair for another 5 to 10 minutes, with the parent returning again once the child is quiet.

Once the child has complied with the initial command, the parent is to respond with a simple statement that the parent likes it when the child does what he or she is asked to do. At no time is the parent to apologize for having had to use time out with the child or for the fact that the child must comply with the command. Following the completion of compliance, the parent is to immediately praise the child for the next desirable behavior that is displayed. This serves not only to prevent the parent from carrying a grudge about what the child has done earlier that day, but it also insures that the child will never be punished more than he or she is rewarded by the parents for his behavior. Furthermore, the child is likely to learn from this that it is noncompliant behavior that creates difficulty with the parents and compliant behavior that can result in praise and positive attention from them. It is hoped that the child eventually makes the connection between the types of behavior and the types of the consequences that accrue from the parents.

Of equal concern to the parents at this time will be what they should do if the child gets off the chair. Although this is spelled out quite clearly in the handout given to the family, it is necessary that the therapist go over it in detail. First, it is necessary to specify what is meant by "getting off the chair." The definition I employ is that if both buttocks of the child have left the flat surface of the chair, then the child is considered off the chair and the consequence for being off the chair is implemented. According to this definition, the child may move around in the chair, so long as the buttocks do not leave the surface of the chair. If the child does leave the chair, the child is given a warning only once. This warning is never to be repeated to the child under any other circumstances at any other time, should the child leave the chair again. The warning is given loudly, sternly, and with the gesture of the parent clapping their hands loudly in front of the child for dramatic effect. The child is told, "If you get off the chair again, I am going to spank you!" On the word "spank," the parent should clap his or her hands loudly together in front of the child to illustrate the point. It has been our experience that if this warning is given properly and loudly enough, the vast majority of children will not leave the time-out chair again and therefore will never have to be spanked.

However, some children will refuse to heed this warning. At this point, the parent must follow up the warning by spanking the child. This is done very swiftly and in a very businesslike manner; the parent takes a seat in the time-out chair, pulls the child's pants down and places the child over one knee, and delivers two swift firm spanks to the child's buttocks. The child's pants are then pulled back up, and the child is returned to the time-out chair. At this point, the child is told that if the child should leave the chair again he or she will be spanked again. The few children who will continue to leave the chair are spanked by the parents until they have been spanked four or five times in one particular incident. If this should occur with a child, the parents are instructed not to spank the child any more at that particular time. Instead, they are to implement one of several other systems. They can tell the child that time in the chair will be extended by an additional 10 minutes for every time the child leaves the chair. Another possible alternative for the parents is a physical restraint procedure that consists of standing behind the chair and wrapping their arms around the child firmly but gently, locking their wrists to the side, in order to keep the child in the chair. A different version of this restraint procedure is simply to take the child's arms and hold them gently but firmly by the wrists behind his or her back so that the child cannot leave the chair. If neither physical restraint procedure is palatable to the parents, they may employ a response-cost procedure with the child by indicating that every time the child leaves the chair, he or she will have to give back to the parent a certain number of points or tokens previously earned for episodes of positive compliance. Obviously, such a program will not be effective unless the parents have previously implemented a point or token system, as noted earlier, for use with positive compliance.

Some parents will inquire at this point what they should do about children who refuse to go to the time-out chair and simply run away or leave the house. Our advice to the parents has been to tell such children that if they do not go to the chair as requested, then they will have to spend double the amount of time that they normally would have spent in the chair for refusing to go to the chair cooperatively. This is often quite successful at dealing with such children's refusal to go to a time-out chair.

In our opinion, it is extremely important to explain to the parents at this time that the spanking, if it is to be used, is probably a more humane and better controlled procedure than the physical discipline that most parents implement with their hyperactive children prior to coming to the training program. Many hyperactive children are spanked on a frequent, if not daily basis, for their noncompliance. The spanking that parents implement is often done after they have repeated their commands 7 to 10 times and when they are quite emotionally distraught. This is absolutely the wrong time to employ a physical disciplining procedure, because the parents are so close to losing control that they may actually physically harm the children out of frustration over their noncompliance. In contrast, the present program involves consequating hyperactive children's noncompliance within 10 to 15 seconds after they have failed to follow an initial command. The physical disciplining occurs only if the children leave the time-out chair. In this instance, the time-out chair is actually the first line of disciplining, while the spanking is used only to back up that disciplinary measure. Once such a child learns to stay in the chair, spanking can be eliminated from the family's style of management, as the time-out chair will be sufficient to manage noncompliance. Thus, the current procedure is likely to result in an actual reduction in the frequency with which a child is spanked, and those spankings that do occur will be given under more controlled, less emotional circumstances than would have been likely in the family previously.

As the parent handout shown in Figure 7.18 notes, there are several appropriate places for the time-out chair to be located within the family's home. The chair should not, however, be placed in the child's room, in a bathroom, in a closet, or in a living room where a television may be on. Instead, the family should place the time-out chair in a relatively dull corner of a dining room, a foyer, a hallway, or another room in the house in which the child is not likely to find many things to play with. Although the chair is placed facing the wall at a sufficient distance from the wall to prevent the child from kicking the wall when seated in the chair, it is not mandatory that the child actually face the wall. If the child squirms about in the chair, this is considered acceptable so long as the child does not leave the chair. I suggest to parents that the chair be left out constantly for the first 2 weeks of the time-out program to serve as a reminder to a child of what will happen if noncompliance occurs. After that point, the chair may be replaced in its original location and taken out only when it is needed.

Children, being as creative as they are, will often attempt several ploys or tactics in order to get out of the chair prematurely. One of the best examples of this is that a child will ask a parent for permission to go to the bathroom. In almost every instance, the child does not have to go to the bathroom but has found this ploy successful in the past in order to get out of certain circumstances. The parent is to reply that the child can go to the bathroom only after the time is up. The cases in which children may actually have to go to the bathroom and prove unable to control themselves are unfortunate but rare. In fact, these cases are so rare that parents should be told that they are highly unlikely to occur. Thus, it is my opinion that the parents should not acquiesce to the bathroom ploy. In other cases, children may use verbal statements to the effect that they no longer love the parents or will not do any favors for them in the future. Although obviously a reflection of the children's emotions at that particular moment, the parents should be instructed not to construe such statements as reflections of the children's long-term feelings about the use of discipline. Children's emotions are rather capricious in such moments, and so are their statements about their emotions. Should the parents let the children out of the chair when they make such threats, they have only guaranteed that the children are more likely to use such statements in the future when placed on the chair.

The main point of this program is therefore that a child will either have to comply with commands or spend time sitting in a chair. There are no options other than these for the child. This may be quite different from what the child has experienced previously; the child may have had the opportunity to watch television, dawdle, malinger, or generally behave belligerently or obnoxiously toward a parent while engaging in noncompliance to the parent's request. As noted previously, it is quite likely that many children, by stalling, can actually avoid having to comply with a command, because the parents will eventually acquiesce and either perform the requested chore themselves or simply forget about the fact that it was ever asked of the child. This is not the case under the present program. Parents are often quite surprised to find that the use of this simple procedure can result in improvements of up to 80% in their children's rate of compliance to their requests. Obviously, when compliance does occur to the first command, the parents will respond with appropriate praise, positive feedback, and perhaps even tokens or points to reinforce compliance further. This insures that the appropriate alternative behaviors to noncompliance are actually being encouraged with positive incentives. The combination of the positive aspects of this program with the time-out program frequently results in a rapid change in a child's non-compliance during the first week or two in which the time-out program has been implemented.

In our parent training program, I often take the opportunity to explain to the parents that the time-out part of the program is effective not because it is punitive or aversive to the child, but simply because it results in the child's missing out on opportunities to gain positive reinforcement while seated in the chair. To put it another way, it is what the child is missing while seated in the chair that makes the time-out chair an effective disciplinary measure. This should obviously lead the parents to conclude that if the child is not missing very much while seated in the chair, the time-out program is not likely to prove very effective at altering noncompliance. This particular situation arises when time out is used to discipline the child for not going to bed at night. Here the parents need simply ask themselves what it is that the child is missing by sitting in the chair. The answer is obviously "not much." It may therefore be necessary to keep the child on the chair for a somewhat longer period of time than would be normal during the daytime hours in order to make the time-out program sufficiently unpleasant. It is for this reason that the use of the time-out program during the first week after its introduction is restricted from bedtime situations. That is, the parents will be allowed to select any other behavior within the home to use the time-out program with during the subsequent week. They are not, however, to select bedtime or any behavior problems which occur in public places, as both of these situations will be dealt with in subsequent sessions.

This problem with time out arises not only during bedtime but also during mealtimes. Should the child misbehave during mealtime and wind up being placed in time out, the child is to miss the entire meal, or at least that part of the meal during which the child is to remain in the chair. If the child has missed only part of the meal before the time-out period is up, he or she is then permitted to return to the table and continue eating only as long as the rest of the family is eating. When the rest of the family has completed the meal, the child's food is to be removed even if the child has not completed the meal. Should the child miss all or part of a meal, the parents should not make any effort to make up this meal to the child by sneaking food to him or her between meals. This obviously subverts the purpose of time out in that the child has not actually missed anything while seated in the time-out chair. The parents can be reassured that the child is not likely to be harmed simply by missing one meal.

In some instances, the mother may have considerable problems getting the child into the time-out chair, especially if the child is older, as a result of physical aggression and resistance. The father, however, may have no such problems with enforcing time out. When this occurs, the mother should be told to use the time-out procedure at first only when the father is home. In addition, the child can be told that cooperation with a time-out procedure will result in a reduction in the time-out period and perhaps a return of a few of the tokens removed from the child for the misbehavior if the family is using a token system. Once the child becomes more cooperative with the procedure, the mother can use it in the father's absence.

Most parents will be more than willing to implement these procedures with the child during subsequent weeks. Some parents, however, often have concerns about the program or have some reservations about using it. One parental reaction is often that the parent has tried this type of program before but that it has not worked for them. Their attitude is one of "Why should we try it again?" The therapist can explain to the parents that it is quite likely that the earlier version of the time-out program was probably flawed in several respects. First, it is likely that the parents did not implement the time-out program until they were quite frustrated with the child and had repeated their commands many times in order to get the child to comply.

Second, most parents have used a time-out program in a manner that has allowed control of the time-out period to remain in the hands of the child. That is, they have told the child to go to his or her room and to stay there until *he or she* is ready to come out. This obviously leaves complete control over the time-out period to the child. A third mistake that parents have often made is in actually allowing the child to use his or her own room as a time-out location. There are clearly too many positive activities in which the child can engage in this room, and these will make the time-out period ineffective. I therefore believe it is appropriate to use a chair placed in a relatively dull location of the home yet still within plain view for supervision, instead of a chair in the child's own room. A fourth problem that many parents have had is that they have not used a time-out period that is long enough to be sufficiently unpleasant to the child. They often believe that a matter of a few minutes is sufficient for a child to be punished for noncompliance. Time-out intervals of this brief duration, especially with older children, are likely to be extremely ineffective. Finally, it is quite likely that the parents did not use time out consistently for noncompliance. On a day when they are in a certain mood and the child doesn't comply, they may implement time out after several repetitions of their initial command. On another day, they may simply choose to acquiesce to the child's noncompliance and perform the requested task themselves. Such inconsistency only undermines the effectiveness of the time-out program when it is employed.

Another reaction of some parents with which the therapist must be prepared to deal is the fact that certain families will resist the use of the spanking procedure with their child. As described above, there are several other alternatives that the family can employ but that, in my opinion, will prove less effective. Either of the two physical restraint procedures can be used, or the parents can merely increase the amount of time the child remains in the chair for leaving the chair against the parents' wishes. The third alternative is simply to implement a response-cost program in which the child must return previously earned tokens or points as a result of leaving the chair. Related to this parental concern is often a belief that they may have to spank the child quite frequently in order to get him or her to remain on the chair. The parents should be reassured that this occurs very rarely, and that most children usually follow the warning or need to be spanked only once in the entire program before they learn the relationship between staying in the chair and avoiding the spanking. The parents can be told that this will often result in a reduction in the number of spankings being administered to the child over the number of spankings being given before entering this program. Also, as noted above, the spanking is being administered at a time when the parents are quite likely to remain in full control of their behavior. In contrast, the point at which parents have typically implemented spanking in the past is the point in the interaction with the child at which they have repeated themselves quite frequently and become quite emotionally upset over the child's noncompliance; as a result, they may have implemented physical discipline that has gotten out of control.

Some parents will ask what they should do if the child misbehaves when there is a visitor in the home or when the child has friends over to play. Their concern here is that the time-out program may be embarrassing to the child or to themselves. My response is that the child should be placed in time out anyway and that the social embarrassment is simply one of the consequences for the child's misbehavior. If the child has friends over at the house at the time, these friends are simply told that they should go back to their homes and that the child will see them later. Using time out under such circumstances usually results in the child's being much less likely to misbehave when there is company in the home or when he or she is playing with friends. Both of these situations are usually severely problematic for hyperactive children prior to their entry into this program.

As noted earlier, there are several restrictions on this program's implementation during the first week of its introduction. It should not be used at bedtime because of the need to increase the time-out period in order to make the program effective. By waiting to deal with bedtime behavior problems in a later week of the program, the parents may be able to capitalize on improved compliance with the first commands assigned and to generalize this compliance to the child's bedtime behavior problems. In other words, once the child learns that the parents mean business when giving commands, the child may be more likely to comply with bedtime commands without ever requiring a time-out procedure for them. Also noted above is the restriction that time out is not to be used in public places until a subsequent session, at which time the special conditions of the use of time out in public places can be discussed with the family. Obviously, when a parent and a child are in a public place such as a shopping center or a grocery store, there is no time-out chair available for use with the child. In addition, there will be the added problem of public scrutiny of the parent's efforts to deal with the child. The parents will have to be prepared to deal with both of these problems, and this will take up sufficient time in a subsequent session so that it should not be pursued in any detail in the present one. A further restriction on the use of time out during this first week is that the parents should select only one or possibly two situations in which noncompliance occurs for use with the time-out program. This is done to make sure that the child is not receiving a disproportionate amount of punishment during any given week. It also is designed, again, to try to capitalize on possible generalization from one type of command to another type of command that may be given in the future; it is assumed that the child will comply with the new command because of earlier experience with time out for noncompliance.

The homework to be assigned for the subsequent week involves several activities. First, the parents are to continue, as they have previously done, to keep the diary of one or two noncompliant behaviors that they began during the second session of this program. The parents may choose to select one of these two noncompliant behaviors with which to use the time-out program— provided, of course, that these do not include bedtime or public behavior by the child. The second homework assignment involves having the parents select one type of noncompliant behavior with which to employ the time-out program for the subsequent week. They may also choose a second mis-behavior to implement later during this first week, should the use of the time-out program for the first behavior go so successfully that the child has little or no experience with time out. The final part of the homework assignment involves having the parents record their use of the time-out procedure, the noncompliant behavior with which time out is used, and the length of time for which the time-out interval lasts. These records will be reviewed in the subsequent session to insure that the time-out program is being used both ethically and effectively.

SESSION VI: EXTENDING TIME OUT
TO OTHER NONCOMPLIANT BEHAVIORS

This session is begun by a review of the diary kept by the family on the use of time out. If the time-out procedure has been implemented with one of the two noncompliant behaviors that the parents have been charting for several weeks, then the records should indicate that there has been some reduction in these noncompliant behaviors. How effectively the time-out procedure has been employed can be judged by the separate records being kept on when, for what, and for how long the time-out procedure has had to be implemented. The therapist may often be surprised by the fact that some parents will never have had to use the time-out procedure because of the effectiveness of the warnings which they gave to their children for their initial noncompliance. Other children may have had to experience the time-out procedure only once or twice before learning that noncompliance will be dealt with immediately by the use of time out. A good percentage of time in this session should be given to reviewing in detail the way in which the parents have used the time-out procedure and their feelings about its use. When necessary, the therapist can correct any problems the parents have had in implementing these procedures. Of course, the therapist also speaks with the family about the continued use of the "special time" play procedures introduced earlier in the program, as well as about the use of positive reinforcement programs for compliance by the child.

Once the previous week's records have been reviewed and discussed, the therapist can then have the parents select two other situations in which the child is likely not to comply with commands and direct them to extend the use of time out to these problem behaviors. One of these new situations to be dealt with can be bedtime, if it has proven a problem for the family in the past. The therapist need only instruct the parents that the child should remain in the time-out chair somewhat longer than (usually twice as long as) he or she would have had to stay in the chair during the daytime, in order to make the procedure effective in this case. Otherwise, the use of the procedure is identical to its use during the previous week. The only restriction on the use of time out for this subsequent week of the program is that it cannot be used in public situations where the child may not comply. This is done in the hope that positive compliance to commands given at home may generalize to commands given in public situations. The use of time out in public situations will be dealt with in the next session. If it appears that the parents are quite comfortable with and skillful in using time out, then this particular session will prove to be a brief one. The homework for this part of the program consists simply of having the parents select two additional home problem behaviors with which to implement the time-out program. In addition, they are to continue recording the one or two noncompliant behaviors that they began to record during the earlier sessions. Finally, they are to continue to keep a record of their use of the time-out procedure.

SESSION VII: MANAGING NONCOMPLIANCE IN PUBLIC PLACES

Once more, this session begins with a review of the homework assigned during the previous session. The therapist can gain some idea from the family's diary of the child's response to the extension of time out to the additional behaviors selected during the previous week. In addition, the therapist can also review the one or two noncompliant behaviors that the parents have been tracking since the second session. Obviously, these behaviors should have diminished by now as a result of the use of time out for noncompliance and positive attention for appropriate social behavior. Problems with the implementation of the time-out program in other situations around the home can be reviewed, and changes in the parents' style of using time out can be made in order to improve these problem situations. Assuming that the use of time out has been successful up to this point, the parents can be instructed to begin using the time-out program for all episodes of noncompliance within the home during the coming week. The parents need not continue to record any further noncompliant behaviors or the use of the time-out program unless there have been problems with the previous week's homework assignment that require additional attention and charting.

The therapist is now ready to introduce the new material dealing with the management of noncompliant behaviors in public situations. It should be stressed to the family at the outset that the key to success in utilizing disciplinary measures in public is to *anticipate* problem situations and to be prepared to manage them when they occur. The key word here is "anticipation," something most parents rarely exercise in preparing for possible problem behaviors from their children in public situations such as grocery stores, restaurants, churches, or shopping centers. Usually, parents wait until they have gotten into public situations and their children have begun to create problems for them before they begin to consider what they ought to do to manage the children's difficulties. By this time, it is too late—the parents are usually quite upset and are approaching a loss of emotional control, and the children are likely to be using a variety of coercive behaviors in an effort to resist the parents. The therapist should provide the family with a copy of the parent handout as shown in Figure 7.19 and permit them a few minutes to read over the handout before going over it with them in some detail.

Once the parents have finished reading this handout, the therapist can explain to them that there are three essential elements in the successful management of public behavior. First, as noted above, the parents need to anticipate the types of problems they are likely to encounter from this particular child before going into a public situation. The parents should consider the type of situation they are going into, the nature of the problems that the child has presented previously in such situations, and the nature of the behavior they desire from the child.

Second, the parents should be prepared to implement a particular reward system with the child to serve as an incentive for appropriate behavior in public situations. For example, the child can be given a poker chip or token to hold onto during the excursion into a public setting and then permitted to cash in this token for an extra privilege at home upon the family's return. Or, if the parents prefer, they may offer the child a small sum of money prior to going into the public situation, along with the instructions that the child cannot spend the money yet but may hold onto it. If the child behaves well in the public situation, he or she will then be permitted to use the money to purchase something at the end of the trip or to place it in a savings bank upon the family's return home. In either case, an incentive is implemented before entering any public situation to motivate the child further to display the appropriate behaviors in public.

Third, the parents should be prepared for the use of a modified time-out program if it is needed for dealing with child noncompliance. The same rules for time out apply in the store as at home. That is, it is to be implemented immediately when a 10-second period has elapsed following a command and the child has not complied. Whichever form of time out is to be used (different possibilities will be discussed below), the child is not to be removed from time out until he or she is quiet and until enough time has passed to

MANAGING NONCOMPLIANCE IN PUBLIC PLACES

After your child has been trained to comply with commands at home, it will be somewhat easier to deal with noncompliance in public places such as shopping centers, stores, and so on. There are two important aspects of managing your child in public. These are outlined below.

DEVELOPING POSITIVE BEHAVIOR AND COMPLIANCE

As you have learned previously, you must praise and attend to positive behavior by your child if you expect it to continue. This is just as true of behavior in public as it is of behavior at home.

1. When your child complies in public, be sure to praise and attend to his or her good behavior. Sometimes it is necessary to reward the child with money or to permit the child to purchase a small item for being good. This is because shopping centers and stores are designed to get your attention and buy items, and therefore your child's attention is being drawn to these items rather than to you. To keep the child's interest in following your commands, you may therefore have to offer something more than your attention and praise for compliance.

2. Before entering a public place, take your child aside and remind him or her of the rules he or she is to follow in that place. Have the child repeat these back to you. Then, when the child opens the door to the place, begin attending to him or her immediately for complying with the rules. This should help to nip problem behaviors in the bud.

3. Provide the child with responsibilities in helping you shop, if this is possible. Keeping a child busy with these activities can prevent him or her from engaging in undesirable ones.

4. If you are going to reward the child with money or some other tangible reward, it is sometimes helpful to let the child hold the reward while going through the store or public place with you so that the child sees what he or she will be rewarded with. If the child misbehaves, then take the reward away from him or her immediately, telling him or her why you have done so.

MANAGING NONCOMPLIANCE IN PUBLIC PLACES

If your child misbehaves in public, it should be dealt with immediately, just as at home. Instead of using the chair, however, you will have to use one of the following:

1. Stand the child in a dull corner of the store. The child will probably need to spend much less time in this time-out place, since it is clearly more aversive than sitting in the chair at home.

2. Take the child to a bathroom and have him or her stand in a dull corner of that room.

3. Take the child out to the car and have him or her sit on the floor of the back seat while you stand outside the door.

4. Use a black notebook and tell the child that if his or her name is written in it for misbehavior, he or she will have to sit on the chair when the family gets home. Some parents actually take a Polaroid snapshot of the chair to carry with them in public if they elect to use this "black book therapy."

Whether you reward a child for good behavior or discipline the child for negative behavior, it is always important to remember that the consequences should be immediate and should be consistent over time and between the parents.

FIGURE 7.19. Parent handout on ways of managing a hyperactive child's behavior in public, to be introduced during Session VII.

make the punishment unpleasant. Normally, in public places, much shorter time-out intervals can be used because of the heightened aversiveness of being placed in time out when other people are watching the child. In addition, the child is missing out on a great deal of activity in the store or other public situation, and this in itself makes time out more unpleasant.

Let us assume for ease of illustration of these principles that the parents are about to take the child into a grocery store. As the parents approach the store, they should stop outside the store for a moment before opening the door. The parents should then ask the child to repeat the rules about behavior in a public situation that have been explained to him or her; this is especially important if this is the first time the family has used this program with the child. Most often, these rules involve the child's staying within arm's reach of a parent, not touching anything, not asking for anything, and doing as directed at all times. The child must repeat each of these rules verbatim before being permitted to enter the store. If the child does not repeat the rules accurately, the parent can correct any mistakes and can ask the child to repeat the rules again. This form of self-instruction on the part of the child serves to reinforce the memory of the rules in the child's mind just before entering the store. Once the child has accurately repeated the rules that will govern behavior in these circumstances, the parents should then implement some incentive system for the child. As noted above, either money or tokens are acceptable, though I have often found that the use of the token system is obviously much less expensive and much easier to fit in with a home token system if one has been established by this time. At this point, the child can also be told that if the rules are broken, the token or mney will be taken away, and he or she will be placed in a dull corner of the store for several minutes of time out similar to time out in the chair at home. Once the parents have reviewed the rules with the child, established an incentive for following the rules, and explained the consequences for noncompliance, they may then open the door to the store and allow the child to enter.

As soon as the door is open, the parents should immediately scan the store for a corner or dull area of the store that can be used for the time-out program. Often, the area around the frozen food section, the hallway leading back to the bathrooms, or the doorways leading back to the meat-cutting area can all serve as excellent time-out corners. Where no appropriate corner is available, the parents should immediately look to see if there is a restroom in the grocery store. For relatively young children, mothers can use the women's room as a time-out place. Wherever time out is to be implemented in the store, the parents should never leave the child unattended; one parent should stand nearby while the child serves the time-out interval. In department stores, places located near elevators, stairways, or water fountains; restrooms; the credit department; or even those areas where men's and women's coats are on display often serve as relatively good places for the use of a time-out program.

After the parents have identified a time-out location, they should then begin paying positive attention to the child for following the rules. At the end of each aisle in the grocery store, the child is given some positive feedback for compliance with the rules specified outside the store. Simply waiting until the shopping trip is through to bestow praise is not sufficient to control a hyperactive child's behavior. Periodic praise and attention will be required to keep the child following the rules. The parents, as usual, should be very specific with their feedback and praise; they should let the child know that it is his or her compliance with the rules with which they are satisfied. For older children, involving them in some responsibility in helping with the shopping can often help to subvert the development of noncompliance or disruptive behavior.

In many cases, there is no acceptable location for time out in the public situation. In this case, the parents have three alternatives to using the regular time-out program. The first is that of using the car as the time-out location. This, of course, is based on the assumption that the car is within a short distance from the store and is easily accessible. If the car is to be used for time out, the child should be taken there immediately upon the occurrence of noncompliance and requested to sit in the back seat, either on the seat or on the floor, with the typical rules for the use of time out applying in this situation. One parent stands outside the car or sits in the front seat of the car while the child serves the time-out period. If the parent is to remain outside the car, he or she should be sure to retain the keys to the car so as not to be locked out. The child should never be left unattended while serving a time-out period in an automobile.

If the family car is not accessible for time out, then the parents can use a small black spiral notebook to record the child's misbehavior. If this method is to be employed, the parents should go over the use of the notebook with the child before entering the store. In this instance, the parents explain to the child that if he or she misbehaves, the misbehavior will be written in the black book, and the child will have to sit on the time-out chair immediately upon the family's return home. It may take one or two shopping trips involving problems before the child eventually learns that the parents in fact mean what they say. Once the child learns this association, the black spiral notebook often can serve as an excellent intermediary form of discipline when no actual time-out location is available. As noted earlier and in Figure 7.19, one family found it helpful to take a Polaroid picture of the time-out chair at home and to keep it with the black spiral notebook at all times.

If the parents choose not to use the notebook, then simply having a pen or pencil available during any trip to a public place can help as a form of discipline. With this method, when the child begins to resist compliance or to become disruptive, the parents simply place a small hash mark on the child's wrist and tell the child that he or she will have to spend 10 minutes in the time-out chair at home for every mark on the wrist at the end of the trip.

Again, if this method is to be used, the parents should review the method with the child prior to entering the store. In each of these cases, as with the use of time out at home, the key to the program is that the time out or other disciplinary measure is to be implemented immediately upon the occurrence of noncompliance. The parents should not engage in any repeated warnings or repeated commands, and should not fail to follow through with at least one of these consequences when noncompliance occurs.

I have often seen that many child behavior problems can be effectively eliminated with the use of this program if the parents simply spend some time anticipating situations in which they are likely to encounter problems and implementing some incentive system to motivate the child toward greater compliance with commands. In addition, reviewing the rules that will govern the child's behavior in the public situation before entering that situation serve effectively to remind the child what is expected of him or her. These three basic rules, along with the specifics of the program already discussed above, can be used in virtually every public situation in which a family is likely to take a child. This includes a visit with the child to the home of a friend or relative, or even long family automobile trips. In the case of the car trip, the family should also bring several toys with which the child can play during the extended time expected for the trip. Again, using an incentive system and reviewing the rules before entering the car to begin the trip are often quite effective in precluding the development of noncompliance and disruptive behavior.

In analyzing my previous treatment cases, it has been my impression that one of the greatest causes of failure to implement rewards and discipline in public situations is the parents' embarrassment at having to deal with the child in a situation where they are likely to be observed by other adults. This can become especially problematic for a parent when the child is showing extremely disruptive behavior and thus is drawing attention to both the parent and the child in the public situation. Here, the parent may experience a great deal of guilt, embarrassment, and frustration with the child, both because of the behavior problems and because the parent does not know what to do and fears being judged negatively by other adults in the situation. I have often found this to be the case even after we have discussed the methods that the family may use in a public situation if they should encounter problems with the child. Therefore, at this time, it is helpful to review with the parents certain things in their own behavior and in their own way of thinking about the public management of children's behavior in an effort to show them that they are a part of the problem in this situation.

One of the best ways that I have discovered of alleviating the guilt or embarrassment experienced by parents in such situations is a brief review of the principles of rational–emotive therapy as set forth by Albert Ellis and more recently by Wayne Dyer (see Ellis & Harper, 1975, and Dyer, 1977, in

"Suggested Reading"). Briefly, it is necessary to show the parents that it is neither the scrutiny of the other adults in the situation nor the child's misbehavior that is causing them to feel the way that they do (i.e., guilty, embarrassed, or ashamed). It is what they *think* about these events that causes them to experience these negative emotions. Getting the parents to discuss these thoughts and the conclusions about themselves to which they eventually lead is often quite helpful in revealing this point to them. For instance, when many parents note that other people are watching them deal with their child, they begin to engage in a series of thoughts and self-statements that sounds something like this: "This person is looking at me because I am not handling my child properly. Good parents would be able to deal with their children effectively and would not have the problems that I have. The fact that my child is acting up must mean that I am a terrible parent and am not capable of properly raising my child. I am, in short, a failure." These or highly similar statements often run through the mind of parents faced with the public scrutiny of other adults while trying to handle their children in public situations. Once the parents realize that their thinking is creating their emotional reaction to this situation, they can then be shown that changing the way they think about the situation can result in very different emotional reactions to the situation. The indirect result of making such a change in thinking is improved management of the child.

Instead of engaging in a variety of negative self-statements that clearly result in feelings of failure and shame, the parents should replace these self-statements with more positive ones that clearly state that the parents are doing the right thing. For instance, the parents can state to themselves, "I am this child's teacher, and if I do not deal with this behavior immediately whenever it occurs, then I am not being an effective parent to this child. It is therefore important that I deal with this child's inappropriate behavior whenever it occurs. It would be nice if I did not have to deal with my child in public when others are watching me, but I must if I expect him or her to grow up to be a better behaved person who has more self-control. Thus, I am a good parent and am doing the right thing by managing my child's misbehavior in this situation." The therapist should then ask the parents to describe the worst possible things that can happen to them for attempting to discipline their child publicly for misbehavior. By going over these possible consequences, the parents can come to see that all of them are trivial in virtually every instance. This simple review of the manner in which one's thoughts actually affect one's emotions can have a striking influence on a family's success at implementing particular behavior modification programs in public situations.

The therapist then asks the parents whether they anticipate any other problems in implementing the above-noted procedures with the child during the coming week. The therapist can also encourage the parents to plan one or two bogus shopping trips during the coming week; the only purpose of these trips should be to practice this part of the program. In this way, if the child should act up, the parents will be fully capable of dealing with the problem because they will not have any other agenda for that trip. In addition, once the child learns through such a shopping trip that the parents will deal firmly with noncompliance, then when the parents must go out for a shopping trip that has other purposes, the child has already been exposed to the rules of the program. In essence, the homework assignment for the subsequent week is to have the family plan at least several trips out into public with the child, during which they will try to use the above procedures. They are to record these trips, their use of the procedures, and the outcome of the methods in the notebook that they have been keeping to date. The parents need not keep any other records for the coming week than these, unless problems during the previous week with the use of time out in the home situation have been encountered. When no such problems have been encountered, the therapist can ask the family to use the time-out program for all noncompliant behaviors within the home. In addition, if the parents have been continuing to repeat regular household rules to the child on a daily basis, they should be told to stop repeating any of these rules. Instead, once the child is discovered to be violating a household rule that he or she is clearly aware of, the child is to go immediately to the time-out chair without the parents ever repeating the household rule again. For instance, if the family has a rule that the child is not to go to the refrigerator without asking, the parent can warn the child once against this infraction if it should occur. At any future time, should the child be found in the refrigerator without permission, he or she is to go immediately to the time-out chair without any further restatement of the household rule. We have found that this part of the program helps the child to remember and internalize household rules and rules of social conduct with others without needing to have them repeated on a daily basis.

SESSION VIII: MANAGING FUTURE MISBEHAVIOR

For many parents, this will be the last session other than the booster session to take place one month after this one. In this particular session, the therapist again begins with a review of the previous homework assignment and the extent to which it has been successful in its goals. When problems have been encountered in the use of time out or incentive systems in public places, the therapist can correct the parents' style of using these methods and assign further homework in this area, if needed, for the subsequent week. Often, the parents have had little trouble implementing the methods used in public situations, and they are typically quite pleased with the results. The therapist then moves on to the major purpose of this session, which is to teach the parents a general strategy for use with any future misbehavior that may develop.

Instead of introducing any new material at this point, the therapist simply reviews some of the major principles and concepts in which the family has been trained during the previous seven sessions. These basically include providing immediate and consistent consequences to the child, determining the behavior that the parents would like the child to engage in and then designing an incentive system for it, and implementing a disciplinary method for inappropriate behavior when it occurs. The consequences should always be immediate, specific to the appropriate or inappropriate behavior in question, and agreed upon by both parents to enhance consistency in the parents' dealings with the child. It may also be helpful to review some of the conclusions from the first two sessions on hyperactivity in children and on parent–child interactions.

The parents are then ready to be taught by the therapist what they should do if a new behavior problem with which they have had no prior experience develops. First, the family should begin to keep records on the occurrence of the misbehavior, the social contexts in which it is occurring, the number of times it occurs each day, and any events that can be identified as precipitating it. This is a relatively easy step, as the parents have already had practice in keeping records throughout the program. Second, the parents should review the number of times they are repeating their commands to the child in an effort to control this particular problem behavior. They will often be quite surprised to find that they probably have slipped back into the habit of repeating their commands very frequently without consequating the child for the noncompliance. This obviously suggests that they should also review the consequences that are accruing to the child for this new misbehavior. Third, the parents should attempt to define the appropriate alternative behavior they would like the child to display instead of the new misbehavior. Fourth, the parents should then attempt to design an incentive or reward program that will motivate the child to demonstrate this appropriate alternative behavior. Fifth, the parents must also decide what disciplinary program they will implement for the occurrence of the inappropriate behavior. They have already had experience with the use of time-out systems, response cost, and several alternatives to the time-out program for public misbehaviors. Sixth, once the parents have implemented both the reward and disciplinary programs, they should continue to keep records on the occurrence of the inappropriate behavior and to review these records at frequent intervals. The programs can then be altered as needed if it appears that they have not been initially successful. The parents are encouraged to allow their reward and disciplinary programs to stay in effect for at least 2 weeks before judging the effectiveness of these programs. Parents are often very quick to give up programs before the programs have had a chance to demonstrate whether or not they are actually effective at controlling inappropriate behavior. If the initial programs do not appear to be successful, subsequent modifications also prove unsuccessful, and no other ways of changing the program suggest themselves to the parents, then the parents should be encouraged to contact the therapist for a reinitiation of a brief treatment interval. Assuming that the parents follow all of the steps above, it is highly unlikely that they will need to contact the therapist again for the development of minor misbehaviors in the child.

At the close of this session, the therapist should schedule a follow-up session to take place about a month later; at this session, the therapist will review with the parents any problems that have developed over the previous month and the continuing degree of the program's success for the parents. As Patterson (1976) has noted, parents often tend to rely more on punishment methods, even after training in both reinforcement and punishment, once parent training has been completed. This may result partly from the fact that the punishment methods have more immediate success in temporarily elimi- nating inappropriate child behavior. The reinforcement methods, on the other hand, may have less effect in the short run but are more likely to be successful at developing appropriate alternative behaviors to the inappropri- ate one. The therapist will probably have to reiterate the need for the family to continue to develop and use various reward and incentive systems with the child, so as to continue to reinforce appropriate and compliant behavior. During the booster session, the therapist should also discuss with the family his or her "open door policy" if future problems with the child develop. Although the parents have been trained in what to do if a future behavior problem develops, they should also be told that some problems may well occur that they are not capable of handling. In this case, the parents should not feel any qualms about contacting the therapist again for assistance with the new problem.

OUTCOMES OF PARENT TRAINING

This parent training program has a number of effects on various parent and child behaviors, as well as on family functioning in general. Some of these effects are illustrated in a single case study involving two children and their parents who received the parent training program on an individual basis. The two children, Tom and Dave, were observed during a baseline phase in which no treatment was provided to their families and during a parent training phase in which the mothers received individual instruction in the methods outlined in this chapter. The effects of the training program on certain maternal and child behaviors, measured on one scale as well as on several questionnaires, are illustrated in Figures 7.20 through 7.22.

Since the training was intended to have a direct effect on the responses of the mothers to the behavior of their children, it is important to examine first the results for the mothers' behavior. Figure 7.20 shows the percentage of maternal commands given to each child across each of the two phases of treatment. In addition, it illustrates the percentage of positive maternal responses to appropriate child compliance when such compliance occurred. Both of these maternal behaviors were assessed on the Response Class Matrix described in Chapter 4 and in Appendix A of this book. As Figure 7.20 shows, the percentage of maternal commands to both children showed a dramatic decrease throughout the parent training program. Tom's mother's

FIGURE 7.20. Percentages of maternal commands and of maternal positive responses to compliance from two hyperactive boys, measured on the Response Class Matrix during a parent training program for noncompliance.

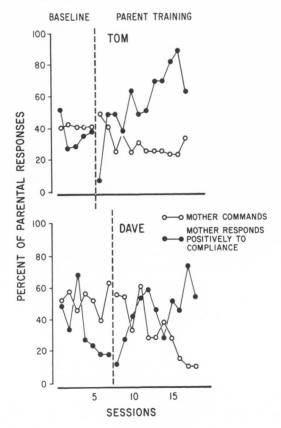

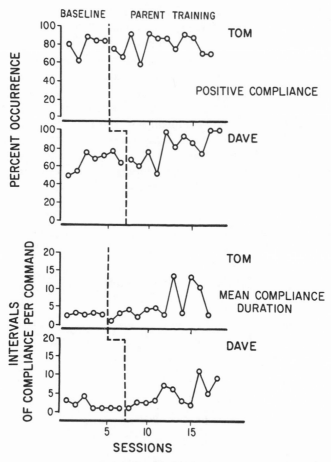

FIGURE 7.21. Percentage of child positive compliance to commands and mean compliance duration for two hyperactive boys, measured on the Response Class Matrix during a parent training program.

baseline level of commands shows that commands initially made up about 40% of the interactions she had with her child. This was reduced to approximately 22% toward the end of the parent training program. This is an 85% improvement in the mother's rate of commands to her son. Similar results are seen for Dave's mother as well, whose pretreatment level of commands shows that commands constituted between 40% and 60% of her interactions with her child; these dropped to between 15% and 20% toward the end of parent training. It can also be seen in Figure 7.20 that the percentage of positive maternal responses to child compliance increased dramatically throughout the parent training program. Both mothers demonstrated a two-

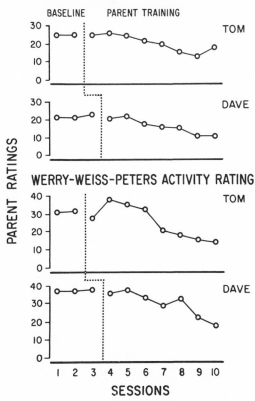

CONNERS PARENT'S QUESTIONAIRE

FIGURE 7.22. Scores on the Conners Parent Symptom Questionnaire and the Werry–Weiss–Peters Activity Rating Scale for two hyperactive boys during a parent training program.

fold to threefold increase in the percentage of positive attention they provided to their children for their compliance as a result of the parent training program. These results coincide with the heavy emphasis placed during the initial sessions of parent training on providing positive attention to appropriate child behaviors.

The rates of positive compliance demonstrated by both boys, again measured on the Response Class Matrix, are illustrated in Figure 7.21. These data indicate that Tom complied with approximately 70% to 85% of his mother's commands during the baseline phase, with little further improvement in this behavior during the parent training program. Although it may seem as if this child was showing normal rates of compliance prior to and during the parent training program, these results should be viewed in conjunction with the level of maternal commands being given during the baseline phases for both boys (see Figure 7.20). An examination of both the rates of maternal directiveness and the rates of child compliance shows that, although the children were demonstrating high rates of compliance prior to treatment as recorded by this observation method, the mothers apparently did not find this level of compliance or its quality especially satisfactory. That is, although the children may have shown attempts to comply with maternal commands prior to treatment, the quality of their compliance and their ability to sustain their compliance were substandard. This is shown in the high rate of maternal commands needed to keep the children on task during these baseline phases, and it was confirmed by the opinions of the observers recording the children's behavior. Thus, although Tom does not show any substantial increase in positive compliance as measured by this coding system, one can obviously assume that the quality of his compliance improved substantially, as the rate of maternal commands decreased during the parent training program by an impressive degree. The results for Dave in Figure 7.21 show more obvious effects of the parent training program on child compliance. Prior to treatment, Dave appears to have shown compliance with approximately 60% to 70% of the maternal commands given. During treatment, especially the latter phases of treatment when the time-out program was introduced, Dave's level of compliance improved to such an extent that he was now complying with 80% to 90% of his mother's commands. These data, when viewed in conjunction with the remarkable decrease in the level of maternal commands seen during treatment (see Figure 7.20), indicate that both Dave's rate of compliance and his quality of compliance must have improved considerably as a result of treatment.

A third way of demonstrating improvement as a result of parent training is to readminister periodically the Conners PSQ and the WWPARS, both commonly used rating scales of hyperactive behavior. These scales are discussed in Chapter 3 of this book. The results for the parent-completed rating scales are shown in Figure 7.22 for both boys. This figure demonstrates that both boys showed pretreatment ratings on both questionnaires that fall well within that range considered to indicate hyperactivity (scores above 15 on the Conners PSQ and scores above 20 on the WWPARS). During treatment, there is a gradual decrease in the level of ratings of behavior problems for these children, with some of the scores eventually falling within the normal range of ratings on these questionnaires. The scores for both boys improved by as much as 60% to 100% over the scores given during the pretreatment phases. These results suggest that in terms of changes in maternal behavior toward the children, child compliance to maternal commands, and parent ratings of hyperactivity, the parent training program is quite effective in rendering improvements in parent–child interactions.

Besides these highly specific changes in parent–child interactions, parents often report other, less easily measured changes in the functioning of the family as a result of the training program. One of these is improvement in the behavior of siblings of a hyperactive child following the training of the parents. It is obvious that the parents are utilizing the techniques with other children in the family besides the hyperactive child, and this often results in remarkable improvements in the behavior of the siblings. Patterson (1976) has reported similar findings as a result of his parent training program, and Forehand (1979) has published data on a similar parent training program that document these chain reaction effects.

Some parents also report improvements in their relationships with their spouses as a function of improvements in their ability to cope with their hyperactive children's behavior. This is probably an indirect effect of the decreased arguing over how to manage the hyperactive children's behavior. In addition, it may also result from improvements in the self-esteem of the parents now that they feel they can competently manage the hyperactive children's misbehavior. For whatever reason, the reduction in the amount of stress within families that can result from the effective use of the principles in this parent training program can have many positive effects beyond those specifically seen in parent–hyperactive child interactions.

One change that is often difficult to measure objectively is that achieved in the parents' attitude toward a child's behavior and toward the reasons for any misbehavior the child may continue to show. As a result of the initial sessions in the parent training program, the parents have come to accept the idea that they must learn to cope on a daily basis with the child's misbehavior, instead of expecting any program to result in "normalization" of their hyperactive child. Even though remarkable improvements may occur in the child's misbehavior following parent training, the parents are told that the child is still at risk for future behavior and academic problems because of the hyperactivity. This attitude seems to cause many of the parents to re-examine their view of the causes of a hyperactive child's misbehavior. Before training, many parents viewed their hyperactive children as intentionally displaying misbehavior in order to disrupt family functioning and irritate the parents. By the end of training, such parents have come to realize that the children may not have complete control over all of their problems all of the time. Thus, they come to expect that the children may remain somewhat impulsive, inattentive, and occasionally noncompliant and that the children cannot necessarily help displaying some of these problems. On the other hand, these parents have learned that through the use of the methods demonstrated during the training program, the children can learn some degree of control over their problems, even if it is not complete amelioration of the problem behaviors.

AMENDING THE CORE PARENT TRAINING PROGRAM

Although the aforementioned program for training parents of hyperactive children is often sufficient to result in remarkable improvements in many child behaviors, other problems that are not directly related to noncompliance may persist. It may therefore be necessary for the therapist to add several extra sessions with the parents in order to focus on these additional problems and their remediation. Some of the problems likely to remain are briefly discussed here; references will be made to articles dealing more fully with the treatment of these additional problems. One problem that often persists beyond the core parent training program is that of getting the child to accomplish homework in a relatively positive atmosphere. While this can obviously be reconstrued as noncompliance, it is sometimes necessary to treat homework accomplishment in a slightly different fashion. Because the accomplishment of school homework often takes an extended period of time, it may be necessary for the parents to break the homework period into shorter intervals, perhaps by using a timer, and to permit the child to have breaks between these work intervals. The parents can be instructed to require that the child accomplish a certain quota of problems during each 15- to 20-minute work period, with praise, positive attention, and rewards contingent upon accomplishing the quota. Often, parents can employ the token or point system discussed earlier with homework accomplishment. Should the child fail to accomplish the assigned tasks in the allotted interval, then tokens or points can be removed as a negative consequence. A number of other guidelines should be given to parents for working with a hyperactive child during homework accomplishment. Some of these are taken from an article by Gerald Spadafore (see Spadafore, 1977, in "Suggested Reading"). These guidelines are as follows:

1. The parents should never attempt to do homework with a child immediately after school. Normally, for any hyperactive child, the stay in school has probably been a quite restrictive one and has taxed the child's self-control. The child should therefore have sufficient time after school to play outside with friends or to engage in other recreational activities. It is often best to leave the homework until after dinner. For those hyperactive children receiving medication, working on homework after school proves additionally problematic because of the side effects often associated with the "washing out" of the medication each day. Hyperactive children are often quite irritable, active, emotionally sensitive, and prone to crying at these periods in the afternoon, and this is not conducive to homework accomplishment.

2. If the parents are angry with the child, they should not attempt to engage in tutoring the child over homework. Nor should the tutoring period be used as a punishment for the child for poor schoolwork that day. The homework time should be relatively positive in nature, with incentives being used as noted above to motivate the child to accomplish a certain quota of problems during small intervals of homework activity. Parents who are impatient, chronically angry with their hyperactive child, or often tired themselves after a day of work should not attempt to engage in working on homework with the child. Such parents are best advised to seek a tutor to help with the child for two to three afternoons each week.

3. The hyperactive child's impulsivity, poor attention span, and difficulty in following rules will often interfere with his or her ability to work on homework independently of adult supervision. Independent work can be greatly facilitated if the parents make up a card containing a list of instructions the child is to follow when working on homework. This, of course, is only suitable for hyperactive children who are already reading. Contained on the card can be several statements dealing with general problem-solving skills. Such statements can include the following:

a.   Repeat the problem out loud or describe out loud what it is you have been asked to do.

b. Ask yourself whether you have seen this problem or similar problems before.

c.   If so, do the solutions which were used with the previous problems seem to apply here?

d. Before working on the problem, describe some of its features.

e. Talk yourself through the problem out loud.

f. When you have reached a solution, check your answer carefully by rereading the description of the problem.

g. Praise or compliment yourself if you think you've done a good job.

By having these statements printed on a card in language geared to that of the child's level of development, the parents can give the child a concrete reminder of problem-solving activities that can be helpful for accomplishing any homework assignment. It may be necessary at first for a parent to remain with the child and periodically to ask the child to restate the descriptions on the card while working on particular problems. Eventually, it is hoped that the child will internalize these problem-solving statements.

4. The parents should be taught never to nag, to lecture, or to insult the child's integrity while the child is working on homework. Such remarks only add a negative atmosphere to what may already be a strained parent–child relationship and are unlikely to motivate the child further to desire to do homework with the parent. The use of the token or point system for reward and punishment is often sufficient to consequate the child's activities.

5. Throughout the homework period, the parent should occasionally use the positive attending skills learned during the initial sessions of parent training. Such remarks as "I really like it that you're paying such close attention to your homework," or "You really seem to be doing a fantastic job getting your homework done," are phrases that can help to motivate the child further to independent homework accomplishment.

6. Homework should be accomplished in a quiet and comfortable location where there are few distractors or interruptions to the child's activities. Televisions, radios, stereos, toys, or other distractors should not be in the setting used for homework because of their high appeal to the child. The child should work at a table with a comfortable chair, good lighting, and appropriate homework supplies, such as paper, pencils, crayons, scissors, and so forth.

7. The parents can be instructed to try to personalize the learning activity whenever possible. That is, when a child requests help with a particular problem, the parent can remark that this problem is similar to one that may arise in an area of greater interest to the child, such as sports, automobiles, models, cooking, fashion, and so on. This can often make it easier for the child to understand the problem, and it can certainly enhance motivation for attending to homework. The same Socratic method of teaching that the therapist has used with the parents throughout the above parent training program can also be taught to the parents for use with the child, especially if the child is older, for use during homework. As before, this method simply means that the parent asks leading questions of the child but permits the child to reach the solution independent of the parent's direct help.

In addition to sessions for homework problems, additional sessions may have to be scheduled in order to treat such frequent problems as enuresis, encopresis, aggression, stealing, or lying. Although some of these difficulties may improve with parent training for noncompliance progresses, others may still remain. Treatment programs that have been effective with enuresis and encopresis are described in a study by C. Eugene Walker (1978; see "Suggested Reading"). While aggression, lying, and stealing can be handled through the core parent training program discussed above, it may be necessary to amend the program slightly for these unacceptable behaviors. Because these behaviors are often low-rate, and frequently unobserved, they are often difficult to treat. Hence, when they do occur, the parents should attempt to make the learning experience surrounding the consequences very salient. This may call for the parents to raise their voices substantially, correct the child immediately, warn the child severely about consequences that will occur in the future if this recurs, and then place the child directly in a time-out location without any repeated commands or warnings. When necessary, the adult neighbors of the family can be asked to help monitor the child's behavior outside the home and to report back to the family when any instance of these inappropriate behaviors occur so that they may be dealt with swiftly. Whatever the target selected for these additional sessions, continued recording of problem behaviors by the parents is an essential part of insuring that the treatment methods are followed outside the sessions, as well as of documenting the changes that may be occurring in the child's behavior.

It is often necessary to combine the parent training program with other treatments for the hyperactive child or for other family members. In some cases, this may involve the use of stimulant medications, despite the fact that parent training may have improved the child's behavior. In cases in which children were on medication before parent training began, the therapist can notify the physician supervising the medication that it might be worthwhile to attempt a reduction in medication following the parent training program. When financial, health, or personal problems continue to plague one or both parents, the family may need to be referred for additional help from other professionals. The therapist should therefore never view the parent training program as the sole intervention needed for hyperactive children or their families.

When resources permit, there are a number of "luxuries" that can be helpful in training parents to manage their hyperactive child. Should a clinic playroom with a one-way mirror be available, this can, as noted earlier, allow the therapist to model the appropriate parental behaviors with the child while the parents observe the interaction. Subsequently, each parent can be placed in the playroom with the child and asked to practice the new skills being taught with the child directly. The purchase of a "bug in the ear" apparatus (available from Lafayette Instrument Company, Lafayette, Ind.) can enhance the usefulness of this playroom further by permitting the therapist to talk to a parent through a small telemetered hearing device so that the child is not aware of the therapist's comments. This can greatly assist the therapist in shaping the parents' behavior directly as they interact with the child and the problem behaviors that the child presents. Should videotaping equipment be available, it is often helpful to videotape each parent's practice session and to review the tape subsequently with the parent, pointing out both the strong and weak points of the parent's use of the technique under instruction. Finally, if small cassette tape recorders are available, one can be loaned to the parents to take home and record certain problem situations with the child. This provides the therapist with even greater information on the manner in which the parents are handling the particular problem situation and on the specific child behaviors that are causing the problem.

Another way of amending the core parent training program discussed above is to train groups of parents rather than individual families. In many clinics, group parent training is necessary because of the high demand for these programs and the small number of therapists available to teach them.

When the program is to be taught to groups, it may be necessary to extend the sessions from 1 hour to 2 hours each week in order to cover the material within each session. The additional time is also needed so that each set of parents has a chance to review the previous week's assignments and activities with the therapist. This can often benefit the other members of the group, who can learn what types of problems the other parents may have and how the therapist recommends dealing with them. In addition, it fosters a sense of cameraderie and group cohesiveness when parents share problems that are common to other members of the group. This group cohesiveness can be fostered in the initial sessions by having each set of parents introduce themselves and describe their child and the nature of the problems that brought them to the parent training program. When this is done in a group of six to eight families, it often clearly demonstrates to each set of parents that they are not alone in the types of problems they have been having with their hyperactive child. The therapist can facilitate this process by directly relating the similarity between one family's difficulties and those of another that have already been brought up within the group. In conducting such parent training groups, it is even more essential that a Socratic style of teaching be used to permit the group to come to the conclusions that the therapist desires. Direct lecturing should be avoided where possible, as it often cuts down on the appeal of the group sessions over time. Since the children of the parents in the group will not be coming for the sessions, it will be necessary for the therapist to role-play those methods under instruction in a given session. This can be done by selecting one parent in the group to serve as a child and modeling the techniques with this parent. Otherwise, the procedures for conducting a group as opposed to those for conducting individual parent training are quite similar to those outlined above.

TREATING HYPERACTIVE ADOLESCENTS AND THEIR FAMILIES

The core parent training program outlined earlier is most effective with children 12 years of age or younger. It can, however, be utilized with 13- or 14-year-old hyperactive children who prove quite socially and emotionally immature. In most cases, once however, a child is older than 12 or 13, the nature of intervention with the family takes a quite different turn. In this case, the therapy sessions must involve the adolescent, and the procedures are quite similar to many behavioral family therapy programs. Such therapy sessions rely quite strongly on the child's motivation for treatment. When the child is unconcerned about the problems or is actually adverse to therapy, it is best not attempted, since it is often likely to prove unsuccessful. However, when there exists even a modicum of interest in treatment, the hyperactive adolescent and his or her family can be started in individual family therapy on a weekly basis. The therapist is warned that such treatments often last considerably longer than the typical training program described earlier. This is true mainly because of the rather long history of problem behaviors for the hyperactive adolescent, as well as the need for involving the adolescent directly in the treatment program. In general, the therapy sessions consist of reviewing the child's responsibilities and the household rules that apply to the child with the child and the parents. The therapist must also serve as a negotiator during these sessions, helping the parents to reach some agreement with the child on the rules that will be applied to the child's behavior. Once some agreement is reached on what is expected of the child, then the parents and child can work together to establish consequences for compliance or noncompliance with the agreements. These most often consist of the awarding or withdrawing of privileges, such as using the telephone, watching TV, using the family car, and so on. They may also include "grounding" for more serious infractions of rules. It is often helpful at this point to use the behavioral contracting procedures outlined by Richard Stuart (1971; see "Suggested Reading"). The therapist, the parents, and the adolescent specify the behaviors expected of the adolescent, as well as the consequences for compliance and noncompliance, in the contract. The parents and child then sign the contract, and the contract is posted in a relatively obvious place in the family home, such as on a bulletin board in the child's room, on the side of the refrigerator, or on a noteboard in the family kitchen. Whether or not the contract has been abided by during a particular week is reviewed in subsequent therapy sessions; the contract may have to be amended, or new contracts may have to be introduced for additional behavior problems.

The procedures outlined in Chapter 6 for the typical approach to behavioral therapy can also be implemented during interventions with adolescent hyperactive children. In brief, these procedures include selecting mutually agreed upon target behaviors of the adolescent; reviewing the precipiting factors of these problem behaviors; discussing alternative appropriate behaviors to the inappropriate behaviors; specifying consequences that will accrue to the child for compliance or noncompliance in a particular situation; and having the family keep records on the subsequent occurrence of the problem behaviors. In subsequent sessions, the efficacy of the intervention is reviewed and amended where necessary. When intervention is first being attempted with a hyperactive adolescent, the likelihood of success in treatment is often quite small. For many years, the child's behavior will have proven quite successful at manipulating the parents, and it will be most difficult to change these coercive strategies in any short-term therapy program. Furthermore, by this age the child has developed a sense of self and a will of his or her own that may often run contrary to the parents' desires and expectations for the adolescent. Attempting at this point to treat an adolescent who does not want help, in spite of the parents' wishes that help be obtained, is quite similar to trying to force any adult into a psychological intervention that the adult does not desire. In short, the outcome is often quite unsuccessful. On the other hand, when the adolescent seems sufficiently motivated for treatment, appears to have some degree of self-awareness as to the nature of his difficulties, and has established a good rapport with the professional, therapy can prove quite successful.

PLACEMENT OF THE HYPERACTIVE CHILD
OUTSIDE THE HOME FOR TREATMENT

On rare occasions, a hyperactive child's behavior becomes so difficult and distressing to the family that the parents are incapable of dealing with it within the context of the home. Children who have become so aggressive that they threaten the physical well-being of other neighborhood children or class-mates; children who continue to violate household rules such as curfews, to steal, or to lie; or children who generally endanger their own lives or those of others may require placement outside the home for treatment. Such treatment can occur either within a residential treatment center or within a group home facility. Sometimes, temporary placement of the child outside the home gives the parents a temporary respite from the child while the child is undergoing closer supervision and treatment in an inpatient facility or group home. During the child's placement, the family can attend parent training and family therapy sessions at the treatment facility to ease the child's transition back into the home.

A number of considerations apply in the decision to remove the child from the home. One of these obviously is the severity, chronicity, dangerous-ness, and resistance to previous treatments of the child's problems. The second is the ability of the family to deal with the child's difficulties. Single-parent families, or families with parents whose own psychiatric difficulties preclude their effective coping with a hyperactive child, may often require removal of the child from the home for temporary treatment. As noted earlier, if children present a danger to themselves or others within the home, the school, or the community at large, this may be legal grounds for placing such children within a residential facility. In some instances, a child may have been resistant to medication trials within the home or school. Such a child may therefore be temporarily placed in an inpatient program where greater supervision of the medication trials can occur.

Of course, in deciding whether or not to place a child outside the home, the therapist needs to consider the possible detrimental effects of such a separation on the child and the family. For instance, removing the child from the home may relieve the parents of any feeling of responsibility for managing the child's difficulties. With the child gone, the family may have little motivation to continue any treatment program. In addition, some residential care facilities might place the child with more "hardened" predelinquent adolescents or with other children who could serve as negative role models for the child. Certainly, these factors must be weighed in any decision to remove the child from the home for treatment purposes.

If the decision to remove the child seems likely, the therapist must consider the resources that are available within the local community to handle the child and the length of the waiting lists for various institutions. In the Milwaukee area, for example, long waiting lists are often encountered, and this fact makes residential treatment an unlikely source of help during any crisis with a child. The therapist must also consider the expense of the treatment facility to the family and the possibility of any subsidizing of the expense by third-party payees or county or state agencies. Whichever facility is chosen, the therapist should insure that the facility will work closely with the family in efforts to ease the child's transition back into the home. Sometimes, only day treatment facilities may be needed if the problems of the child in question have primarily occurred at school; the day treatment facility serves as an appropriate alternative to the school setting. Although generally infrequent, the need to place a hyperactive child outside the home occurs often enough to require that a therapist dealing with hyperactive children have some awareness of the programs that are available within the local community or state to deal with such children when placement outside the home is necessary.

SUMMARY

In conclusion, this chapter has attempted to present a variety of specific approaches toward training parents of hyperactive children to cope with their children's problems. Emphasis has been on objective, empirically demonstrated behavioral methods that are primarily focused on the noncompliance of the child to adult commands, situational rules, or rules governing social conduct. The approach for the parents stresses coping with rather than curing a child's difficulties; while improvements may be made in the child's behavior problems, but some problems are likely to remain, or others are more likely to develop in the future. Whichever methods are employed, the parents are trained to expect that interventions with such a child will often be necessary throughout his or her development, as problems that have not been previously encountered may occur. In many cases, training of the parents will often be combined with psychopharmacologic interventions, training of teachers to handle the child within the classroom, and perhaps additional psychiatric or psychologic help to the parents or siblings for their own behavioral or psychological difficulties.

SUGGESTED READING

Bell, R. Q., & Harper, L. *Child effects on adults.* New York: Wiley, 1977.

Dyer, W. *Your erroneous zones.* New York: Avon, 1977.

Ellis, A., & Harper, R. A. *A new guide to rational living.* North Hollywood, Calif.: Wilshire Book Co., 1975.

Forehand, R., Sturgis, E., McMahn, R., Aguar, D., Green, K., Wells, K., & Breiner, J. Parent behavioral training to modify child noncompliance: Treatment generalization across time and from home to school. *Behavior Modification*, 1979, *3*, 3–25.

Hanf, C. *A two-stage program for modifying maternal controlling during mother–child interaction.* Paper presented at the Western Psychological Association Meeting, Vancouver, B.C., 1969.

Mash, E. J., Hamerlynck, L. A., & Handy, L. C. (Eds.). *Behavior modification and families.* New York: Brunner/Mazel, 1976.

Mash, E. J., Hamerlynck, L. A., & Handy, L. C. (Eds.). *Behavior modification approaches to parenting.* New York: Brunner/Mazel, 1976.

Patterson, G. The aggressive child: Victim and architect of a coercive system. In E. J. Mash, L. A. Hamerlynck, & L. C. Handy (Eds.), *Behavior modification and families.* New York: Brunner/Mazel, 1976.

Patterson, G. R. *Families.* Champaign, Ill.: Research Press, 1979.

Patterson, G. R., Reid, J. B., Jones, R. R., & Conger, R. E. *A social learning approach to family intervention.* Eugene, Ore.: Castalia, 1975.

Ross, D. M., & Ross, S. A. *Hyperactivity.* New York: Wiley, 1976.

Spadafore, G. A guide for the parent as tutor. *The Exceptional Parent*, 1977, *9*, 17–18.

Stuart, R. B. Behavioral contracting within the families of delinquents. *Journal of Behavior Therapy and Experimental Psychiatry*, 1971, *2*, 1–11.

Walker, C. E. Toilet training, enuresis, and encopresis. In P. Magrab (Ed.), *Psychological management of pediatric problems.* Baltimore: University Park Press, 1978.

CHAPTER EIGHT

BEHAVIOR THERAPY IN
THE CLASSROOM

He that has found a way to keep a child's spirit easy, active, and free, and yet at the same time to restrain him from many things he has a mind to, and to draw him to things that are uneasy to him, has, in my opinion, got the true secret of education.—John Locke

One area in which hyperactive children present with considerable problems is that of their functioning within the educational setting. The problems presented in the classroom are often similar to those that the parents are experiencing at home. In some cases, however, hyperactive children may not show difficulties in classroom functioning, partly because of the nature of particular classroom programs, the ability of particular teachers to spend additional individualized time with these children, and the degree to which certain teachers incorporate effective child behavior management principles into their interactions with the children. Most hyperactive children, though, will have difficulties with restlessness, attention span, and impulse control in their school classrooms. These problems frequently manifest themselves in specific difficulties with remaining in their chairs when requested to do so, completing assignments, and generally refraining from disrupting the classroom. Hyperactive children are often seen to engage in substantial out-of-seat activity at inappropriate times and to have difficulties completing assignments in class or during homework. they are frequently noisy, disrupting the classroom by talking to other students at inappropriate times or by generally making noises while they work. They often show poor social skills in their interactions with other children, and they are frequently aggressive toward those children. As with their home behavior, they often show very poor awareness of the possible consequences of their behavior for themselves and for other people. Furthermore, as noted in Chapter 1, hyperactive children are more likely to show specific learning disabilities in selected areas of classroom achievement. These learning disabilities will further compound these children's already difficult behavior and will frequently lead the children to experience further conduct problems and depression. After several years of failure in behavioral manageability and academic achievement in the classroom, such children may be placed within a special educational setting for learning-disabled, behavior-disordered, or emotionally disturbed children.

Recent research has shown that these behavior problems of hyperactive children in school settings often lead teachers to respond to the children in ways similar to those seen in parents of hyperactive children. The teachers may become quite frustrated over their inability to manage such children's behavior appropriately. They may also become angry over the children's frequent disruptions of their daily routines and of their attempts to educate the other children in the classroom. The teachers, like parents of hyperactive children, are not immune to feelings of inadequacy and incompetency when their typical methods of managing child behavior break down with moderate to severely hyperactive children. Sometimes, this may lead such teachers to blame the parents for their children's behavioral difficulties in the classroom. In other instances, it will result in the teachers' referring these children for evaluation to determine whether placement within a special educational setting is required. Specifically, in the classroom, research has shown that teachers are more likely to respond to hyperactive children with commands, punishment, and generally negative interactions than they are to respond in this way to normal children. Such teachers are often also less likely to praise or to have positive interactions with hyperactive children than they are to do so with normal children. Over time, the teachers may come to change their strategies of managing these children in a sequence similar to the parental response hierarchy outlined in Chapter 2. That is, the teachers may attempt to ignore the children's behavior initially, after which they will begin to resort to numerous restrictive commands in an effort to control the children's behavior. Should this fail, they are likely to resort to increasingly negative interactions and social disapproval with the children. In addition, they may remove activities and privileges from the children as punishment for their continued misbehavior. With continued failure at managing the children, the teacher may acquiesce to such children, permitting them to fail to comply with commands given in the classroom. Because of professional, ethical, and legal restrictions over their behavior, teachers may not resort to physical discipline as often as parents would when frustrated with hyperactive children's behavior. Instead, they may employ social isolation or send the children to be dealt with by their school principals. The final result is often a generally negative tone of interactions between the children and their classroom teachers. It is therefore frequently necessary to intervene in such children's classrooms in order to improve their academic performance and classroom behavior.

It is the purpose of this chapter to present various methods of behavior modification that have proven helpful in controlling the problems of hyperactive children in the classroom. As explained in Chapters 6 and 7, however, it is not the intention of these intervention methods to cure the children's hyperactivity. Instead, their purpose is to reduce the children's inappropriate behavior and to improve the occurrence of more appropriate behavior in the classroom situation. In spite of these intervention methods, it is quite likely that these children will continue to experience periodic problems in academic performance throughout their educational careers.

ISSUES IN UTILIZING BEHAVIOR MODIFICATION IN THE CLASSROOM

Before reviewing the specific methods that have proven helpful in managing hyperactive behavior in school settings, it should be noted that several issues must be confronted by therapists attempting to implement such programs. Chief among these is an issue of practicality—the question of whether teachers will have sufficient time to implement many of these programs. Many teachers have 20 to 25 children in their classrooms for whom they are responsible. This often means that teachers will not have the time to observe and record hyperactive children's behavior, to implement multiple behavior management programs for controlling such children's inappropriate behavior, or to meet regularly with therapists in order to review and modify these programs. It is essential, therefore, that therapists recommend programs to classroom teachers that are well within the constraints of the teachers' time and responsibilities.

Another problem with implementing behavior therapy in the classroom is similar to a problem seen in training parents to manage child behavior. That is, once teachers have been trained in the methods of management, there is no guarantee that they will continue to utilize them after therapists cease their active involvement in the program. It may therefore be necessary to schedule booster sessions at periodic intervals with teachers to determine whether or not and how effectively the behavior management principles are continuing to be utilized.

Should hyperactive children be functioning within regular school classrooms, one issue raised by many teachers about behavior modification methods is whether these methods draw undue attention to the children for their misbehavior. Some teachers believe that such methods may result in increased harassment for these children from their peers, or in depression in the children as a result of being stigmatized as requiring special educational methods. Although the issue is often raised, there is little if any evidence to support or refute the occurrence of such phenomena at this time. In my experience, few children experience any increase in the amount of peer harassment or ostracism over the amount they are currently receiving because of their high rates of inappropriate social behavior. On the contrary, the behavior therapy methods often lead to greater peer acceptance. Another concern about behavior modification in a classroom setting is that hyperactive children should not be provided with special reinforcement programs because other children in the classroom whose behavior is normal are not receiving such incentives. Normal children may become jealous of hyperactive children because of the increased rewards the latter are receiving, or normal children may in fact begin to misbehave themselves in an effort to gain access to the reinforcement programs that the hyperactive children are receiving. Again, in spite of numerous studies of the effects of behavior management on the classroom functioning of behavior-disordered children, there is little if any evidence available to show that this is in fact a problem. One way of circumventing this problem is for a teacher to employ group rewards contingent upon appropriate behavior from a hyperactive child. This intervention strategy will be discussed later in this chapter. Suffice it to say here that the procedure results in normal children in a classroom receiving the same rewards as the hyperactive child, provided that the hyperactive child demonstrates improvements in particular target behaviors. This sort of procedure would seem to alleviate the problem of the increase in attention to hyperactive children for their behavior problems.

Another issue of importance in implementing classroom behavior management programs is the determination of the most appropriate target behavior for treatment. Early studies in behavior modification in the classroom selected the children's off-task, inattentive, and generally disruptive behavior as the focus of intervention. In other words, the goal of behavior management was to have the children sit still and pay attention while in the classroom. Although these studies demonstrated great success in achieving these goals, they were not able to show any appreciable increase in the children's academic achievement or productivity as a result of the improvements in in-seat or on-task behavior. Later studies focused on applying behavior modification programs to areas of academic achievement and productivity. In these programs, the children received consequences for achieving certain quotas of completing assigned problems or for achieving a certain degree of accuracy in the problems completed. These studies indicated not only that the children's level of functioning in these areas improved, but that the children were often better behaved as an indirect result of these treatment programs. This latter result is obviously based upon the fact that in order for children to accomplish a certain quota of assigned problems, they are going to have to display certain levels of on-task behavior and self-control. More recent studies of behavior modification methods have come to employ programs to improve the social skills of hyperactive children in their interactions with their peers during both free-play and lesson periods. It is therefore possible to conclude that if the goal of behavior therapy in the classroom is to improve these children's academic performance and productivity, then the target of intervention must be more than getting the children to sit still and pay attention in the classroom. Instead, behavioral contingencies and consequences will have to be applied directly to academic accuracy, productivity, and achievement. When interactions with peers are the primary difficulty, then behavior modification programs will have to be aimed directly at those aspects of the children's social skills that are proving problematic.

One factor that has been shown to be related to the successful implementation of behavior management programs in the classroom is that of teachers' orientations to or philosophies about child psychology and education. Teachers who believe in a nondirective, laissez-faire approach to educating and managing children are not likely to adopt or implement behavior management programs based upon a belief that it is the environment and its consequences that substantially determine children's behavior in the classroom. Such teachers often believe that children contain within themselves all that is necessary for successful academic achievement, and that the role of teachers is to provide a relatively nurturant, nondirective, and relaxed atmosphere in which the children's basic learning skills will manifest themselves. These teachers often view behavior modification techniques as mechanistic, lacking in humanism, simplistic, and often symptomatic in the treatment of hyperactive children's difficulties. They are more likely to endorse individual psychotherapy or play therapy for such children and to view the parents and the general home atmosphere as the main contributors to the children's difficulties. In some cases, discussion with individual teachers espousing this philosophy can often lead to a change in their attitudes and hence to successful implementation of behavior management programs. When their attitudes remain essentially unchanged after such an exchange of ideas, it is unlikely that they will use the suggested behavior modification programs consistently or effectively in coping with the children's classroom problems. It is at this point that parents may have to decide whether a change in classroom teachers for their children, or in some cases a change in schools, would be desirable. Nonetheless, most teachers are quite able and willing to implement behavior management programs that have previously proved successful, if for no other reason than the fact that they are, like the parents of these children, at their wits' end in trying to find methods that successfully control the children's behavior. Once implemented, the success of the behavior modification program is often the most persuasive evidence for its continued use in the classroom.

GENERAL APPROACH TO BEHAVIOR THERAPY IN THE CLASSROOM

As noted in Chapters 6 and 7, there is a general set of procedures that is followed in the successful implementation of behavior modification programs. The first step involves identifying the target behavior that will be the focus of the intervention methods. This means that the behavior in question must be specifically defined so that it can be observed and recorded on a reliable basis. Second, the behavior selected should be observed and recorded for a sufficient period of time to permit an analysis of the antecedent and consequent events surrounding its occurrence. These records are then studied to help determine the changes that should be made in a child's environment to bring about improvements in the target behavior. This may involve changing the nature of the commands or tasks given to the child in question, the nature of the physical environment in which the tasks are being accomplished, or the consequences being provided to the child for the occurrence or nonoccurrence of the target behavior. Throughout this process, the therapist must also determine the appropriate alternative behavior that the child should show in the classroom in place of the inappropriate behavior selected as the target. The next step of the approach involves implementing the suggested changes in the environment and evaluating their effectiveness at changing the target behavior. Records continue to be kept on the occurrence of the behavior, and these will be used for further analysis of and changes in the manner in which the child is being managed in the classroom. The specific types of changes that can be made in the child's environment to facilitate improvements in target behaviors are similar to those that have been discussed in Chapter 6; these will also be briefly discussed in this chapter.

INDIVIDUAL PROGRAMS

With but a few exceptions, most of the individualized behavior therapy programs that can be used in classrooms with hyperactive children are similar to those outlined in Chapter 6. The difference between the methods used at home and those used at school is primarily in the target behaviors that are selected for modification. At home, these targets may primarily be such behaviors as performing assigned chores or complying with parental commands. In the classroom, they may include accomplishing individual assignments at one's desk, sitting quietly without disrupting the class, or obeying teacher commands. As a result of the similarities in methods, only brief attention will be given here to a review of classroom management techniques.

Positive Reinforcement Methods

Like home reinforcement methods, behavior modification in the school can capitalize upon the highly reinforcing value of adult attention and praise in increasing appropriate behavior among hyperactive children in school. The use of this method does not require that teachers exert any more time and effort in managing such children than they are already displaying. Studies with disruptive children indicate that teachers spend approximately 77% of their interactions with these children in negative, controlling behaviors, while spending only 23% of their interactions in positive attention toward the children. These studies clearly suggest that negative behavior in the classroom produces more attention from the teacher than positive behavior does, even though the teacher attention may be somewhat controlling and directive in its manner. The use of positive social attention and praise in the classroom would merely require that the teachers shift the emphasis of their interactions with these children from negative to positive ones. That is, instead of giving all of their attention to disruptive behavior when it occurs, they should ignore the inappropriate behaviors or engage in less controlling interactions when they occur, and should instead provide a substantial increase in the amount of positive attention and praise upon the occurrences of more appropriate classroom behavior.

That even negative teacher attention can actually be reinforcing to children was demonstrated in a 1968 study. This study involved recording the amount of time that children spent out of their chairs in the classroom and the effects that teacher commands to sit down had on out-of-seat behavior. The findings from this study are illustrated in Figure 8.1, which clearly shows that the more the teachers stated the command "Sit down" to try to control child out-of-seat behavior, the more time the children spent out of their seats. Hence, although teachers may think they are actually disapproving of and punishing out-of-seat behavior by providing reprimands and restrictive commands, they may actually be encouraging the very behavior they are attempting to restrict.

Some research is available to suggest that there are positive spill-over or chain reaction effects upon other children in a classroom when a teacher begins to engage in providing positive attention and praise to one child for appropriate classroom conduct. The children in the class who are not the focus of the behavior management program will begin to improve their own classroom conduct as a result of vicarious learning. That is, upon seeing that the target child is receiving increased praise and attention for appropriate behavior, the other children increase their rates of appropriate conduct on the assumption that similar consequences will accrue to them as well. All of this is by way of saying that a mere shift in the emphasis of teacher attention from providing substantial controlling and negative interactions for inappropriate behavior to providing positive praise for appropriate behavior can result in dramatic improvements in the conduct not only of hyperactive children, but of their classmates as well.

In addition to using praise and attention, teachers can also employ high-rate or intrinsically rewarding activities (often called privileges) when hyper-

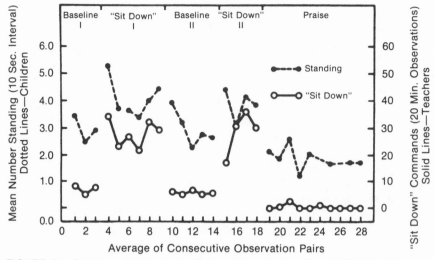

FIGURE 8.1. Out-of-seat behavior by first-graders as a function of "Sit down" commands and praise given by teachers. (From "An Analysis of the Reinforcing Function of 'Sit Down' Commands" by H. Madsen, Jr., W. C. Becker, D. R. Thomas, L. Koser, and E. Plager. In R. K. Parker (Ed.), *Readings in Educational Psychology*. Boston: Allyn & Bacon, 1968. Copyright 1968 by Allyn & Bacon. Reprinted by permission.)

active children display appropriate classroom behavior. These activities may include access to games in the classroom, availability of free play or recess time, permission to assist teachers in performing what to the teachers may be menial classroom activities, or other such typically rewarding activities for children. Most teachers already employ methods similar to this when they single out children for extra privileges because of good behavior over a particular period of time in school. The problem here is that the teachers do not employ the method consistently or immediately upon the occurrence of appropriate classroom behavior. Instead, these privileges are most often given to children who are typically not having difficulties in classroom behavior to begin with.

A program that employs secondary reinforcers for appropriate child behavior, similar to that used in the home, can be instituted in school. Such programs, as noted earlier, are commonly known as token or point systems; tokens, poker chips, bingo chips, or other symbolic reinforcers are provided to children as rewards for appropriate conduct. These tokens or points are then exchanged periodically for tangible rewards or for intrinsically rewarding high-rate activities that the children desire. In setting up such a system, teachers need only decide what type of token or secondary reinforcer they wish to use, make up a list of 10 or 12 activities for which the children can exchange the tokens, and then assign a point value or a cost to each activity. The cost is simply the number of tokens required by a child in order to engage in that activity or acquire that particular reward. As noted in Chapter 6, the use of token systems has numerous advantages over other positive reinforcement methods. Primary among these is the fact that the tokens are convenient to carry, easily utilized across numerous situations, and maintain a relatively constant reinforcing value for children because they can be exchanged for any activities that happen to be reinforcing to the children at the moment. Unlike tangible reinforcers or even social praise, token systems are less subject to fluctuation in value as a result of children's satiation with or deprivation of particular reinforcers. Rather than attempting to second-guess the types of activities which a particular child finds rewarding, a teacher may schedule time during a recess period or after school to meet with the child and determine the activities that the child would prefer to have listed on his or her reinforcement "menu."

   That token systems can be effective in modifying both classroom behavior and academic achievement has been demonstrated in several studies. Probably one of the most widely cited studies demonstrating this effect is that made by Teodoro Ayllon, Dale Layman, and Henry Kandel (1975), in which a token reinforcement system was contrasted with stimulant medication in the control of classroom hyperactivity and academic performance. In this study, three hyperactive children who were receiving medication were observed during both their math and reading classes, and the occurrences of three different classes of phenomena were recorded. One of these was the percentage of math problems assigned that were correctly completed by the child; the second was the percentage of reading problems assigned that were correctly completed by the child; and the third was the occurrence of deviant classroom behaviors, such as gross motor movement, noisiness, disturbance of others, talking out of turn, and other behaviors felt to be incompatible with learning. All three children were observed while they were on medication during a 17-day baseline phase. Following this time, the children were removed from medication for varying lengths of time, with no behavior modification program being implemented. Subsequently, a token reinforcement system was put into effect in which the teacher reinforced the children with checkmarks on index cards for each correct academic response occurring during math and reading periods. These points could then be exchanged for various activities and tangible rewards, such as candy, school supplies, free time, and occasional picnics in a neighborhood park.

   The results for one of the children involved in the study are shown in Figure 8.2. These results are typical of those seen for the other two children involved in the study. As can be seen in this figure, the percentage of occurrence of behaviors considered hyperactive during the medication phase of the study as compared to the percentage when medication was removed

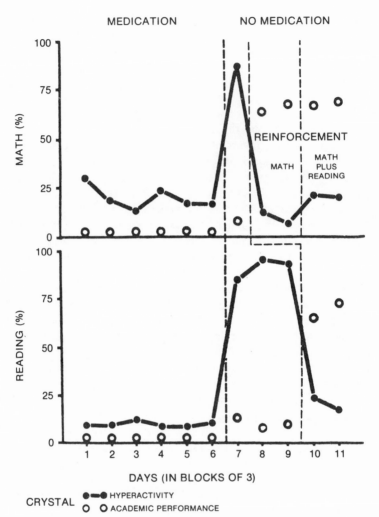

FIGURE 8.2. The percentage of intervals in which hyperactivity took place and the percentage of correct math and reading performances for one of three hyperactive children observed. The first and second segments, respectively, show the effects of medication, and of its subsequent withdrawal, on hyperactivity and academic perform-ance. Multiple-baseline analysis of the effects of reinforcement on math and reading performance and of concurrent effects on hyperactivity is begun in the third top segment. The last segment shows the effects of reinforcement on math plus reading and the concurrent effects on hyperactivity. (The asterisk indicates one data point averaged over 2 rather than 3 days.) (From "A Behavioral–Educational Alternative to Drug Control of Hyperactive Children" by T. Ayllon, D. Layman, and H. J. Kandel, *Journal of Applied Behavior Analysis*, 1975, *8*, 137–146. Copyright 1975 by The Society for the Experimental Analysis of Behavior. Reprinted by permission.)

indicates that the stimulant drug was in fact reducing the occurrence of deviant behavior in this child. However, in spite of this relatively low rate of occurrence of hyperactive behaviors, the child's percentage of correct academic performances remained quite low. This illustrates the point made earlier in the chapter that simply improving a child's attention span and behavior, by whatever means, do not automatically result in improvements in that child's academic performance. This figure also shows that when the reinforcement program was instituted for math, the percentage of correct mathematics problems completed increased significantly, while the percentage or occurrences of deviant behaviors showed a corresponding decline. It should be remembered that the deviant behaviors were not the direct target of the intervention system; only the percentage of correct problems accomplished by each child was being reinforced. The lower graph in this figure shows that when reinforcement was implemented for math only, the child's performance in reading did not change from its relatively low rate of correct occurrence, nor did the incidence of hyperactive behaviors in the reading class show any change from the relatively high levels of occurrence during the no-medication phase. In the final phase of intervention, the reinforcement system was applied during both the math and reading classes, producing changes in academic performance and hyperactivity in reading class similar to those previously demonstrated in math class when reinforcement was contingent only on the performance of correct math problems.

The results for this token reinforcement program underscore the point made earlier in this chapter that improvements in deviant classroom behavior can be brought about by reinforcing correct academic performance without ever focusing on the deviant behavior itself as a target of intervention. These results suggest that if the goal of behavior modification programs in the classroom is the improvement of academic performance, then the occurrence of academic accuracy and productivity must be one of the targets of intervention. In selecting such targets, therapists may find that there is no need to single out other forms of behavior in the classroom for intervention, as these may be indirectly controlled by the application of reinforcement methods to measures of academic performance.

Another type of positive reinforcement system that can be used in the classroom is the application of tangible rewards or edible substances as rewards for appropriate behavior. Such methods have numerous disadvantages, as noted in Chapter 6, and they should only be employed when other reinforcement systems have failed to improve a child's behavior. I have found that tangible or edible rewards are rarely needed beyond the preschool years as part of an effective positive reinforcement system within a classroom. For hyperactive preschoolers, tangible or edible rewards may be necessary, since these children may not have the cognitive skills necessary for effective use of a token system. Older hyperactive children are more likely to respond to reinforcement methods employing praise and access to privileges, or to token reinforcement systems in which tangible or edible rewards either serve as backup reinforcers to the token system or play no role at all in the program.

Another reinforcement method that seems to have equal efficacy at home and at school is the use of contingency contracting with children. While not itself an actual reinforcer of child behavior, contingency contracting can serve as a nice vehicle for the formal arrangement of reinforcement contingencies for hyperactive children. The target of a contract can be disruptive or inappropriate classroom behavior, poor academic productivity or accuracy, or both. The contract may actually specify several types of reinforcers that can be earned by correct completion of the agreement made in the contract. Such a reinforcement method often works well with older hyperactive children, for it is highly desirable to have such children participate in the specification and implementation of behavior modification programs.

In some instances, teachers may have no idea as to what to employ as an effective reinforcer for hyperactive children. When this is the case, it is often helpful to have such teachers keep written records of how the children spend their free-play time so as to determine what high-rate activities may be used as reinforcers. Talking with the children about possible activities or rewards may also help to reveal previously unknown sources of reinforcement for them. Should both of these fail, the teachers may wish to discuss the program further with the parents in order to obtain their opinions as to what reinforcement methods have worked successfully with the children at home. When even this fails, the teachers may have to implement home-based reinforcement systems, such as daily report cards; these systems are discussed later in this chapter.

Punishment Methods

Many of the methods of punishment discussed in Chapter 6 for use at home can also be applied to children in a classroom situation. Some, such as corporal punishment, cannot be used or must follow strict guidelines for utilization because of ethical and legal constraints placed upon their use in the classroom. It seems that those methods of punishment employing the withdrawal of positive activities from children upon the incidence of inappropriate behavior are those with the greatest applicability to the classroom setting. Those that involve the introduction of aversive stimulation upon the occurrence of deviant behavior are the ones that are limited for obvious ethical and legal reasons. Therefore, more attention will be given here to the former methods than to the latter ones.

One method that teachers often employ, sometimes inadvertently, is the withdrawal of social attention and praise, or ignoring, whenever children engage in unacceptable behavior. When combined with the provision of positive attention and other rewards for the occurrence of alternate appropriate behavior, this method can often be used quite successfully to modify the hyperactive behavior of children in the classroom. This method, known as the differential reinforcement of other behaviors, is simply the systematic application of both reinforcement and punishment methods to develop acceptable behavior more rapidly in these children. Nonetheless, with many seriously hyperactive children, the use of ignoring alone may prove ineffective. In fact, as Patterson (1976) has shown in families of aggressive children, ignoring may serve as a cue to the child to increase more high-rate, aversive, and coercive forms of behavior.

One method of punishment that has received widespread utilization in the classroom is time out from reinforcement, or social isolation. In the classroom, as at home, there are various degrees of time out that can be employed, depending upon the severity of the deviant behavior for which it is being administered and on the cooperativeness of individual children with the procedure. In many cases, time out may simply involve having children place their heads down on their desks for brief periods of time upon the occurrence of unacceptable behavior. In other cases, it may involve placing a child at the back of the classroom or in a chair located in a relatively dull part of the classroom. In some instances, when a child is likely to leave the time-out location repeatedly without permission, some method of physical restraint may have to be employed, such as a harness or seat belt. In certain cases, the time-out location has been a three-sided cubicle placed in a dull corner of the room where a child is sent either to sit quietly or to accomplish individual academic work. Should this fail, some teachers may employ a method whereby children are sent to sit out in the hallway as a form of punishment. This, of course, assumes that the children will remain seated in the hallway instead of wandering about, as many hyperactive children are prone to do. In a few schools, it may be acceptable for children to be isolated within a small time-out room separate from the classroom. When such a method is to be employed, certain legal and ethical guidelines will have to be followed. Since each school district varies in its requirements for the use of such restrictive methods of social isolation, the school principal, the district supervisor of special education, or the school superintendent's office should be consulted before any program that involves the use of a separate room for time out is implemented. Some of the issues involved in the use of time out in school are similar to those that must be considered at home, such as the location where the time-out period is to be served, the length of time to be spent in time out, and the criteria that must be fulfilled before a child can leave time out, as well as the type of behavior upon which time out will be made contingent.

If a child leaves the time-out location prematurely, or actively resists the implementation of the time-out procedure, then several alternative methods may have to be used. These may include extending the time-out interval for every incident of resistance or of leaving the time-out location without permission. In addition, when a classroom token system is employed, the teacher may wish to use a response-cost procedure in which a child is penalized a certain number of tokens or points for uncooperative behavior during the time-out period. In any case, it is highly unlikely that the teacher will be able to use a spanking procedure like that described in the parent training program in Chapter 7 in order to maintain a child within the time-out location.

As suggested above, another procedure of punishment that can be used within the classroom is the response-cost method. This merely involves taking away tokens or some reinforcer, such as a high-rate or intrinsically motivating activity, upon the occurrence of undesirable behavior. Like the token reinforcement system upon which it is typically based, response cost is quite convenient to implement in virtually any situation and can be employed with virtually any type of target behavior. Some studies have suggested that the addition of a response-cost method to a token system adds very little to the efficacy of a behavior management program. The few studies that have found this to be the case were not dealing with highly disruptive or hyperactive children, and this may explain why only a positive reinforcement method was needed to improve the children's behavior. I am in agreement with Patterson and many other investigators that highly disruptive and seriously deviant children, such as those who are hyperactive, may require the use of some punishment method to achieve acceptably low rates of deviant behavior and high levels of desirable behavior within the classroom.

That social reprimands can serve as an effective deterrent to deviant classroom behavior has been demonstrated in many studies. This research appears to indicate that when social reprimands involve direct eye contact with the children who have committed undesirable acts, and when such reprimands are given in a loud, stern voice that surprises the children, the reprimands can prove an effective method of managing some forms of deviant classroom behavior. Again, it is my experience that hyperactive children are not likely to respond as successfully as other children to the use of social reprimands alone, because many hyperactive children have a prior history of chronic exposure to the ineffective use of these methods at home. Such reprimands will probably have to be combined with other forms of punishment, such as time out or a response-cost procedure in a token system, in order to back up the threats made as part of the reprimands.

Although the use of physical discipline or corporal punishment in schools is not entirely illegal or unethical, the circumstances under which it can be employed are often restricted by legislation or by public school policy. Such restrictions often prevent the use of physical discipline immediately upon the occurrence of unacceptable behavior, and this lessens its effectiveness even when it is employed following acceptable guidelines. Many successful intervention programs for hyperactive children that have not included any element of physical discipline have been designed; such programs make it unlikely that therapists will ever have to consider the incorporation of such methods into a planned behavior modification program. In fact, a school suspension procedure is probably more desirable than a corporal punishment procedure if a child's behavior should prove so serious or so deviant as to warrant extreme methods. Suspension alone, however, may prove ineffective because it is often delayed in its implementation as a result of certain school policy procedures, and because for some hyperactive children the opportunity to leave school may actually be reinforcing. The effectiveness of the suspension procedure depends partly on the manner in which parents deal with children upon their return home following a suspension.

For the therapist who desires to incorporate a punishment procedure, it is essential that a reinforcement procedure for appropriate alternate behaviors be designed and implemented prior to or in conjunction with the punishment procedure. This will sometimes indicate that the punishment procedure is unnecessary, as the reinforcement method may be all that is needed to improve classroom behavior. If not, the use of a positive reinforcement procedure in conjunction with some method of punishment, such as time out or response cost, may actually accelerate the improvement in a child's behavior to such an extent that the punishment procedure only rarely needs to be employed.

GROUP PROGRAMS

Probably one of the best procedures that can be used with an entire classroom of children is the token reinforcement system discussed earlier as an individual program. When it is used with a group, a greater variety of activities is made available to the children; as with the individual procedure, each activity requires a certain amount of tokens or points in order to be attained. The teacher dispenses tokens or points to each child in the classroom, including the hyperactive child, for the occurrence of desirable academic or social behaviors. The use of group reinforcement procedures such as this one avoids the criticism often raised about behavior modification programs that involve only one child. In this case, all children are capable of earning rewards for appropriate behavior, not simply the hyperactive or target child. Some studies have also been conducted in which the peers of the hyperactive child also dispense points or tokens to the child for the occurrence of appropriate class conduct. There is no reason that this system could not be extended so that all children in the classroom have the capacity to reinforce one another for the occurrence of acceptable behaviors. Such a token reinforcement system could also involve the use of a response-cost procedure in which tokens or points are taken away upon the occurrence of unacceptable behavior. Under these circumstances, it would not seem advisable to have peers be given the responsibility for a response-cost method, as this could lead to indiscreet or unacceptable occurrences of punishment from peers.

The research literature seems to suggest that a number of factors affect the degree to which a token system can be effectively employed in a classroom situation. One of these appears to be the ability of teachers to use praise, ignoring, rules and commands, and firm individual reprimands in addition to the token system with children in a classroom. This seems partly related to the ability of teachers to continue to monitor the behavior of various students within the classroom, instead of becoming so preoccupied with teaching agendas that they are essentially unaware of the occurrence of appropriate or inappropriate behavior. In addition, it may also be related to teachers' basic philosophies about the manner in which children should be educated. As noted earlier, a teacher who believes that all that needs to be provided for children is a safe, secure, and relatively nurturant yet nondirective classroom environment is unlikely to employ reinforcement and punishment methods as consistently or contingently as a teacher with a different philosophy.

A second factor affecting the success of token systems in classroom situations is obviously the quality and quantity of training that teachers have received in the use of the token system and other behavior modification methods. Regardless of these factors, however, it seems that if a teacher has a number of other problem children in the classroom besides the hyperactive child, the effectiveness of a token system may be less. Certainly, the severity of the problem behaviors with which teachers must deal must also have some influence on the effectiveness of a token system in the classroom. Other research also suggests that the amount of peer support that hyperactive children receive for their disruptive behavior may serve to counteract the effects of a token system. One way of dealing with this is to employ a group token economy or to coach peers in ways of reinforcing more acceptable behavior in target hyperactive children. Finally, no matter how favorable the above factors may be, the antagonism of parents, or at least their lack of support for the programs which teachers are attempting to implement, are likely to lessen the effectiveness of those programs with any behavior problem children.

When a teacher elects to establish a group token system in the classroom, several cautions must be heeded. One of these is that the teacher must be sure not to focus entirely upon inappropriate behavior to the exclusion of appropriate alternative behaviors that deserve reinforcement. Giving the teacher the ability to penalize or fine students in a token system for their misbehavior may serve inadvertently to focus undue attention upon the children's negative behavior, with the result that less positive reinforcement or fewer tokens are given for acceptable behaviors in the classroom. A second issue to be concerned with is the timing of the use of response cost following an inappropriate behavior by a child. If the unacceptable behavior has had a certain negative emotional effect on the child, it is probably worthwhile to implement a "cooling-off period" before taking away points or tokens for the unacceptable behavior. Otherwise, if the child should be emotionally upset and the teacher should implement a response-cost procedure at that time, the procedure might serve to enrage the child further. The result of this might be progressive escalations in the child's fine for the ever greater pitch and intensity of the negative behavior. This "punishment spiral" is often seen in conduct-disordered or impulsive children, who, when emotionally upset or frustrated, do not appear to care much about any further punishment they may receive once punishment has been implemented. It is probably best, therefore, to allow a child a brief period of time to regain emotional composure before discussing with that child the loss of points to which his or her behavior has led.

SELF-CONTROL PROCEDURES

Although discussed in Chapter 6 as methods for use with hyperactive behavior at home, self-control procedures have probably been more thoroughly studied as classroom management methods and educational procedures. The reader will recall that self-control techniques can be broken down into four separate components: self-observation and monitoring, self evaluation or standard-setting, self-instruction, and self-consequation (reinforcement or punishment) contingent on whether the behavior has achieved the set goals or standards. In most cases, previous studies have involved most, if not all, of these components in their intervention programs. The results of the research suggest that the self-control methods are just as effective as externally imposed methods of behavior modification for improving disruptive behavior and academic performance in the classroom.

One of the earliest studies involving the use of self-control procedures with disruptive children was that made by Orin Bolstad and Stephen Johnson

(1972). This study involved the assignment of between five and nine children to each of five treatment groups in order to compare the effects of external regulation or reinforcement programs with those of self-regulation and reinforcement programs, as well as with the effects of no treatment at all. One of the five groups received an external regulation treatment consisting of the implementation of a typical classroom token system. In this case, the teacher dispensed reinforcement contingent upon her evaluation of the children's behavior and its level of disruptiveness. The two groups of children assigned to the self-regulation procedures received training in the observation and recording of their own behavior and in the administration of points to themselves for the occurrence of appropriately designated classes of behavior. In earlier phases of the program, the children in the self-regulation groups had their self-monitoring and self-reinforcement checked by observers to ensure its accuracy. In later phases of the program, the children were permitted to monitor and reinforce themselves without any checking of their accuracy by the observers. As noted, the remaining two treatment groups involved essentially no treatment controls; the children received typical classroom instruction and management procedures.

The results of this study are graphically depicted in Figure 8.3. Here it can be seen that the children in one of the two no-treatment control groups showed an increase in disruptive behavior over time. Children in the second no-treatment control group showed a mild reduction in disruptive behavior, although this reduction was not nearly as large as those seen in any of the actual treatment groups. Children who participated in the externally regulated classroom showed significant reductions in disruptive behavior over time, but their disruptive behavior tended to return to its original baseline levels when the token economy was discontinued in Phase V of the program. As this figure shows, the children assigned to the two self-control classes showed reductions in disruptive behavior equal to if not greater than those of the children in the externally regulated classroom. In addition, during the extinction phase (Phase V), when no points were awarded for appropriate behavior, the children in the self-control classes did not show as much of a return to original baseline levels of behavior as the children in the externally regulated treatment program. This is probably in part the result of the fact that the children in the self-control classroom were continuing to record and report their disruptive behavior, even though there was no reinforcement involved for doing so. This study clearly demonstrates, then, that the use of self-control procedures is both practical and effective in the modification of inappropriate classroom behavior in children.

Similar results were obtained in a study conducted by myself, Anne Copeland, and Carol Sivage (1980). In this study, six hyperactive boys participated in an experimental classroom at the University of Oregon Health Sciences Center: all of the procedures in the classroom involved

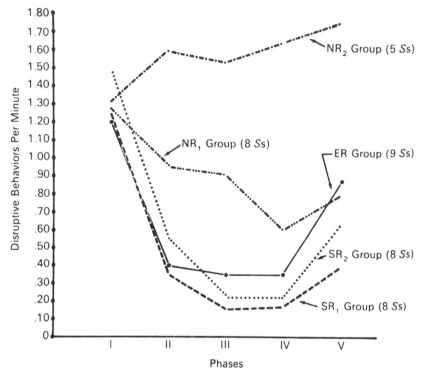

FIGURE 8.3. Average disruptive behavior per minute for children in each of five experimental of groups. During Phase I (baseline), disruptive behaviors were observed in class. During Phase II (external regulation), children in all experimental groups (ER, SR_1, and SR_2) were awarded points after class for fewer disruptions. During Phase III, the children in the ER group remained on external regulation, while those in the self-regulation groups (SR_1 and SR_2) were trained to record and report their own behavior and were given points for accurate reports of fewer disruptions. Phase IV was the same as Phase III, except that points were given for children reporting fewer disruptions, regardless of the accuracy of their reports. In Phase V (extinction), no points were given, and only the children in the SR_1 group were still required to record and report on their disruptive behavior. (From "Self-Regulation in the Modification of Disruptive Classroom Behavior" by O. Bolstad and S. Johnson, *Journal of Applied Behavior Analysis*, 1972, *5*, 443–454. Copyright 1972 by The Society for the Experimental Analysis of Behavior. Reprinted by permission.)

training in various aspects of self-control. A matched group of six hyperactive children was assigned to a control group and remained within their regular public school classes during the 8 weeks of the study. Briefly, the classroom procedure involved having the boys come to the special classroom for 2½ hours each day for 4 school days each week. During each class period, the boys spent the initial 15 minutes in free play and then participated in a large-group instruction period that lasted for approximately 30 minutes. Three of the children were then given individual academic assignments to accomplish at their desks, while the other three participated in a small-group instruction period. This part of the classroom lasted 30 minutes, after which there was a 10- to 15-minute snack time. Following the snack period, the three children working on individual academic tasks then moved into the small-group treatment procedure, while those who had previously been receiving small-group instruction were now given individual seat assignments to accomplish. Again, these procedures lasted 30 minutes. At the end of this time, the boys were given a 15-minute free-play time before they went home for the day.

The first week of the program consisted of a baseline or no-treatment phase, during which the classroom teacher and her aide used typical methods of classroom instruction and classroom behavior management for dealing with the six hyperactive children. During the next 3 weeks, the self-control procedures were implemented. During the large- and small-group activities, the self-control treatment consisted of having the teacher model methods of problem-solving and self-instruction in the solution of various academic and social problems. Each boy was then brought before the group to solve a problem by the method that was modeled by the teacher. The teacher also dispensed tokens for the boys during the performance of the self-instruction procedure. During the individual seat work, the children were trained to follow a set of guidelines for appropriate, on-task behavior. These guidelines were set forth on an easel before the children during their individual seat work. Each boy also had a small plain card on his desk; this was used to record the self-awarding of points for appropriate behavior. A tape recorder was used to sound a tone at various unpredictable intervals for the boys. When the tone sounded, they were to ask themselves if their behavior was in accordance with the guidelines set forth on the easel. If it was, they could administer themselves a token for on-task behavior. During the early phases of this procedure, the tone sounded an average of once every minute. Some intervals were longer than this, while others were shorter. The timing of the tones was increased to a variable-interval 3-minute procedure during the second week and to a variable-interval 5-minute procedure during the third week in an effort to wean the boys from frequent self-reinforcement. During the fourth week of the class, all treatment procedures were discontinued as a reversal phase in the experiment. In the next 3 weeks of the program, all treatment procedures were reinstituted. The only change in treatment procedures involved the variable interval of self-reinforcement that was being used by the children working on individual seat activities. This time, during the first week of treatment, a variable-interval 1-minute procedure was used for sounding the tone on the tape recorder. For the second week, this was increased to a variable-interval 1.5-minute procedure. In the third week, this was increased to a variable 3-minute procedure. This change in the sequence of intervals from the sequence used in the first 3-week treatment phase was implemented because the boys showed a marked deterioration in their on-task behavior when the variable interval was increased from 1 minute to 3 minutes. It was felt that a smaller increase during the second treatment phase would assist the boys in maintaining high rates of on-task behavior while gradually weaning them from frequent self-reinforcement. The eighth and final week of the treatment program consisted of posttreatment testing of the children on various measures of academic achievement.

The results for this self-control classroom are displayed in Figures 8.4 and 8.5. In the first figure (Figure 8.4), each individual child's percentage of on-task behavior is shown for each of the treatment phases. The measure of on-task behavior was taken during the individual academic work time. This figure indicates that the children were working at extremely low rates of on-task behavior during the initial baseline phase. When the self-monitoring and self-reinforcement phases of the study were implemented, on-task behavior increased to a level between 90% and 100% for most of the boys. The fading out of the frequent reinforcement intervals resulted in a deterioration in some of the children's behavior in the later phases of the first 3-week

FIGURE 8.4. The percentage of time on task (× 10) during individual work time for each of six hyperactive boys across baseline (A), treatment (B), and reversal (A) phases. Data were collected on each boy for each day of the program. The graphs are in order of highest to lowest mental age (MA) (upper left to lower right) for the boys: Brad (MA = 10 years, 2 months), Seth (MA = 10 years, 1 month), Karl (MA = 8 years, 6 months), Gene (MA = 8 years, 1 month), Jim (MA = 6 years, 9 months), and Tim (MA = 6 years, 6 months). (From "A Self-Control Classroom for Hyperactive Children" by R. A. Barkley, A. Copeland, and C. Sivage, *Journal of Autism and Developmental Disorders*, 1980, *10*, 75–89. Copyright 1980 by Plenum Publishing Corp. Reprinted by permission.)

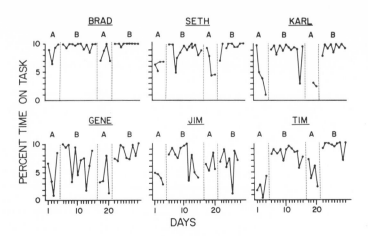

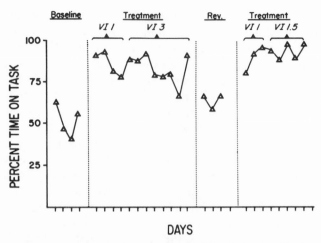

DAYS

FIGURE 8.5. Mean percentage of time spent on task by six hyperactive boys during all treatment conditions. (From "A Self-Control Classroom for Hyperactive Children" by R. A. Barkley, A. Copeland, and C. Sivage, *Journal of Autism and Developmental Disorders*, 1980, *10*, 75–89. Copyright 1980 by Plenum Publishing Corp. Reprinted by permission.)

treatment period. During the "no treatment" reversal phase, on-task behavior dropped to its initially low levels. Once treatment was reimplemented, the self-monitoring and self-reinforcement procedures resulted in a return to the high levels of on-task behavior seen during the first treatment phase. The shift to a procedure that involved more gradual weaning from the frequent reinforcement intervals enabled most of the boys to maintain relatively high levels of on-task behavior in the face of progressively longer intervals of self-reinforcement. The effects of the treatment procedure are more apparent when the results for all six boys are averaged together, as depicted in Figure 8.5.

One of the findings shown in Figure 8.4 is that children of younger mental age were less able to tolerate the shifts in the self-reinforcement schedule than children of older mental age were. The individual graphs in this figure are ordered according to the mental ages of the boys, beginning with the highest in the upper left-hand corner of the graph and progressing to the lowest in the lower right-hand corner. As noted in Chapter 6, the effectiveness of self-control procedures must depend to some extent on the level of cognitive development of the child with whom the procedure is being used. Younger children, whose verbal ability is limited, will probably have greater difficulty utilizing self-monitoring and reinforcement procedures than will older children, whose verbal skills are better developed and who are more capable of following a self-instruction and self-control procedure. Although the findings for the six hyperactive children in the control group are not shown here, they continued to show relatively low rates of on-task behavior and high rates of disruptive behavior in their regular classroom throughout all phases of this study. In addition, observers also recorded the behavior of the six boys in the experimental classroom while they attended their regular public school classes in the mornings. These observations indicated that there was no generalization of treatment effects from the experimental classroom to the boys' regular classroom in any phase of the treatment program. Nonetheless, these data and those of other studies suggest that self-control procedures can be an effective treatment package for improving disruptive classroom behavior. In addition, the use of self-instruction and problem-solving procedures, as discussed in Chapter 6, can also serve as an excellent vehicle for teaching various academic subjects.

Despite these positive findings for self-control methods, there remain several problems with the use of these procedures with hyperactive children. First, if the procedures are to remain effective, there must be some degree of supervision over the children's self-monitoring and self-reinforcement in order to insure that the children remain honest in the awarding of consequences for particular behaviors. In studies that have evaluated this problem, it has been shown that once external supervision for self-control is discontinued, rates of inappropriate behavior gradually return to baseline or no-treatment levels. Another problem with the self-control procedures is one that plagues all forms of psychological interventions with hyperactive children at this time—that is, the lack of generalization of treatment effects to settings in which treatment has not been implemented. As noted in my study with Copeland and Sivage, the self-control procedures work well within the treatment setting in which they are implemented, but are unlikely to affect the children's behavior outside of that situation, where no treatment procedures are being implemented. Thus, only when efforts are made to program for generalization of treatment effects are improvements in other situations likely to be found. Finally, there is no evidence to suggest that the self-control procedures are consistently superior to the results obtained by more traditional behavior modification programs. In fact, it is quite likely that the costs of the training and monitoring involved in implementing self-control methods may be somewhat greater than the costs incurred by traditional behavior therapy procedures in the classroom. Thus, at this time, although self-control methods offer an exciting and intriguing alternative to traditional behavior therapy methods for hyperactive children, their cost-effectiveness in comparison with these traditional procedures remains to be thoroughly evaluated.

HOME-BASED REINFORCEMENT METHODS

The method of home-based reinforcement for controlling classroom behavior merely involves the provision of consequences within the home setting for behaviors that have occurred at school on any particular day. Communication between a child's parents and teacher on a regular basis, frequently daily, serves as the vehicle by which the child's school behavior is evaluated and consequated within the home. Many teachers already employ a similar system albeit inconsistently, with children in their classes who have behavior problems. Notes are often sent home on a regular basis, usually for inappropriate behavior in the classroom. This often results in the children's being frequently punished at home for what has happened in school on some days, yet rarely being reinforced on those days when no notes are sent home. This system could certainly be improved by having the notes sent home on a more regular basis, and also by requiring that notes dealing with positive classroom behavior as well as notes dealing with inappropriate behavior be sent home.

Probably a better device for utilizing home-based reinforcement is a formal daily report card for specific child behaviors in each subject or in the class of each teacher whom a child interacts with on any given day. One such daily report card is displayed in Figure 8.6. On this card, there is room for a child's name and the date, as well as for an explanation of the ratings that the child can receive for his or her behavior. The ratings range from 1 to 5, with the child receiving a rating of 1 for excellent behavior, 2 for good behavior, 3 for fair behavior, 4 for poor conduct, and 5 for seriously inappropriate behavior. The teacher simply places the appropriate number beside each specific area of behavior listed on the left-hand side of the card. There is enough room across the card for up to six teachers to rate the child, or for the child to receive ratings in six different subjects from the same teacher. The teacher or teachers initial the card at the bottom of each column to ensure against forgery of the numbers. The bottom and back of the card can be used for additional comments or for specifying the child's homework assignment that day.

The child using such a card takes it to school from home each day and returns it to the home at the end of the school day. At this time, one of the parents reviews the card and assigns a certain number of points or tokens for each rating on the card. The child receives 25 points for every rating of 1, 15 points for every rating of 2, 5 points for every 3, −10 points for every rating of 4, and −25 points for every rating of 5 on the card. The positive and negative points are then added for the total of points awarded to the child that day. The child may then use these points to purchase various privileges within the home. In addition, the child can also save up the points for activities outside the home or for the purchase of toys or other tangible

DAILY STUDENT RATING CARD

NAME _____ DATE _____

Please rate this child in each of the areas listed below as to how he performed in school today using ratings of 1 to 5.   1 = excellent, 2 = good, 3 = fair, 4 = poor, 5 = terrible or did not work.

AREA	CLASS PERIODS / SUBJECTS					
	1	2	3	4	5	6
participation						
class work						
handed in homework						
interaction with other children						
teacher's initials						

Place comments on back if needed:

FIGURE 8.6. Daily school report card for use with home-based reinforcement system. Each teacher in up to six different classes (or the same teacher for six different subjects) rates the child's behavior in each area on a scale of 1 (excellent) to 5 (terrible) and then initials the card. At home that day, the ratings are converted to points, which are then used to purchase various privileges and rewards. A rating of 1 = +25 points, 2 = +15 points, 3 = +5 points, 4 = –15 points, and 5 = –25 points.

rewards. When the system is first implemented, the parents sit down with the child to make up a list of privileges and to decide how many points each will cost.

In some cases, children attempt to circumvent this treatment procedure by forging the ratings on the card, by failing to get certain teachers to fill out the card at the end of that class, or by forgetting to bring the card home altogether at the end of the day. Various levels of response cost, or negative point values, are assigned for these infractions. For every forged number that is on the card, a child may be penalized 25 points. For every teacher whose evaluation is absent from the card, the child may be fined 100 points. And, if the child fails to bring the card home from school that day, he or she may be grounded for that day and fined 250 points. This method of response cost frequently discourages children from attempting to circumvent the reinforcement procedure.

Home-based reinforcement by means of a daily report card system such as that discussed above has several useful features. First, children receive immediate evaluations from their teachers at the end of each class or each subject. Studies have shown that this evaluative encounter between teachers and children is in many cases sufficient to help the children maintain appropriate classroom behavior without the need for reinforcement at home. A second advantage of this system is that it provides families with daily information about the children's classroom performance. Often, families are not aware of children's difficulties in school until the end of the typical 9-week grading period. At this point, it is often too late to go back and correct for difficult behavior shown earlier in that grading quarter. Under the present system, such families can determine immediately whether the children's performance in class is deteriorating and can take steps to meet with teachers in order to correct for this deterioration. Finally, the daily report card system capitalizes on sources of motivation and reward for the children in the home that may be more potent than those sources of motivation available to teachers within a classroom. Research has indicated that most children above a preschool level can respond quite favorably to the use of this daily report card system. Such daily report card systems can also often serve as effective counterparts to other classroom management methods. Finally, over time, the children can be weaned from the daily report card system by increasing the intervals at which report cards are sent home from daily, to every other day, to weekly, then to biweekly, and finally to monthly evaluations or no evaluations whatsoever.

Obviously, the effectiveness of this procedure depends largely upon the accurate assessment of the children's behavior in the classroom when their teachers evaluate their performances, as well as upon the consistent and contingent use of consequences by parents upon their children's return home from school. The program is not likely to work successfully if teachers overestimate the children's class performances or if parents inconsistently apply the token system at home, so that children are able to gain access to rewarding activities in spite of poor performances at school that day. Nonetheless, with minimal supervision, this program can serve as an effective behavior management program for hyperactive children.

STANDARD PROGRAMS FOR CHANGING CLASSROOM BEHAVIOR

Some attempts have been made recently to develop a standard series of treatment approaches contained within a treatment package for use with behavior problem children in classroom settings. Probably the most rigorously developed and thoroughly tested of these programs is the one developed by the Center at Oregon for Research in the Behavioral Education of the Handicapped (CORBEH). CORBEH has developed a series of treatment packages entitled CLASS, PASS, PEERS, and RECESS. The CLASS program (Contingencies for Learning Academic and Social Skills) is the program of greatest interest here, because it has been designed to deal with acting-out and hyperactive-like behaviors in the classroom. The treatment packages have been developed for use with children between kindergarten and third grade. Although they are primarily intended for children within regular classrooms or mainstream settings, there is no reason they could not be used in special educational programs, such as classes for the learning-disabled, the behavior-disordered, or the emotionally disturbed. The CLASS and PASS programs are primarily intended for use within classroom settings, while the PEERS and RECESS programs are designed for the development of appropriate social conduct in playground and recess situations. These programs were designed primarily by Hill Walker and Hyman Hops of the University of Oregon and the Oregon Research Institute. Information about the packages and the supporting research can be obtained by writing to CORBEH, Clinical Services Building, Center on Human Development, University of Oregon, Eugene, Ore. 97403. Approximately 5 to 6 years of research and development have been invested in these programs, with substantial improvement being shown in the behavior of children with whom the program has been applied. (See Walker & Hops, 1979, in "Suggested Reading" for a more thorough review of this research.)

The CLASS program, of particular interest here, is composed of a variety of behavior modification procedures that have proven useful in managing disruptive classroom behavior. These include a token economy or point system, with both positive-reinforcement and response-cost components; contingency contracting procedures; teacher praise and attention; school and home rewards; and the occasional use of a systematic suspension procedure for certain types of disruptive or destructive school behavior. There are two general phases in the implementation of the CLASS program: an initial consultant-implemented phase is followed by teacher implementation of the later phases of the program. Days 1 through 5 of the program consist of the consultant's implementation of the procedures, with days 6 through 30 of the program being used for the teacher's implementation of the procedures begun by the consultant. The program further divides the teacher's phase of implementation into two parts: during days 6 through 20, all components of the program are operated, while days 21 through 30 are designed to maintain treatment gains from the first phase of the program. During the second phase, the token economy within the classroom, as well as the school and home rewards, are eliminated. Certain procedures from the CLASS program can be implemented indefinitely, or as long as necessary, and reinstitution of the formal program components can occur as "booster shots" if needed. Reintroduction of the program is often required when children do not meet satisfactory levels of appropriate behavior during the maintenance phase of the program. The CLASS program has been designed to keep costs relatively low, to avoid overwhelming teachers with the implementation of the program during the initial phases, and to be capable of being easily taught to school psychologists, teachers, social workers, classroom aides, and other school personnel.

The problem discussed earlier of singling out children with behavior problems for special rewards for appropriate behavior is dealt with in this program by insuring that the rewards earned by the children in school are administered on a group basis. That is, the children's classroom peers participate fully in the rewards or classroom privileges that the target children have earned. Of course, the privileges and rewards earned at home are given on an individual basis and are contingent on the children's performance at school.

In the first 5 days of the program, considered the consultant phase, the individual trained as the consultant to a classroom teacher operates the program within the daily routine of the classroom for two periods of approximately 20 to 30 minutes each during each class day. One period occurs in the morning, while the other occurs in the afternoon. Appropriateness in 80% or more of the target child's behavior is made a criterion for a group reward on each day of the training session; the reward for the entire group is contingent upon the target child's achieving this criterion each day. As part of this phase, the consultant sits near the target child's desk and uses a red and green index card located on the desk. This card is used to provide feedback to the child on the appropriateness of his or her behavior, and to award points or take away points as needed during the morning or afternoon sessions. Every 30 seconds, the consultant selects a 10-second block randomly from the 30-

second interval and awards a point on either the red or the green side of the card. Points earned on the green side are for appropriate behavior and are used to earn the group activity or reward, while points earned on the red side are considered a response cost for inappropriate behavior. If the target child achieves 80% of the possible total of points during the morning or afternoon session, the reward is given to the class. A reward at home is also earned by the child for achieving this criterion each program day. If not, both rewards are withheld for that particular classroom day. In addition to administering points, the consultant also frequently praises the child for appropriate behavior.

Beginning on day 6, the teacher begins to operate the program, and the use of the consultant is phased out of the procedure. At this point, the teacher has observed the consultant's behavior and the manner in which the program has been implemented. Of course, the teacher does not monitor the child's behavior as closely as the consultant has, but in this case he or she selects a 5-second block of time out of each 10 minutes of class time and awards the child a point on the red or green side of the point card on the basis of the child's behavior during that randomly selected 5-second block of time. The criterion for delivering the reinforcement to the child is the achievement of 80% appropriate behavior during the available 10-minute class periods each day. On day 11, the daily group rewards are terminated in an effort to begin phasing out the program. At this time, rewards of higher magnitude are made contingent upon the child's achieving the criterion for 2 program days in a row. If the child has not been successful at this during the first days of the program, the first stage is maintained until success is achieved before further phases of the program are implemented.

Throughout the program, if the child emits any of the following behaviors, the therapeutic suspension procedure is implemented: harming or attempting to harm another person; stealing or destroying property; or repeated disobedience to a staff member. When suspended, the home and school rewards are forfeited by the child, who must also complete all assigned work for that day in order to return to the school the following day. The research indicates that this aspect of the program is highly effective in managing those classes of misbehavior listed above. Under circumstances when it is impossible for a child to return home for the suspension, the suspension occurs at an in-school location arranged in advance with school staff.

By day 21 of the program, the child's behavior is being maintained by praise alone, and the token system is no longer used. Should the child be unable to maintain formerly high rates of appropriate behavior without the token system, it is reimplemented for a period of time, and then an attempt is made to withdraw it again to see if the child can be successful without it. As noted above, research suggests that the CLASS program can produce substantial changes in the appropriate behavior of many acting-out children within public school settings.

The PASS program is designed primarily to remediate low academic performance within the classroom, while the PEERS program is a treatment package designed for children who are socially withdrawn. The RECESS treatment package was developed for the treatment of socially negative and aggressive behavior outside the classroom. The reader is encouraged to write for further information on these four packaged treatment programs because of their ease of implementation and previously demonstrated success.

REDUCING CLASSROOM DISTRACTIONS AND STIMULATION

Probably one of the most widely recommended treatment programs for inattentive children in the classroom is an attempt to reduce those factors in the classroom felt to be distracting to such children. Many times, this is accomplished by having children work within three-sided study cubicles or place their desks in a location within the classroom, typically a corner, where they face the wall rather than the open classroom. In the 1950s, when this program was first suggested, it was common for teachers to be asked to reduce the number of colorful and stimulating pictures and posters within the classroom; to wear subdued jewelry, if any; to avoid wearing brightly colored clothing; and to reduce nonessential auditory stimulation. These recommendations, which were initially taken from the work of Strauss and Lehtinen, appeared to have some intuitive support for them. However, experiments attempted at several public elementary schools were not able to find any convincing evidence of the efficacy of the reduced stimulation programs. Similar research on the use of study cubicles for highly distractible and inattentive children also has not found any evidence to suggest that they are beneficial to improving the classroom behavior, academic productivity, or accuracy of such children. Thus, although these practices tend to be used quite frequently within many public schools, there is very little research to support their utility.

Research on the issue of whether hyperactive children are more distractible than other children continues to be quite controversial. At this time, there are probably as many studies suggesting that reducing distractions with hyperactive children is not effective as there are studies to support its efficacy. Some of the more recent and more rigorous research tends to suggest that hyperactive children are more distractible when distractors of very high appeal occur within a particular academic task. With distractors of low appeal, hyperactive children have not been found to be more distractible than normal children. At this point, it is probably best to conclude that there probably exist certain classes of high-appeal distractors that are more likely to draw hyperactive children off task than they are to distract normal children. However, a program that focuses solely on the reduction of distractors is quite unlikely to bring about any substantial improvement in the behavior or academic performance of hyperactive children.

ISSUES IN MAINTAINING PARENT–SCHOOL–THERAPIST RELATIONS

A variety of problems and issues arise in attempting to coordinate educational programs for hyperactive children. The utilization of classroom behavior management programs requires that there be appropriate channels and opportunities for communication between parents and schools. Periodic meetings should be held involving parents, school staff, and therapists consulting to the schools to review the goals of the children's educational programs and the degree to which they are being achieved by current programming.

Some problems that develop in the maintenance of cordial yet effective relations between parents and schools are those having to do with the expectations of the parents for the educational program. Many parents tend to believe that the ultimate purpose of special programs within the public schools is to "cure" children's difficulties, be they problems in behavior, in emotional adjustment, or in academic achievement. As the early chapters in this book have indicated, such goals are rarely achieved and should never be promised to parents by school staff. Often, if parents are told plainly from the beginning that the purpose of school programs is to attempt to minimize the difficulties their children are having at school and to optimize their academic achievement—not necessarily to "normalize" the children—the parents are much more likely to cooperate with school programs. They will also be more empathetic with the difficulties teachers may be experiencing in dealing with their children.

A second, though related, problem seen in the relationship between many parents and their school systems is the belief that the schools should maintain more frequent communication with families about the children's performance than that which typically occurs. Certainly, for hyperactive children, classroom teachers need to communicate more frequently with parents than the typical 9-week grading evaluation allows. On the other hand, to expect teachers to maintain daily contact, or even contact several times per week, by telephone or by personal meeting, results in an exorbitant demand on the teachers' time and detracts from their responsibilities to the other children in their classes. Obviously, therapists must see that some reasonable balance is struck between the parents' need for communication and the teachers' responsibilities in the classroom if cordial relations between parents and teachers are to continue.

A third problem often witnessed with parents of hyperactive children occurs in those cases when parents are having few if any difficulties managing the children's behavior at home during a particular academic year, while teachers are having considerable difficulties doing so in the classroom. Often, in these circumstances, the parents cannot believe that the teachers are having as much difficulty as they report, since they themselves do not see problems occurring to this degree within the home. Parents may tend to blame schools for the problems the children are having within the classroom, to accuse teachers of inadequate or incompetent teaching or behavior management methods, or, in some cases, to accuse teachers outright of fabricating problems about the children because of a presumed "personality clash" with them or a desire to have them removed from the classroom. In many cases, this problem can be alleviated if therapists explaining to both teachers and parents that hyperactive children are likely to show great variability or inconsistency in their behavior problems from one situation to the next or from one day to the next during any given period of time. Hence, it is not inconceivable that such children could be having significant problems in the school and yet could remain more manageable within the home circumstances. Where facilities permit, having parents come in to observe their children unobtrusively—without the children's awareness, if possible—may allow them to witness the difficulties the teachers are having with the children and therefore to gain a better appreciation for the basis for the teachers' complaints.

Similar problems may arise from the teachers' perspective in dealing with parents of hyperactive children. Some teachers tend to believe that the children's difficulties within the classroom are the result of deep-seated emotional problems or unmet emotional needs for which their families, the parents in particular, are responsible. This belief implies that the primary cause of the children's hyperactivity is functional or emotional, rather than organic, physiologic, or temperamental. This may sometimes lead teachers to accuse the families of creating the children's problems, or to encourage the families to enroll the children in long-term psychotherapy in the belief that this will somehow resolve the children's emotional difficulties. The function of therapists in this situation must be to provide adequate reading material and opportunity for discussion with the teachers in order to educate them about the nature of hyperactivity and its causes, as well as to assist them in making more appropriate recommendations to families for obtaining help for their children.

A second difficulty that teachers may have pertains to the limited time available to them to implement additional behavior management programs with the hyperactive children in regular classrooms. As noted above, the teachers are likely to have numerous other responsibilities to the other children in her class, as well as to school administrators, and they may not be able to provide as much time with the children as the parents or behavior modification programs demand. Here therapists must weigh carefully the time involved in implementing and maintaining particular behavior management programs in the classroom before making recommendations to the teachers. If this is not done, a situation may arise in which a therapist recommends a particular classroom program, the teacher does not have time to implement it, and the parents become angry with the classroom teacher or the school staff in general because of their failure to follow through on recommendations made by an outside professional consultant. By showing compassion for the many responsibilities teachers must have in the course of personal meetings with parents and teachers, it is quite possible for therapists to avoid these sorts of pitfalls in maintaining professional relations.

One of the easiest ways to avoid the above difficulties is for consultants or therapists to make a habit of visiting hyperactive children's classrooms and to discuss the children's programming and progress periodically with their teachers. Involving the parents in these meetings in many cases allows for open, candid communication about the children's responses to programs that have already been implemented, and it allows all parties to suggest ways in which they feel the programs might be changed for the children's betterment. At times, this may mean that therapist–consultants will have to admit that they do not have all the answers or all the programs that are guaranteed to improve the children's behavior. Instead, the consultants will make available to the schools and the parents certain programs that have previously demonstrated effectiveness with similar children. When initial programs fail, they can be amended or others can be substituted for them, with input from parents and teachers. In this way, all parties to the programs are made responsible for their success or for their revision, and hence no one is to blame if the programs do not live up to their desired goals. This simply necessitates that the programs be revised or that new programs be designed to meet particular children's needs more successfully.

When difficulties between parents and teachers that do not seem to be capable of solution in personal meetings develop, then it may be necessary to go to administrators higher up in the echelon of responsibilities within the schools to attempt resolution of the problems. When this is not successful, it may be necessary to bring formal legal appeals on behalf of the children under Public Law 94-142, the federal legislation dealing with the education of handicapped children. This, however, should remain the absolute last resort, to be employed only when it is obvious to consultants that schools are not meeting children's needs as dictated under this public law and similar statutes in state law. In my experience, however, this rarely needs to be done, because very nearly all school staff members are quite responsive to making those changes within their power for the betterment of hyperactive children's education.

SUMMARY

This chapter has reviewed a number of methods that can be used to manage hyperactive behavior within the classroom. In most cases, the methods described have a substantial amount of scientific research supporting their efficacy in managing disruptive behavior. In addition, when the methods are applied to various aspects of academic performance (i.e., accuracy and productivity), improvements in these parameters have also been witnessed. Like the management of hyperactive behavior in the home, the management of hyperactive children in the classroom is approached with an attitude of attempting to cope with and diminish the children's problems rather than to cure them. It is expected that the children will present with periodic management problems throughout their educational careers, and that therefore periodic psychological and educational assistance will be required. Nonetheless, through the use of the methods outlined here, substantial improvements in classroom behavior and achievement can occur. In some cases, these methods can be combined with psychopharmacological treatment in order to cope more effectively with the problems presented by particular hyperactive children. Whichever methods are chosen, care must be taken to insure that they are cost-effective, that they are well within the teachers' time and ability to implement in the classroom, and that they are periodically reviewed for their ongoing efficacy and need for revision. Some attention also needs to be given to maintaining cordial and responsive relations between parents, school staff members, and therapists in the day-to-day and year-to-year management of hyperactive children. No matter how much evidence may exist to support the effectiveness of a particular behavior management method in the classroom, it is unlikely to prove so in an individual child's case if communication, rapport, and general working relationships are impaired among the parents, school staff, and outside consultants.

SUGGESTED READING

The readings listed at the end of Chapter 6 would also be appropriate for obtaining information on classroom behavior management. In addition, the following are of particular interest:

Atkinson, B. M., & Forehand, R. Home-based reinforcement programs designed to modify classroom behavior: A review and methodological evaluation. *Psychological Bulletin,* 1979, *86,* 1298–1308.

Ayllon, T., Layman, D., & Kandel, H. J. A behavioral–educational alternative to drug control of hyperactive children. *Journal of Applied Behavior Analysis,* 1975, *8,* 137–146.

Ayllon, T., & Roberts, M. Eliminating discipline problems by strengthening academic performance. *Journal of Applied Behavior Analysis,* 1974, *7,* 71–76.

Ayllon, T., & Rosenbaum, M. S. The behavioral treatment of disruption and hyperactivity in school settings. In B. Lahey & A. Kazdin (Eds.), *Advances in child clinical psychology* (Vol. 1). New York: Plenum, 1977.

Barkley, R. A., Copeland, A., & Sivage, C. A self-control classroom for hyperactive children. *Journal of Autism and Developmental Disorders,* 1980, *10,* 75–89.

Bolstad, O., & Johnson, S. Self-regulation in the modification of disruptive classroom behavior. *Journal of Applied Behavior Analysis,* 1972, *5,* 443–454.

O'Leary, K. D., & O'Leary, S. G. Behavior modification in the school. In H. Leitenberg (Ed.), *Handbook of behavior modification and behavior therapy.* New York: Appleton-Century-Crofts, 1976.

Patterson, G. The aggressive child: Victim and architect of a coercive system. In E. J. Mash, L. A. Hamerlynck, & L. C. Handy (Eds.), *Behavior modification and families.* New York: Brunner/Mazel, 1976.

Walker, H., & Hops, H. The CLASS program for acting-out children: R & D procedures, program outcomes, and implementation issues. *School Psychology Digest,* 1979, *8,* 370–381.

CHAPTER NINE

OTHER TREATMENT
APPROACHES

Nothing can be more unphilosophical than to be positive or dogmatical on any subject.—When men are the most sure and arrogant, they are commonly the most mistaken and have there given reins to passion without the proper deliberation and suspense which alone can secure them from the grossest absurdities.—*David Hume*

The most common and most effective treatment approaches for hyperactive children have been described in earlier chapters of this text. There are, however, a number of lesser known and less well substantiated treatment approaches that deserve at least passing reference in this manual for the clinician, if only because of the public controversy and popularity that surrounds them. Attention will not be given to every type of treatment recommendation that has been made for hyperactive children. Such an examination of unsubstantiated treatment programs would require a volume in itself. Instead, this chapter will briefly examine those treatment approaches that seem to be receiving large amounts of public attention at this particular time. These include dietary and nutritional regimens, treatment of allergic reactions, experiments in limiting fluorescent lighting, and biofeedback treatments.

DIETARY AND NUTRITIONAL TREATMENTS

Probably the most popular dietary approach to the management of hyperactive children is the Kaiser–Permanente diet described by Benjamin Feingold in a book published in 1975. At the outset, it should be noted that Feingold's idea can hardly be considered original, as papers have appeared since 1922 that have asserted that behavior problems and hyperactivity could result from allergic or toxic reactions to various substances. Nonetheless, it is the Feingold diet that has received the most vocal popular support and the greatest scrutiny among scientific studies.

Feingold's thesis, simply stated, is that hyperactivity and other childhood disorders are frequently caused by intolerance to food additives and salicylates. The latter compounds tend to occur naturally in some fruits and vegetables. He insists that food additives are a major cause of hyperactivity in children in this country—in fact, that they may account for as much as 40% to 50% of the hyperactive population. Feingold believes that certain children have a natural toxic reaction or intolerance to artificial colors, flavorings, antioxidants, preservatives, and other substances added to foods to enhance their attractiveness or to increase their shelf life. The regimen proposed by Feingold attempts to eliminate these substances as much as possible from a child's diet in order to improve the child's hyperactive behavior. While this chapter focuses on Feingold's claims that his diet reduces hyperactivity, it is worth noting that Feingold has also advocated his diet as a primary treatment for mental retardation, vandalism, delinquency and crime, learning disabilities, and early infantile autism. Feingold argues that dramatic clinical responses are evidenced in these groups of children when they are placed on additive-free diets, such as the one he advocates. Because of the hypothesized widespread involvement of food additives as causative agents for the aforementioned problems, Feingold has advocated that school districts should establish highly controlled school lunch programs, using foods free of the toxic substances that supposedly lead to hyperactivity and the other childhood problems. The reader wishing to obtain greater detail about the foods and medicines that Feingold claims should be eliminated from children's diets is referred to Feingold's book (1975; see "Suggested Reading").

There are a number of case reports appearing in quasiscientific publications that claim dramatic improvement in children's hyperactive symptoms as a result of putting such children on the Feingold diet. The reader who takes the time to track down the more rigorously controlled scientific studies will find little evidence to support the dramatic claims made by Feingold. Nonetheless, some of the scientific reports have found that perhaps a *small* percentage of *younger* hyperactive children may display a *mild* exacerbation of their symptoms when given single doses containing moderate to large amounts of food additives. Clinicians would be well advised to become acquainted with the scientific literature in this area because of the frequent requests from many parents of hyperactive children for professional advice about the Feingold diet. This literature would permit a more balanced viewpoint about the efficacy of the diet, as opposed to one based simply upon uncontrolled case reports provided by the highly vocal advocates of this dietary regimen.

One of the first studies to attempt a more rigorous evaluation of influence of food additives on hyperactive behavior was conducted in 1976 by C. Keith Conners and his colleagues of that time at the University of Pittsburgh. This experiment was a double-blind crossover treatment program comparing a control diet with a diet that eliminated artificial flavors, colors, and naturally occurring salicylates, as recommended in Feingold's book. The study involved 15 hyperactive children, who were rated at various times on teacher and parent rating scales (the Conners PSQ and TRS, described in Chapter 3 of this book). The children were rated during a 2-week baseline period while all stimulant medication was withheld and before either of the diets was implemented. The children were then randomly assigned to either the control diet or the experimental diet for a period of 4 weeks, with parents and teachers completing the rating scales each week. In addition, a global indicator of improvement was made by the principal investigators on the basis of parental interviews and school reports. The children then "crossed over" to whichever treatment procedure they had not yet received for an additional 4-week period. Again, the PSQ and TRS were completed weekly during the last 4 weeks of this program.

Although the parents' and teachers' ratings reported fewer hyperkinetic symptoms while the children were on the experimental diet, only the ratings noted by the teachers were statistically significant. The reduction in symptoms noted by parents and teachers was one of approximately 15% from the original baseline ratings, with the most dramatic improvement being evidenced in those children who received the control diet first and the Feingold diet second. Despite the statistically significant reductions noted in the teacher ratings for the hyperactive children while they were receiving the Feingold diet, the degree of change in these ratings can hardly be considered clinically significant. The teacher ratings while the children received the control diet had a mean of 17.18, while the mean for teacher ratings during the Feingold diet was 13.93. This mean difference of slightly more than 3 points on the Conners TRS can hardly be viewed as dramatic, considering that the range of scores on the rating scale may vary from 0 to 30. In addition, drug and behavior therapy procedures typically produce reductions in these ratings of at least 50% from the initial baseline ratings. The results of the study for the clinicians' global ratings of improvement similarly reflect this fact; 10 of the 15 children were rated as showing minimal change, as showing no change, or in fact as worsening as a result of the Feingold diet. Only one of the 15 children was actually rated as showing any marked degree of improvement as a result of the dietary treatment.

There are a number of problems with the study noted above; foremost among them is the fact that the two diets were not necessarily adequately matched, making it quite possible for the experimental diet to be differentiated from the control diet by the nature of the foods used within it. A second problem with the study was its reliance on only the subjective judgments of parents and teachers as indicated in rating scales completed on a weekly basis. Such rating scales are known to be highly sensitive to the effects of expectation and to show a large amount of variation over time. Obviously, the marked order effect found in this study, in which the experimental diet showed its primary benefits only after it followed the control diet and not when it preceded the control diet, may well support the contention that parents could detect differences between the experimental and the control diets on the basis of their content. In any case, the order effect found in this study has been found in subsequent studies as well and has yet to be adequately explained. The most that could be concluded from the study, then, is that fewer than 30% of the children showed any clinically noticeable change in their symptoms in response to the Feingold diet, and that only one of the 15 children demonstrated what could be considered a clinically significant improvement in behavior.

In a subsequent paper reported by the same research group (1980), 16 hyperactive children were selected for study on the grounds that they had shown previous improvements in behavior in response to the Feingold diet. These 16 children were then challenged at various times throughout the course of the study to determine whether the food additives in fact worsened their behavior. The study involved having the 16 children remain on the Feingold diet, but periodically challenging them with chocolate cookies containing large amounts of dyes or with placebo cookies containing no dyes. The results of the study indicated no significant effects of the food dyes on the hyperactive children, either as measured by parent and teacher rating scales or as noted by a visual–motor tracking task presumed to measure distractibility. Upon closer inspection of individual subjects' responses, the investigators found that three of the 16 children may have shown a deterioration in behavior in response to the food dyes. These children tended to be the youngest among the subjects (between 6 and 7 years of age) and tended to show their behavior changes on the measure of attention span and distractibility within several hours after receiving the challenge cookies. In a second phase of this study, eight younger subjects (mean age, 5.3 years) who were also previously shown to be diet-responsive were combined with five other children (mean age, 7 years) who were considered borderline responders to the diet. These subjects were taken through the same treatment procedures as those used in the first phase of this study. The food dyes were noted to have a significant effect on their behavior as rated by parents; the effect was primarily limited to a 3-hour period immediately following ingestion of the food dyes.

A major problem with this series of challenge studies and with many to be discussed subsequently lies in their application of a single-dose administration of food dyes to children as part of the experimental procedures. The doses that are used in these and in subsequent studies are considered equal to if not greater than the average daily amount of food additives that children are likely to consume, as estimated by various Federal or commercial agencies. The major difficulty here is that the amount of dye a child may consume during a given day is spread out over the course of the child's waking day—not consumed in a single acute dose. The challenge studies, however, are giving the children this amount of dye, or in some cases more, in a single dose. Hence, the challenge studies cannot be taken as representative of the reactions a typical child would show to food dyes if small amounts of the dye were consumed over a long period of time.

In 1978, Terry Rose of Northern Illinois University published another study that tended to support the idea that food additives may exacerbate the behavior of some hyperactive children. This study involved two 8-year-old hyperactive girls who had been previously shown to be responsive to the Feingold diet. The children participated in a single-case, reversal design under double-blind conditions. The procedures involved maintaining the children on the Feingold diet and then periodically challenging them with cookies containing food dyes or with placebo cookies that contained no food dyes. One advantage of this study over the studies previously reported is that objective observations were made of the children's classroom behavior throughout the course of the study. The results for one subject in the study are displayed in Figure 9.1; these indicate that this child showed significant worsening in measures of on-task time and out-of-seat time in the classroom as a result of the challenge periods. As with the previous studies, these findings indicate that a small group of hyperactive children may in fact have their symptoms made worse by the ingestion of artificial food dyes. They do not speak to the issue of whether food dyes are in fact primarily responsible for causing hyperactivity in the 40% to 50% of hyperactive children claimed by Feingold.

Similar results were obtained in a study reported by James Swanson and Marcel Kinsbourne (1980). The children in this study were given two different doses of dyes estimated to be at the 90th percentile or higher for daily consumption of artificial food dyes by children; the dyes were administered as part of this study in a single acute dose. Only one dependent measure was taken, a laboratory learning task believed to reflect attention span and simple verbal learning. The results found that either dose of food dye could significantly impair the performance of the 20 hyperactive children and 20 nonhyperactive children used in this experiment. The maximum effect of the food dyes occurred within approximately 1½ hours after ingestion of the dye and lasted at least 3½ hours in most of the children. Again, while this study suggests that some children, either hyperactive or normal, may show exacerbation of their behavior in response to food dyes, the conditions of the study are highly questionable as to their representativeness of the typical eating habits of most children. That is, the children in the Swanson and Kinsbourne study received extremely high doses of artificial food dyes in a single acute dose, whereas children are typically likely to consume much smaller quantities of food dye in many more doses over the course of an entire day. In other words, it is highly unlikely that a child would consume

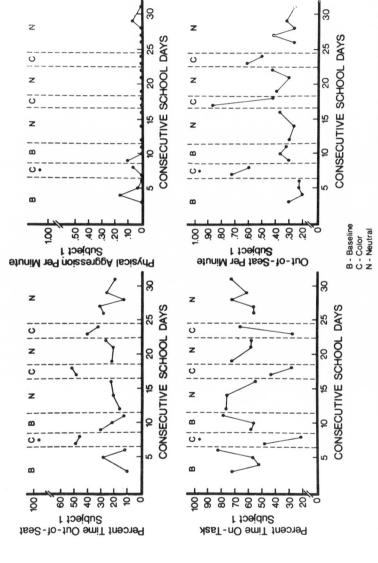

FIGURE 9.1. A comparison of typical hyperactive responses during periods when artificial food colors were ingested and not ingested by Subject 1. Asterisk denotes dietary infraction wherein artificial colors were not experimentally introduced, but were reportedly consumed. (From "The Functional Relationship between Artificial Food Colors and Hyperactivity" by T. L. Rose, *Journal of Applied Behavior Analysis*, 1978, *11*, 439–446. Copyright 1978 by *The Society for the Experimental Analysis of Behavior*. Reprinted by permission.)

amounts of food dye estimated to be at the 90th percentile for daily consumption of most children in a single acute dose in the course of his or her normal dietary habits.

Many studies have found virtually no positive effects of the Feingold diet on hyperactive behavior. Probably the most rigorously conducted of these, or of any of the studies, were those reported in 1978 by J. Preston Harley and his colleagues at the University of Wisconsin. These scientists conducted a two-phase experimental program evaluating the effects of the Feingold diet and of food additives on the behavior of hyperactive children. The studies are noteworthy because of their extremely rigorous efforts to prevent families participating in the study from being able to detect in which phases of the study the children were receiving control diet substances. In addition, the studies used a substantial battery of teacher ratings, objective classroom and laboratory observational data, measures of attention span and concentration, and other neuropsychological measures. In the first phase of the program, 36 hyperactive boys were tested in a crossover procedure in which half received the experimental diet first and the control diet second, while the other half received the experimental and control diets in the opposite order. Only the measure of parental ratings of behavior revealed any positive behavioral changes as a result of the experimental diet, and these seemed to occur primarily in the group which was given the control diet first and the experimental diet second. Again, this finding is similar to that obtained by Conners and his colleagues, as noted above. The 10 hyperactive children who showed improvements in behavior as rated by their parents were primarily preschool hyperactive boys. Examination of their results on the laboratory measures of classroom behavior, attention, and neuropsychological measures showed no changes as a result of the diet. The results can therefore hardly be construed as impressive evidence for any treatment effects of the Feingold diet, especially since drug treatment and behavior modification procedures typically produce substantial improvements in most of the measures used in this study.

In the second phase of the Wisconsin program, nine hyperactive boys were selected on the basis of having shown a favorable response to the Feingold diet in the previous study. These children were maintained on a strict Feingold diet for 11 weeks and were then given multiple challenges with placebo and food dye materials, with measures of their behavior being taken in parental and teacher ratings, classroom behavior observations, and neuropsychological test scores. Nine normal children, matched with the hyperactive children on the basis of sex, grade, and academic ability, were also studied and were rated on the same measures. The results did not show any adverse effects of the artificial food colors on any of the measures of behavior for either the hyperactive or the control subjects. The results for the nine hyperactive children are depicted in Figure 9.2. These graphs demonstrate

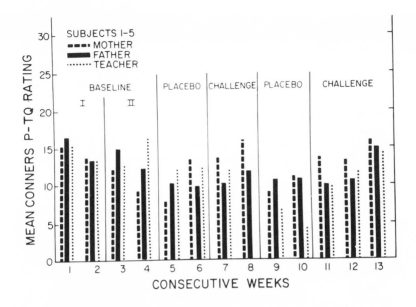

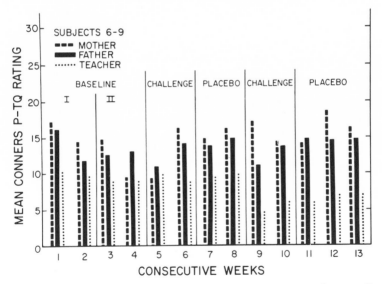

FIGURE 9.2. Upper figure: Mean weekly Conners parent and teacher questionnaire ratings for five hyperactive subjects receiving placebo–challenge–placebo–challenge sequence. Lower figure: Mean weekly Conners parent and teacher questionnaire ratings for four hyperactive subjects receiving challenge–placebo–challenge–placebo sequence. (From "Synthetic Food Colors and Hyperactivity in Children: A Double-Blind Challenge Experiment" by J. P. Harley, C. G. Matthews, and P. L. Eichman, *Pediatrics*, 1978, *62*, 975–983. Copyright 1978 by the American Academy of Pediatrics. Reprinted by permission.)

the results for the parent and teacher questionnaires for the five subjects
receiving the placebo and challenge materials in one experimental order and
for the four hyperactive subjects receiving the materials in the opposite order
of administration. In addition, Figure 9.3 shows the results for the hyperactive and control children on the measure of average disruptive classroom
behavior as recorded in objective observations of classroom conduct. The
figure shows virtually no difference between the placebo and challenge
phases of the study for either the hyperactive or the control children.

In 1980, Bernard Weiss, a highly vocal advocate of the Feingold diet,
reported a study in which 22 young children were maintained on the Feingold
diet and periodically challenged with artificial food colors. Double-blind
procedures were used, and behavioral observations made by the parents
of the children served as the dependent measures. The results indicated that
only two of the children showed any changes in behavior in response to the
challenge with food dyes; one of these children showed a mild response to
the challenge, while the other showed a "dramatic" response. Like the
Wisconsin studies, even this study conducted by an acknowledged advocate
of the Feingold diet produced no clinically significant findings for the effect
of artificial food colors on the behavior of most children.

FIGURE 9.3. Mean disruptive classroom behavior index for hyperactive and control
groups by condition. (From "Synthetic Food Colors and Hyperactivity in Children: A
Double-Blind Challenge Experiment" by J. P. Harley, C. G. Matthews, and P. L. Eichman,
Pediatrics, 1978, *62*, 975–983. Copyright 1978 by the American Academy of Pediatrics.
Reprinted by permission.)

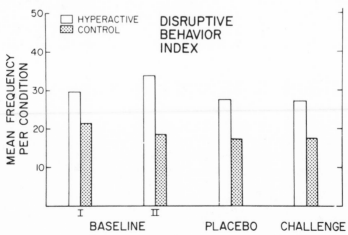

In 1978, J. Ivan Williams and his colleagues at the University of Toronto conducted a comparison study of the effects of stimulant medication and the Feingold diet on hyperactive behavior. Each of 26 hyperactive children was randomly assigned to receive either an active or a placebo medication, and both groups were subsequently challenged with cookies containing artificial food colors or control cookies without these food additives. The primary dependent measures were behavior checklists completed by teachers and parents. The findings indicated that the stimulant medications were substantially more effective than the diet in controlling hyperactive behavior. The effects for the diet were described as "inconclusive." The examination of the individual responses of the children indicated that the behavior of perhaps three to eight children might be considered diet-responsive on the basis of teacher ratings. Nonetheless, the results can hardly be considered impressive evidence for treatment effects of the Feingold diet on hyperactive children. This is especially true when the diet effects are contrasted with those obtained by the stimulant medications typically administered to hyperactive children, which in this case produced their typically dramatic and clinically effective changes in both parent and teacher ratings of hyperactive behavior.

Another study of the effects of food additives on hyperactive behavior was conducted by F. Levy and his colleagues in Sydney, Australia (1978). This study utilized 22 hyperactive children, who were tested before and after 4 weeks on the Feingold diet and after a series of challenges with both a food dye and a placebo substance. The measures used were the Conners PSQ and TRS, objective measures of attention span, standard tests of perceptual–motor ability, and selected subtests from the WISC. Although the results showed a statistically significant improvement in the mothers' ratings of the children's behavior after 4 weeks of the diet, none of the results for the objective measures showed any statistically significant effects throughout any phase of the study. Like previous studies, this study found that the subjective ratings of parents show some improvement when children are placed on an elimination diet, but that these changes are not corroborated by objective behavioral or laboratory measures.

The foregoing brief review of the studies that have attempted to examine the effects of the Feingold diet on the behaior of hyperactive and normal children can hardly be considered persuasive evidence for the adoption of the Feingold diet as a primary treatment for hyperactive children. None of the studies found a dramatic inprovement in the behavior of 40% to 50% of hyperactive children, such as Feingold claims occurs when such children are placed on his diet. At best, one can conclude that a small percentage of hyperactive children (perhaps less than 10%) show a mild exacerbation of their hyperkinetic symptoms as a temporary reaction to single doses containing moderate to high amounts of food dyes. These children tend to be primarily in the younger age groups (6 years of age and younger) and to show a prior history of responding to the diet as determined by subjective parental ratings. Certainly, none of these studies finds any evidence that food additives are a major cause of hyperactivity in children, as hypothesized by Feingold. When effects of food additives are found on children's behavior, the degree of adverse reaction is quite small and can hardly be considered clinically significant.

A number of issues in the research on this treatment procedure must be addressed before the procedure can be taken seriously as an effective treatment for hyperactive children. First, future studies of a highly rigorous and scientific nature are going to have to find a more dramatic change in behavior as a result of the Feingold diet. Second, future studies must address the issue of whether treatment by the Feingold diet produces any adverse effects on children's nutrition and health. Many investigators have now recognized that the foods that Feingold suggests should be eliminated from children's diets are often high in Vitamin C and carbohydrates. Placing children on the Feingold diet may result in less than desirable levels of Vitamin C and carbohydrate intake for them. Third, the proponents of Feingold's theories have yet to give any adequate explanation for the mechanism of the effects of food additives on behavior. Fourth, the proponents of the Feingold diet will have to propose their hypotheses with greater specificity, so that tests can be run to determine which of the 200 or more food additives in existence are in fact being proposed as the causes of difficult behavior in children. These last two issues are even more problematic when one considers Feingold's rather grandiose and unsubstantiated claims that additives not only contribute to hyperactivity, but are also major causes of learning disabilities, retardation, crime and delinquency, and autism in children. A fifth issue is that of whether or not families can be expected to make children adhere rigorously to a diet that eliminates such a wide variety of substances normally found in children's nutritional intake. No study has yet to show that the diet is especially cost-effective in terms of the hours required for preparation of the food and supervision of a child's eating habits, especially in view of the minimal or nonexistent effects that such dietary regimens produce. Obviously, the Feingold diet has yet to show improvements in behavior comparable to those achieved by more traditional methods of therapy, such as behavior modification, educational management, and stimulant medication. At present, many of the scientists conducting research on hyperactive children do not take seriously the extravagant claims made by Feingold for his treatment approach for hyperactive children; nor do most of them consider the Feingold diet an effective alternative to the more traditional therapies for coping with hyperactive behavior.

VITAMIN DEFICIENCIES AND FOOD ALLERGIES

It has been proposed that vitamin deficiencies or imbalances, as well as artificial additives and flavors, can lead to hyperactive behavior. The most vocal proponent of this treatment program is Lendon Smith, a pediatrician in private practice in Portland, Oregon. His ideas have received wide publicity through various media and have prompted a number of parents to pursue the use of vitamins, among other things, as treatments for their hyperactive or behavior-disordered children. Unlike Feingold, Smith has not put forth a well-articulated or unitary etiology of hyperactivity. Instead, he merely proposes that a variety of foodstuffs can create hyperactivity in children and that an equally varied number of vitamins and foods can be used to treat children with behavior problems. In his public interviews, Smith is rarely called upon to document the evidence for his proposals, and they are often taken by parents as authoritative scientific gospel, when in fact many of his ideas have virtually no scientific evidence to support their efficacy. For instance, Smith has proposed that temper tantrums in young children may be a result of a zinc or protein deficiency in the diets of these children. His recommendations for temper tantrums or behavior problems in children may range from suggesting that they have zinc or other vitamins added to their diets, to recommending that parents give their misbehaving children peanut butter upon the occurrence of these misbehaviors in order to increase the amount of protein in their diet and hence to control the number of temper tantrums. A reading of Smith's book, *Your Child's Behavior Chemistry* (1976; see "Suggested Reading"), reveals many contradictory statements and recommendations that are unsubstantiated or that in fact are in striking contrast to well-known principles of learning and behavior in children. Other than case reports from his own private practice, Smith presents no scientific data to support the contention that removing certain foods while introducing other foods or vitamin supplements actually improves the behavior of hyperactive and conduct-disordered children. Probably as a result of Smith's grandiose claims and vague and often contradictory hypotheses, reputable medical and psychological scientists have given little if any research attention to this treatment approach. Clinicians are well advised to follow a similar course until the advocates of Smith's treatments and those of other megavitamin and dietary treatments for misbehavior produce objective scientific data to support their claims.

Ronald Trites and his colleagues (1980) have conducted a series of studies with hyperactive children that indicate that these children do show a greater number of allergies to food substances than matched groups of normal children have. Removing these food substances from their diets has shown a mild degree of improvement in the hyperactive children's behavior, but has not resulted in a complete or even a clinically significant improvement in their hyperkinetic symptoms. The research of Trites on food allergies remains to be replicated by other scientists.

SUGAR

Besides food additives and vitamins, current research has begun to explore the effects of refined sugar on the behavior of hyperactive and normal children. Some clinicians have suggested that hyperactive children consume large amounts of sugar, which leads to hypoglycemia, irritable moods, and restless behavior. Currently, there is little evidence to show either that hyperactive children are more likely to be hypoglycemic or that they ingest large amounts of sugar. Nonetheless, interest in the effects of sugar on children's behavior remains high.

In a recent study, Ronald Prinz, William Roberts, and Elaine Hantman at the University of South Carolina (1980) studied the relationship of sugar consumption to behavior in hyperactive and normal children. A total of 28 hyperactive and 26 control children were followed in the study, which monitored their food consumption through diaries kept by parents for a week. The children's consumption of foods that did or did not contain sugar was correlated with observations of the children's behavior in a clinic playroom for 15 minutes. Measures of three behaviors were also taken: aggression-destruction, restlessness, and locomotor activity.

Comparisons of the two groups of children on seven measures of dietary intake revealed no significant differences in the children's consumption of sugar products or in the ratio of sugar products to other nutritional foodstuffs, such as protein or carbohydrates, in the children's diets. However, the normal children were found to consume significantly more food in general than the hyperactive children. The study reported that 15 of the hyperactive children had a history of stimulant medication, but it does not indicate how many of these were on medication at the time the observations were made. If a large number were medicated, then the known anorexic effects of these drugs could account for the lower food consumption in the hyperactive group.

Correlations were made between the measures of diet and of playroom behavior in both groups. Results for the hyperactive group revealed significant correlations between the various amounts of sugar products consumed and destructive-aggressive behavior and restlessness in the playroom. No correlations with locomotor behavior were significant. These results suggest that children with higher rates of aggressive-destructive behavior and restlessness consume more sugar. In the control group, this pattern of relations was not found. Instead, more consumption of sugar correlated significantly with greater locomotor activity, but not with the other two measures of behavior. Because these results are only correlational, they do not indicate whether high levels of sugar produce greater destructive–aggressive behavior or restlessness—only that the two are related. It is equally possible that more aggressive and restless children are likely to consume more sugared foods as a result of poor impulse control, in which case the higher sugar intake would be viewed not as the cause of their behavior problems but as the result of them. Either explanation is quite tenable at this point.

Several problems exist with this study; its results require cross-validation before much confidence can be placed in them. First, the pattern of correlations was not found to be the same for both groups of children. While this might suggest that hyperactive children respond differently to sugar intake than normal children do, other explanations are possible. For one thing, the correlations between total amount of food consumed by both groups and their behavior were not reported, nor were they partialled out of the other correlations reported between sugar intake and behavior. It is possible that higher consumption of food in general is related to greater behavior problems. This becomes important if we remember that up to 50% of the hyperactive children may have been on medication during the study and that these drugs can reduce both food intake and misbehavior. In this case, the fact that both medicated and unmedicated children were in the same hyperactive group would produce spuriously high correlations between misbehavior and sugar intake in that group but not in the control group; precisely these results were indeed produced. Second, the age ranges in both groups were large (ages varied from 3 to 8 years), and this suggests that age as a variable should also have been partialled out of the correlations between food intake and playroom behavior. Again, this becomes important with respect to medication status in the hyperactive group. Younger hyperactive children are not as likely to eat as much food as older medicated children do. Younger hyperactives are also known to be more destructive and restless than older hyperactives, especially if the younger ones are not on medication. Again, spuriously high correlations between diet and behavior would be expected only in the hyperactive group because of this age $\times$ medication status $\times$ symptom severity interaction. Finally, the study would have been more convincing in addressing these issues if actual sugar intake had been manipulated as part of this study so that its causal role in behavior could be studied.

In conclusion, there appears to be some evidence that high levels of sugar intake may be related to greater amounts of aggressive and restless behavior in hyperactive, but not in normal, children. The causal direction of this relationship is far from clear and requires much further study. What is clear is that sugar is unlikely to be a major etiology of hyperactivity in children, as the rates of sugar consumption do not appear to differ between hyperactive and normal children.

OTHER ALLERGIES

John Taylor, a private practicing psychologist in Salem, Oregon, has proposed in his recent book (1980) that another cause of hyperactive behavior may be allergic reactions to various substances in the environment. He lists well over 50 possible sources of irritants that may produce allergic reactions in some children, and proposes that if hyperactive children do not respond to the Feingold diet, it may be because these other sources in the children's environment are so exacerbating their behavior that they cannot show a positive diet response. Although some evidence is beginning to accrue to the effect that hyperactive children show more allergies to various substances than other children do, there is virtually no evidence to show that these allergic reactions are in fact the cause of the children's hyperactive behavior, or in fact that they even exacerbate the children's hyperkinetic symptoms. In view of the fact that there is virtually no evidence at this point to support the claims of Taylor and others that hyperactivity results from these potential allergens, clinicians are advised to avoid the use of treatment procedures that involve eliminating potential allergens from a child's environment.

FLUORESCENT LIGHTING

In 1974, John Ott, a cinematographer formerly with Walt Disney Productions, proposed that the emission of soft X rays and radio frequencies from fluorescent lighting and television created hyperactive behavior in children who were exposed to such lighting sources. Ott and his colleagues then went on to report the results of an experiment in which children exposed to fluorescent lights that purportedly emitted mild amounts of X radiation showed more disruptive and off-task behavior in the classroom than did groups of children exposed to fluorescent lighting that was shielded for the purported source of radiation. The study suffered from methodological flaws too numerous to mention here. What is worth mentioning is the fact that a more controlled, scientific study of the effects of fluorescent lighting was attempted by K. Daniel O'Leary and his associates (1978). In this study, seven first-grade children with conduct problems and hyperactivity attended a laboratory school classroom for an 8-week period. During this time, the classroom lighting conditions were alternated at the end of each week, and observers unaware of the change in lighting conditions recorded the extent of on- or off-task behavior and completed activity rating scales on the children. On odd-numbered weeks during the program, the classroom was illuminated by standard cool-white fluorescent lighting systems. During even-numbered weeks, the classroom was illuminated with a daylight-simulating fluorescent system with controls for the purported emission of soft X rays and radio frequencies. The results of the study revealed no differences in the effects of the two lighting conditions on measures of disruptive behavior in these first-grade children. Not only do the results of this study call Ott's rather ludicrous hypothesis into serious question, but several physics and medical research scientists wrote to the journal *Pediatric News* shortly after hearing of Ott's hypothesis to explain that fluorescent lighting is incapable of emitting the soft X rays and radio frequencies proposed by Ott.

PROGRESSIVE RELAXATION AND BIOFEEDBACK TRAINING

A few researchers in recent years have attempted to train hyperactive children in the use of progressive deep muscle relaxation procedures in order to reduce the hyperactive behaviors of these children. The resulting studies have generally indicated that, although hyperactive children can be successfully trained to relax various muscle groups, there is no evidence of any simultaneous reduction in hyperactive behaviors outside the laboratory settings in which the relaxation training has occurred. In addition, there has been no effort to correlate changes in muscle tension during treatment with changes in behavior in the treatment situation. At this point, progressive muscle relaxation therapy is not viewed as an effective treatment program for hyperactive children.

Other researchers have attempted to train hyperactive children to alter various parameters of psychophysiological responding through the use of electronically amplified feedback from the psychophysiological systems. In some cases, hyperactive children have been taught to relax the frontalis muscle by using electromyographic (EMG) feedback of frontalis muscle tension. As with the progressive relaxation training procedures, hyperactive children can successfully learn to relax their frontalis muscles, but this has not shown any corresponding improvement in their behavior in the laboratory or natural settings. A few clinicians have attempted to use biofeedback from the alpha rhythms on the electroencephalograms (EEGs) of hyperactive children to alter their hyperkinetic behavior; alpha activity, like muscle tension, is often used as a gauge of the degree to which an individual is in a relaxed state. The resulting studies must be viewed as inconclusive at this time. Some researchers were successful in training hyperactive children to increase their amount of alpha activity, but this did not result in any corresponding improvements in their hyperactive behavior in situations outside the laboratory. Another study was not able to show conclusively that hyperkinetic children could in fact alter the level of alpha activity on their EEGs in response to training. One recent study attempted to teach hyperactive children to alter the sensory–motor rhythms on their EEGs in response to training. The article states that the sensory–motor rhythm is a correlate of attentional processes, and that therefore altering the rhythm should produce improvements in the children's ability to pay attention to assigned tasks.

Like the other studies described above, this study in fact showed that hyperactive children could successfully alter their sensory–motor rhythms; in addition, there was some suggestion that attention span was improved within the laboratory setting. However, none of these studies has produced any conclusive evidence that improvements in attention span, impulse control, or other symptoms of hyperactivity outside the laboratory setting are achieved by the treatment procedures. Hence, at this time, efforts to train hyperactive children in progressive muscle relaxation or in biofeedback-assisted manipulation of various physiological or psychophysiological functions have not produced any improvement in hyperactive symptoms that could be considered at all clinically significant.

CONCLUSION

At present, a number of treatment approaches have been recommended by various individuals for improving the behavior of hyperactive children. Most of these treatment approaches involve the manipulation of such children's diets, whether this be through the elimination of food additives, salicylates, or other supposedly toxic substances, or through the alteration of vitamin or sugar content in the diet. Presently, there appears to be very little if any scientific support for the use of these treatments as part of an intervention program for hyperactive children and their families. Most of the proposed treatment programs, such as vitamin therapy or experimentation with fluorescent lighting, have received little scientific investigation, and the little research that has been done has produced no clinically impressive results. It is therefore suggested that clinicians who are seriously interested in the welfare of the hyperactive children within their clinical practice should avoid the use of these fads, fancies, and other unproven remedies for hyperactive children. Instead, it is best to view hyperactivity as a developmental disorder of attention span and self-control. At present there is no cure, but the disorder can be improved through the use of stimulant medication, the training of parents in effective child behavior management methods, the use of educational interventions, and the counseling of parents on the need to cope with, rather than cure, the symptoms of hyperactive children.

SUGGESTED READING

Conners, C. K. *Food additives and hyperactive children.* New York: Plenum, 1980.
Conners, C. K., Goyette, C. H., Southwick, D. A., Lees, J. M., & Andrulonis, P. A. Food additives and hyperkinesis: A controlled double-blind experiment. *Pediatrics,* 1976, *58,* 154–166.

Feingold, B. *Why your child is hyperactive*. New York: Random House, 1975.

Harley, J. P., Ray, R. S., Tomasi, L., Eichman, P. L., Matthews, C. G., Chun, R., Cleeland, C. S., & Traisman, E. Hyperkinesis and food additives: Testing the Feingold hypothesis. *Pediatrics*, 1978, *61*, 818–828.

Harley, J. P., Matthews, C. G., & Eichman, P. L. Synthetic food colors and hyperactivity in children: A double-blind challenge experiment. *Pediatrics*, 1978, *62*, 975–983.

Levy, F., Dumbrell, S., Hobbes, G., Ryan, M., Wilton, N., & Woodhill, J. M. Hyperkinesis and diet: A double-blind crossover trial with a tartrazine challenge. *Medical Journal of Australia*, 1978, *1*, 61–64.

Mash, E. J., & Dalby, J. T. Behavioral interventions for hyperactivity. In R. Trites (Ed.), *Hyperactivity in children: Etiology, measurement and treatment implications*. Baltimore: University Park Press, 1978.

Mayron, L. M., Ott, J. N., Nations, R., & Mayron E. L. Light, radiation, and academic behavior: Initial studies on the effects of full spectrum lighting and radiation shielding on behavior and academic performance of school children. *Academic Therapy*, 1974, *10*, 33–47.

O'Leary, K. D., Rosenbaum, A., & Hughes, P. C. Fluorescent lighting: A purported source of hyperactive behavior. *Journal of Abnormal Child Psychology*, 1978, *6*, 285–289.

Prinze, R. J., Roberts, W. A., & Hantman, E. Dietary correlates of hyperactive behavior in children. *Journal of Consulting and Clinical Psychology*, 1980, *48*, 760–769.

Rose, T. L. The functional relationship between artificial food colors and hyperactivity. *Journal of Applied Behavior Analysis*, 1978, *11*, 439–446.

Smith, L. *Your child's behavior chemistry*. New York: Random House, 1976.

Stare, F. J., Whelan, E. M., & Sheridan, M. Diet and hyperactivity: Is there a relationship? *Pediatrics*, 1980, *66*, 521–525.

Swanson, J., & Kinsbourne, M. Food dyes impair performance of hyperactive children on a laboratory learning test. *Science*, 1980, *207*, 1485–1486.

Taylor, E. Food additives, allergy, and hyperkinesis. *Journal of Child Psychology and Psychiatry*, 1979, *20*, 357–363.

Taylor, J. F. *The hyperactive child and the family*. New York: Everest House, 1980.

Trites, R. L., Tryphonas, H., & Ferguson, H. B. Diet treatment for hyperactive children with food allergies. In R. Knights & D. Bakker (Eds.), *Treatment of hyperactive and learning disordered children*. Baltimore: University Park Press, 1980.

Weiss, B., Williams, J. H., Margen, S., Abrams, B., Caan, B., Citron, L., Cox, C., McKibben, J., Ogar, D., & Schultz, S. Behavioral responses to artificial food colors. *Science*, 1980, *207*, 1487–1488.

Wender, E. Food additives and hyperkinesis. *American Journal of Diseases of Children*, 1977, *131*, 1204–1206.

Williams J. I., Cram, D. M., Tausig, F. T., & Webster, E. Relative effects of drugs and diet on hyperactive behaviors: An experimental study. *Pediatrics*, 1978, *61*, 811–817.

THE RESPONSE CLASS MATRIX: A PROCEDURE FOR RECORDING PARENT-CHILD INTERACTIONS

ERIC J. MASH

LEIF TERDAL

KATHRYN ANDERSON

The University of Oregon Medical School

GENERAL CONSIDERATIONS IN RECORDING BEHAVIOR

A strong emphasis on the systematic observation and recording of specific behaviors is inextricably bound to the growing body of treatment techniques that fall under the behavior modification rubric. Behavior modification as a clinical approach may be characterized by the following: a strict emphasis on observable (measurable) behavior, a stress on current environmental events as they relate to maintaining both adaptive and maladaptive behavior, control of behavior through the systematic arrangement of environmental contingencies (reinforcers), and objective evaluation of treatment through demonstration of behavior change.

These characteristics place certain demands on the behavior therapist. Specifically, the behavior therapist must define the behavior that he or she is dealing with, must plan for unbiased observation and recording of these behaviors, and must demonstrate that his or her observations and recordings attain at least some minimal level of interrater reliability (Gelfand & Hartmann, 1968; Kanfer & Saslow, 1968).

One advantage of providing for objective observation and recording of behavior is that such records make it possible to pinpoint specific treatment goals. The therapist is often given an ambiguous or distorted account of the presenting problem. This may be especially true when dealing with children, where secondary sources such as parents or teachers are involved (Yarrow, Campbell, & Burton, 1968). For instance, pre-existing biases may cause the one presenting the problem to give an inaccurate account of the actual behaviors that are occurring. Also, there may be a tendency to under- or overestimate the frequency with which certain behaviors occur, as well as difficulty in trying to relate the occurrence of certain behaviors to specific environmental events. For example, a mother may give an inconsistent account on two occasions, even when talking with the same therapist. Furthermore, two parents may present different accounts, and the nature of the problem may be quite different depending upon who is presenting the problem. The information reported to a therapist may also differ as a function of the setting in which the informant had contact with the child (e.g., school vs. home).

Yarrow *et al.* (1968), in a study on research methodology in child rearing, reported finding little relationship between a mother's verbal report of dependency and a teacher's rating of dependency ($r = .29$). They also reported a correlation of only .33 between a combined teacher rating on child aggression with a rating based on mother's interview. Yarrow *et al.* (1968) also challenge the current trend to base treatment and research strategies on verbal report: "There is little comfort for assuming that ratings *labeled* the same in a parental interview and in direct observation are calibrating the same aspects of behavior" (p. 119). Through an objective observation and recording system, the therapist should find it easier to delineate treatment objectives.

The recording of behavior provides the therapist with a technique for monitoring the effectiveness of his or her treatment procedures. When early goals are reached, the therapist and client can plan an approach to new goals. Should initial goals be elusive, the therapist's records provide immediate feedback information with which decisions can be made about the readjustment of goals to more obtainable targets. An objective recording system minimizes the possibility that the particular biases of the therapist will cause him or her to see changes, when in actuality none have occurred. Too often, the success or failure of a treatment procedure is based upon the therapist's selective perception and use of limited amounts of information obtained from the client. Objective records help to circumvent this problem, since the treatment goals are directly reflected in the behaviors recorded, and the success or failure of treatment is evident from changes in the record.

In addition to the monitoring of treatment procedures and pinpointing of treatment goals, behavior observation and recording assist the therapist in choosing those procedures which might be most effective in producing behavior change. Observation and recording may provide information about the particular environmental stimuli which are maintaining certain behaviors. The therapist is given details as to how the environment represents a context for the client's behavior, some of the situations in which the behavior appears, and some of the events which may be reinforcing maladaptive behaviors or limiting the opportunity for more adaptive behaviors to occur (Kanfer, 1967).

Bierman (1969) has pointed out the "relative neglect of research in the parent–child therapy area" (p. 349). He indicates that "this neglect is probably due to the complexities of controlling for the simultaneous impact of two parents, teachers, and also the two different therapists who typically collaborate on a child guidance clinic case" (p. 349). On the positive side he indicates that "twin issues are opening up for investigation: the modification of interpersonal behavior repertoires of child case agents via modeling and behavior-shaping procedures and the effect of the modified behavior repertoires on children" (p. 349).

The procedures and rationale to be described were developed to meet the observing and recording needs of professionals involved in parent–child therapy, both in an applied and research context. As with most procedures, it reflects the efforts of other workers in the field. Theory and techniques concerning the observation and recording of behavioral interactions draw heavily on the work of Gerald Patterson and his coworkers (1968, 1969) and Sidney Bijou (1955, 1957, 1958). The idea for reproducing analogs of parent–child interactions was suggested by Constance Hanf, who has extensively studied such interactions (1969).

Although the particular recording procedures to be described were developed specifically for the study of parent–child interactions, with some modifications they have a more general applicability within any context in which the therapist is concerned with dyadic dimensions.

RATIONALE FOR PRESENT PROCEDURES

Behavioral recording procedures have varied along the following dimensions: recording discrete responses versus recording general classes of responses; recording behaviors continuously versus sampling; and recording behaviors in isolation versus recording responses within the context of antecedent and/or consequent events.

Discrete versus General Response Classes

Human social behavior is sufficiently variable and complex that it presents the observer–recorder with the problem of what to record and how to conceptualize the behavior that he or she is recording. Some researchers (Lewis, 1959) have employed narrative approaches in which they observe and record in idiosyncratic detail all they can of an individual behavior and its context.

Most behavior therapists, however, employ a laboratory model in which they record presence or absence of selected behaviors (Gelfand & Hartmann, 1968). Presumably the selected behaviors have relevance to treatment goals.

While basically adhering to a procedure of recording selected behaviors, some therapists define behavior in discrete detail, such as time out of seat, head banging, placing pegs in peg board, or responding with a vocalized imitative response to a vocalized model sound ă (Marshall & Hegrenes, 1970). Other therapists define behavior in terms of response classes such as destructiveness, play, noncompliance, etc. (Patterson et al., 1969).

The decision to utilize either discrete behavioral categories or general response classes should, in part, hinge on whether the information is to be used to evaluate results on one case alone (discrete categories would suffice) or used to evaluate results across cases. The present procedure employs response classes in order to facilitate comparisons across cases and to evaluate the relationship between demographic variables and parent–child interactions. Such comparisons would be impossible if the topographic features of the behavior categories were too specific.

The specific classes in this procedure were arbitrarily selected because they provided relevant information about classes of behaviors that were frequently reported as concerns by parents, and had been observed to occur in naturalistic settings. The behaviors that fall into a particular class all possess some common features which are described below in the definitions of the behavior categories. For example, a particular child may bite, another may bang his or her head on the wall, and another may whine. All of these behaviors are recorded in the response class of "negative behavior."

The utilization of a response class recording procedure assumes that contingencies maintaining behaviors in a certain response class are similar. From a treatment standpoint, the question may be posed as follows: if one educates a parent to extinguish a child's negative behavior in the form of hitting, would the parent also respond appropriately to decrease the child's rate of biting and head banging? If, indeed, behaviors within a certain class are similar in terms of the relationship they have with certain features in the immediate environment, then the use of response classes provides a way of ordering and describing seemingly dissimilar contingency relationships within that environment.

Continuous Recording versus Behavior Sampling

Recording of behaviors was facilitated in the present procedure through the use of a behavior sampling technique. Many recording procedures denote the frequency with which all designated behaviors occur during a specified time interval. Such continuous recording becomes difficult when there are many high-frequency behaviors that have been selected for recording.

An alternative to continuous recording is that of behavior sampling (Wright, 1960; Allen, Hart, Buell, Harris, & Wolf, 1965). In the present procedure the time spent observing is divided into equal units, each unit of 10 seconds' duration. If more than one response occurs in that interval, only the last response to occur is recorded. No effort is made to record every response. The assumption behind behavior sampling is that those behaviors that are recorded will, over a period of time, be a representative sample of all the behaviors that occur in that observation period.

Behavior in Isolation versus Behavior in Context

Wright (1960), in a review of observational studies from 1890 to the late 1950s, reported that most observational studies involving children failed to relate the child behavior to a context of child-care agent behavior. He called for recording behavior in context: "Common psychological theory now says that for every response there is a corresponding stimulus and vice versa. It would seem to follow that the way to link actions with situations is to divide the behavior continuum . . . into integral units of behavior with its context" (p. 101).

Holland and Skinner (1961) have distinguished three possibilities for focus and recording. One can record only the response, for instance, of the child. Response records, or one-term contingencies, do provide a measure of a response, but omit accounts of the context in which the behavior is emitted. Two-term contingency records provide a measure of responses as well as either a measure of antecedent events or a measure of consequent events. The present procedure uses a three-term contingency record, providing descriptive accounts of antecedent stimuli, consequent events, and responses.

DESCRIPTION OF THE MATRICES FOR RECORDING PARENT-CHILD INTERACTIONS

The present recording procedures make possible the recording of behaviors in relation to specified antecedent and consequent events in the environment. Records of a particular mother–child interaction are obtained by using the two matrices shown in Figures A.1 and A.2. Figure A.1 shows the child's matrix, with seven possible antecedent mother-behaviors as row headings and six possible consequent child-behaviors as column headings. Figure A.2 shows the (m)other's matrix, with six possible antecedent child-behaviors as row headings and seven possible consequent mother-behaviors as column headings.

Two recorders are used, one recording the mother's behavior as an antecedent and the child's behavior as a consequent (Figure A.1), and the other recording the child's behavior as an antecedent and the mother's behavior as a consequent (Figure A.2). Each recorder makes one mark in one of the matrix cells every 10 seconds, with only the last scorable behavior unit to occur during the interval being recorded. Following the recording for a 10-second interval, there is a 5-second pause, and then the behavior occurring during the next 10-second interval is recorded. For example, consider a mother–child interaction in which the following sequence of behaviors occurred:

	(1) Mother commands		(2) Child complies		(3) Mother praises		(4) Child plays		(5) Mother ignores	
Ready	→	10 seconds		→		Mark		→	5 seconds	→

	(6) Mother questions		(7) Child interacts		(8) Mother questions
	Ready	→	10 seconds	→	Mark

FIGURE A.1. Child's matrix.

During the first 10-second interval, the mother gave a command (1), the child complied (2), and the mother praised (3). The recorder on the child's matrix would make a hash mark in the cell corresponding to Mother Commands–Child Complies. The recorder on the mother's matrix would make a hash mark in the cell corresponding to Child Complies–Mother Praises. At the end of the second 10-second interval, the child's matrix recorder makes a mark in the cell Mother Questions–Child Interacts, and the mother's matrix recorder makes a mark in the cell Child Interacts–

FAMILY NAME_____

(M)OTHER'S CONSEQUENT BEHAVIOR RECORD

CHILD'S ANTECEDENT BEHAVIOR	Command	Command Question	Question	Praise	Neg.	Inter. 10 sec.	No Response 10 sec.
Compliance							
Independent Play							
Competing Behaviors							
Negative							
Interaction							
No Response							

Date   Mo Da Yr ☐ ☐ ☐   Participant ☐   Others Present Not Recorded ☐

Location   LAB - 1; HOME - 2; SCHOOL - 3   Session Length   Hr Min ☐ ☐

Session No.   ☐   Situation Code ☐   Matrix Type 1   Family ID ☐☐☐☐

Recorder   _____

FIGURE A.2. (M)other's matrix.

Mother Questions. This scoring procedure continues for the duration of the designated observation period, and the two matrices taken together give an account of the three-term contingency shown for this mother–child interaction.

In order for the present recording system to be meaningful, it was necessary to decide upon certain functional definitions for each of the mother and child behaviors included in the matrices. These functional definitions draw on the experience of Hanf (1968).

Standard Behavior Categories for the (M)other

COMMAND

In this category are direct commands, or statements which include *imperatives*:

1. "Come. . . . "
2. "Let me. . . . "
3. "Put this. . . . "
4. "I want you. . . . "

A direct command may be either *specific*:

5. "Write your name."

or *general*:

6. "Go and play."

In either case, they are scored as commands.

Note: Unless there is an accompanying verbalization, a gesture will not be scored as a command. Thus, motioning for a child to come without saying to come will not be scored as a command.

COMMAND–QUESTION

A command–question is a suggested or "implied" command which includes an *interrogative*:

1. "Will you hand me . . . ?"
2. "Shall we . . . ?"
3. "Why don't you . . . ?"
4. "Can you . . . ?"
5. "Would you like to . . . ?"

As with direct commands, in order for a command–question to be scored, there must be an accompanying verbalization.

QUESTION

Scored in this category are any direct questions not of the command–question type.

1. "What . . . [color is this]?"
2. "What . . . [would you like to do]?"
3. "Where is . . . ?"
4. "Who . . . ?"
5. "How does . . . ?"
6. "When did . . . ?"

PRAISE

The praise category includes both verbal statements and nonverbal actions indicating encouragement, acceptance, and/or approval of the child's behavior.

1. Verbal:
   a. "O.K."
   b. "Good. . . . "
   c. "That's fine. . . . "
   d. "I like that. . . . "
2. Nonverbal:
   a. Pat on back.
   b. Hug.
   c. Kiss.
   d. Clap.
   e. Head nod.
   f. Smile.

Some judgment can be used in interpreting context and tone of voice in scoring praise. A general rule of thumb is that most of the above statements when they follow a *specific* task of behavior on the part of the child, are scored as praise. For example, if on completion of a task the mother says "O.K.," score as praise. If, on the other hand, the child asks if he or she can play, and the mother says, "O.K.," score as interaction for the mother.

NEGATIVE

The negative category includes both verbal statements and nonverbal actions indicating discouragement, nonacceptance, and/or disapproval of the child's behavior.

1. Verbal: Negative verbal statements may take two forms. They may be either
   a. direct disapproval or criticism:
      i. "No, don't. . . . "
      ii. "Stop. . . . "
      iii. "Quit. . . . "
      iv. "Bad boy [girl]. . . . "
      v. "That's not right. . . . "
      vi. "That's all wrong. . . . "
      vii. "You can do better than that."
      viii. "Don't do it that way."
      ix. "You make me sick."
      x. "I don't like that."
   b. or implied criticism or threat:
      i. "You're acting like a 2-year-old!"
      ii. "If you don't stop . . . you'll get it!"
      iii. "You'd better watch it!"

   iv. "One more time and you're in trouble!"

   v. "Your father won't like that when he hears about it!"

 2. Nonverbal: May be either

  a. direct:

   i. Spank or hit.

   ii. Pinch.

   iii. Yank.

   iv. Shove back in chair.

   v. Shake head "no."

   vi. Frown.

  b. or a threat:

   i. Raised hand.

   ii. Shaking of finger at child.

Note: Negative behavior on the part of the mother takes precedence over commands or question–commands; that is, if the mother says, "You get over here!" in a quite threatening manner, this is scored as negative behavior on her part, rather than a command.

INTERACTION

Interaction is an attempt to *initiate* or *maintain* some type of mutual contact. Interaction may be either verbal or nonverbal.

 1. Verbal: Comments that may be neutral, positive, or descriptive but that contain no criticisms, commands, or questions. The mother in some way communicates attention or expresses interest.

  a. "That's a big bridge you're building."

  b. "You sure are running fast."

  c. "There are some toys in the box."

  d. "We'll be going home when we're finished."

  e. "Mmm-Hmm."

 2. Nonverbal:

  a. Holding parts of the same toy.

  b. Handing an object to the child.

  c. Smiling at the child. (In this case, eye contact with the child must occur; if the child does not look at the mother when she is smiling at the child, her response is scored as "no response.")

  d. Physical contact other than negative.

NO RESPONSE

No response is scored when, during the 10-second interval, there is no occurrence of responses in any of the above categories.

1. Mother plays silently with a toy while child plays with another toy.
2. Mother looks out the window.
3. Mother sits and smokes while child plays on floor.
4. Mother looks at child, who does not look at her.

Standard Behavior Categories for the Child

COMPLIANCE

Compliance is scored for the child only when his or her behavior is in response to the mother's command or command–question. Thus, a child's answering a mother's question should not be scored as compliance, but as interaction. Any response ranging from approximation to full compliance may be classified as compliance. Even if a child is having a tantrum, if he or she is complying at the same time, the response is scored as compliance.

1. Mother tells child to pick up the toys and child walks toward the toy.
2. Mother tells child to draw a man and child seems to be trying to draw a man, and not his or her name, numbers, etc.

If the child is given a command or command–question relating to a specific defined *task* (i.e., "Pick up those toys!"), then compliance is coded every 10 seconds for the duration of the task.

However, if the command or command–question is not specifically task-oriented, but rather *play*-oriented ("Why don't you play for awhile?"), then compliance is coded for the 10 seconds only in which the command–question was given. After this, the child's behavior should be classified as independent play, or contingent upon new cues from the mother.

If several commands are given during the 10-second interval, the child's response to the last command given is the response recorded.

COMPETING BEHAVIORS

Noncompliance, or competing behavior, may take several forms. It will be noted that on the child's form there is no category for competing behavior as such. It is assumed that any of the child's behaviors following a command or a command–question that are not compliance are behaviors competing with compliance. The child's form facilitates recording of what the child does when not complying (i.e., plays, asks questions, has a tantrum, suggests another activity, doesn't respond, etc.).

On the (m)other's form, competing behavior as a child-antecedent response is scored only once during the 10-second interval in which the command or command–question is given. Following that, noncompliance is scored as competing behavior only if:

1. The mother gives another command.
2. The mother gives an antecedent which, although not a command, is task-related:
   a. "Isn't it fun to pick up the toys?"
   b. "If you hurry with your pictures, we can go home."
   c. "The toys are waiting for you."
3. In session c (task session), when the mother has given a command specified by the clinician, then the command holds without time limit until the mother clearly changes the requirements or the child completes the task.

INDEPENDENT PLAY

Independent play is recorded when he or she is playing alone and not interacting with the mother. The child must be engaged in some form of *play* for the response to be recorded as independent play. Independent play following a command or command–question is scored as independent play as a child-consequence and as competing behavior as a child-antecedent.

1. Child sits with back to mother and plays with a toy.
2. On child's matrix: Mother gives a command, child continues to play with toy as before.
3. Child silently rummages through box of toys.
4. Child, ignoring mother's questions, plays with the light switch.

Note: Parallel play between parent and child is scored as interaction on the part of the mother if her behavior is interpreted as an attempt to initiate or maintain an interaction with her child. Unless the child responds to the mother or specifically to her play activity, his or her behavior is scored as independent play and not interaction.

NEGATIVE

The negative category for the child includes both verbal statements and nonverbal actions indicating anger, refusal, or discouragement. Negative behavior may be either nonvocal or vocal.

1. Nonvocal:
   a. Tantrum—lie down on the floor and kick.
   b. Hit self, other person, object.
   c. Kick.
   d. Push.
   e. Throw something at something or at someone else.
   f. Bite self or someone else.
   g. Pull away from someone's grasp.

2. Vocal:
   a. Tantrum with screaming.
   b. Refusal—"no . . . !" (In order for "no!" to be scored as negative, it must follow either a command or a command–question.)
   c. Verbal abuse—swearing, name calling, etc.
   d. Crying, whining.

If the child is engaging in any of the above types of behavior following a command or a command–question, but is actually complying at the same time, then compliance and not negative behavior is scored.

On the (m)other's form, negative takes precedence over competing behaviors as a child-antecedent. Example: During the 10-second interval, the mother gave a command and the child responded by turning from her and whining, "I don't want to." This is scored as a negative child-antecedent for the mother's next response in that 10-second interval.

INTERACTION

Interaction is an attempt to *initiate* or *maintain* some type of mutual contact. It should be noted that interaction need not be two-way. The child may be attempting to interact with the mother, but she may not reciprocate. Interaction may be either verbal or nonverbal.

1. Verbal: Comments that may be neutral, pleasant, or descriptive.
   a. The child's answering a question.
   b. The child's giving the mother a command.
   c. The child's naming pictures while mother and child "read" a story book.
2. Nonverbal:
   a. The child's smiling at the mother. (In this case only, she must either initiate or reciprocate the eye contact; otherwise, the child's response is not scored as interaction.)
   b. The child's handing an object to the mother.
   c. Physical contact other than negative.
   d. The child's holding on to same object as mother or playing with same toy as mother. (If mother and child are in close proximity, but they are playing independently from each other, this is not scored as interaction.)

QUESTION

The question category, as a child response, appears only on the child's form. If one is recording the child's antecedent behavior on the (m)other's form, a child's question is recorded as competing behavior if it follows a command or command–question, or as interaction if it does not follow a command or command–question.

NO RESPONSE

No response is scored when, during the 10-second interval, there is no occurrence of responses in any of the above categories.

1. Mother asks child a question and child does not answer, just looks at mother.
2. Mother tells child to do something and child wanders aimlessly around the room.
3. Mother talks to child and child looks away.

The matrix system just described groups specific behaviors into broad response classes. For a more detailed and useful clinical report, it is valuable for the observer to describe some detail after a session to clarify the behaviors that were recorded. For instance, it might be important to note that the majority of a child's negative behavior was biting him- or herself on the hand, rather than hitting or biting someone else.

It will be noted that at the bottom of each behavior record form there are spaces for identifying the particular observation period. On the child's form, "Participant" refers to the person whose behavior is being recorded as a consequent (usually the child). On the (m)other's form, the space for "Participant" is for identifying the person whose behavior on that form is being recorded as consequent (usually the mother, but could be the father, a sibling, a therapist, etc.).

For some purposes it is desirable to ask individuals other than those being recorded to be present in the room with those being recorded; that is, a record may be kept of the mother–child interaction when a therapist is in the room, etc. The space marked "Others Present Not Recorded" is for indicating this kind of situation.

The space labeled "Situation Code" is for designating which of a number of commonly used standard situations was chosen for this particular session. It has been found useful to employ certain standard situations in the clinic where this recording system was developed. Any number of such situations could be designated for use in any setting. Asking the mother and child to interact in the same kind of situation before and after therapy provides information with which to evaluate the success of the therapy. Standard situations are necessary if one is to evaluate the interaction of the same pair over time, or if one is to compare one pair's interaction with other parent–child pairs.

The "Location" label at the bottom of the forms indicates in which of three likely observation areas the particular observation is made. Locations other than Lab, Home, or School are, of course, possible.

The space marked "Session Number" is for indicating in which session the observation is being made, given the same participants, location, and situation.

"Matrix Type 0" and "Matrix Type 1" are simply identification statements for computer analysis. Matrix Type 0 indicates that this is the seven-by-six record form, and identifies it as the child's form. The "Family ID" notation is, similarly, to identify the particular case for computer analysis.

The particular matrix forms described here were designed for use in a particular clinic setting; they are presented as examples of possible ways to implement the general recording principles described earlier.

RELIABILITY

The traditional procedure for analyzing reliability between two observers is percent agreement (Wright, 1960). The formula used in this report is 2 times numbers of agreement/sum of tallies from both coders.

This report on reliability was obtained using three trained coders paired as follows: coders A and B, A and C, and B and C. These coder pairs observed 22 mothers and their normal preschool children in a free-play situation for intervals of 10 minutes each. The percent agreement figures are based on a total of 1536 observations on the child's consequent behavior record, and 1078 tallies on the mother's consequent behavior record.

Combining the agreement figures of the three coder-pairs and evaluating the percent agreement per category on the child's consequent behavior record, the range of agreement was as follows: compliance, 93% from a total of 328 tallies; independent play, 87% (256 tallies); questions, 31% (13 tallies); negative behavior, no tallies; interaction, 95% (932 tallies); no response, 0 agreement from a total of 7 tallies.

It is clear that three categories (question, negative behavior, and no response) represent very low child response rates among our reliability sample. This raises questions about coder reliability for low-rate behaviors. However, the bulk of the analysis for our sample involve the categories in which the percent agreement was 87% or better.

Essentially, similar results were obtained from a total of 1087 tallies on the mothers consequent behavior record. Combining the tallies of the two coder pairs who recorded with the mother's consequent behavior record, the percent in each of the categories was as follows: commands 92% (from a total of 166 tallies); command-question, 78% (54 tallies); questions, 94% (179 tallies); praise, 84% (76 tallies); negative, 79% (20 tallies); interaction, 93% (352 tallies); no response, 96% (321 tallies).

The matrices were constructed to evaluate contingent relationships between consequent and antecedent behaviors. Percent agreement based on matrix cell concordance evaluates antecedent categories and consequent categories as a unit. In this way matrix cell agreement for a given tally is obtained when two coders agree on both a given consequent behavior category and a corresponding antecedent behavior category. On the child consequent behavior record, the overall matrix cell agreement was 81% for coders A and B, 87% for A and C, and 83% for coders B and C. On the mother's consequent behavior record the matrix cell agreement was 84% for coders A and C, and 78% for coders B and C.

AN EXAMPLE OF DATA UTILIZATION FOR AN INDIVIDUAL CASE

The Case of John Jones

Mrs. Jones was referred to the clinic by John's nursery school teacher, to whom Mrs. Jones has gone for help in finding an agency that would do something with John's behavior. When interviewed at the clinic, Mrs. Jones reported that her son, John, age 4 years and 2 months, was impossible to manage at home, although the nursery school teacher has told Mrs. Jones that John is no problem at school, rather, he is a "delight." Mrs. Jones, when asked to describe in what ways John is impossible, said that John is very disobedient; that he has a "mind of his own"; that when she tries to get him to mind her, he screams and hits at her. She elaborated by reporting that he sometimes looks at her daringly when he decides he doesn't want to obey; and at other times he acts as if he doesn't hear her. She asked if he got his bad disposition from her side of the family and mentioned that she had a father who was an alcoholic. She also asked if some children are just born bad and have a mean streak in them.

Mrs. Jones was asked to play with John in a playroom setting in the clinic, just as she would do "at home when the two of your are alone and have a few minutes to play together." Recorders observed the interaction through a one-way mirror.

Several observations can be made about this interaction. The majority of John's responses were characterized as independent play, with some negative behavior. He showed nearly no compliance, although his mother gave many commands. Although Mrs. Jones asked John many questions, he seldom answered (interaction), but continued playing.

Turning to Mrs. Jones, her most typical way of relating to John in this session was to give a command or a command–question, or to ask a question. Since this session was structured by the therapist to be a play session, the large number of commands given by the mother indicated excessive directiveness. Although the behavior record did not clearly pick up this point, the interaction was frequently that of John beginning to play with something and Mrs. Jones then telling him to put it somewhere or her asking him a question about it. This could be seen on the record form as the child's independent play being typically followed by a command or question from the mother. Some of Mrs. Jones's questions were of the kind that a 4-year-old would find difficult to answer (i.e., "What kind of a shoe lace is that?"). Mrs. Jones used no praise with John, either contingently or noncontingently. When John engaged in negative behavior, Mrs. Jones interacted with this by giving more commands or by criticizing and/or threatening him. Mrs. Jones also interacted with competing behaviors, which may partially explain why John does not obey commands from his mother. Her firing one command after another also does not allow John time to comply. It is important to note that John's teacher does not have difficulty in getting John to comply at school. From the records, it is clear that John is beginning to "tune his mother out," and that she is responding to this by increasing her efforts to make him respond to her.

Initial treatment goals would include the following:

1. Teaching Mrs. Jones how to interact with John in a play situation by describing, commenting, or silently playing with John, keeping questions and commands at a minimum. Mrs. Jones should be taught to praise John's play products or processes, letting him take the lead.
2. Mrs. Jones should be taught to ignore John's tantrum behavior when it does occur and not to chase after him in a provoking manner.
3. Mrs. Jones should be taught how to stimulate John's talking to her and initiating approaches to her.
4. A later treatment goal would be to teach Mrs. Jones how to give a command and how to follow through in such a way to secure compliance from John.

Midtherapy, posttherapy, and follow-up sessions should be planned with Mrs. Jones for the purpose of monitoring the progress and outcome of treatment.

SUMMARY AND CONCLUSIONS

The matrix form described here provides a way of recording the behavior of one person in the context of the behavior of another member of a dyad. The use of standard behavior observation recording procedures in the study of parent–child interactions may facilitate the development of therapy and intervention programs. Some of the reasons are as follows:

1. The actual record of an interaction may provide more reliable information about how a parent and child behave in relation to each other than the parent's report.
2. Recording the interaction helps to pinpoint strengths and weaknesses of the parent–child interaction.
3. A record of the initial interaction facilitates the establishment of treatment goals.
4. Interactions subsequent to the pretherapy interaction can be used to monitor ongoing treatment.
5. A record of the interaction at the conclusion of therapy, and at some later follow-up check point provides data by which to evaluate the short-range and long-range effectiveness of the treatment procedure.
6. A standard record allows for comparisons and study across cases, and the identification of relationships between demographic variables and patterns of parent–child interaction.

ACKNOWLEDGMENTS

The above is reprinted with permission of the authors. The study was supported by Health Services and Mental Health Administration, Maternal and Child Health Services Project #920.

REFERENCES

Allen, K. E., Hart, B. M., Buell, J. A., Harris, F. R., & Wolf, M. M. Effects of social reinforcement on isolate behavior of a nursery school child. In L. P. Ullmann & F. Krasner (Eds.), *Case studies in behavior modification.* New York: Holt, Rinehart & Winston, 1965.

Bierman, R. Dimensions of interpersonal facilitation in psychotherapy and child development. *Psychological Bulletin,* 1969, *72,* 338–352.

Bijou, S. W. A systematic approach to an experimental analysis of young children. *Child Development,* 1955, *26,* 161–168.

Bijou, S. W. Methodology for an experimental analysis of child behavior. *Psychological Reports,* 1957, *3,* 243–250.

Gelfand, D. M., & Hartmann, D. P. Behavior therapy with children: A review and evaluation of research methodology. *Psychological Bulletin,* 1968, *70,* 204–215.

Hanf, C. *Modification of mother–child controlling behaviors during mother–child interactions in standardized laboratory situations.* Paper presented at the meeting of the Association of Behavior Therapies, Olympia, Wash., 1968.

Hanf, C. *A two-stage program for modifying maternal controlling during mother–child (M–C) interaction.* Paper presented at Western Psychological Association Meeting, Vancouver, B.C., June 1969.

Holland, J. G., & Skinner, B. F. *The analysis of behavior.* New York: McGraw-Hill, 1961.

Kanfer, F. H. *Directions in behavior modification research or where the insufficiencies are.* Paper presented at the Second Annual Institute of Man's Adjustment in a Complex Environment: The Behavior Therapies. Veteran's Administration Hospital, Brecksville, Ohio, 1967.

Kanfer, F. H., & Saslow, G. Behavior therapy: In C. Franks (Ed.), *Appraisal and general status of the behavior therapies and associated developments.* New York: McGraw-Hill, 1969.

Lewis, O. *Five families.* New York: Basic Books, 1959.

Marshall, N. R., & Hegrenes, J. R. Programmed communication therapy for autistic mentally retarded children. *Journal of Speech and Hearing Disorders,* 1970, *35,* 70–83.

Patterson, G. R., & Harris, A. *Some methodological considerations for observation procedures.* Paper presented at the meeting of the American Psychological Association, San Fransciso, September 1968.

Patterson, G. R., Ray, R. A., Shaw, D. A., & Cobb, J. A. *Manual for coding of family interactions.* Unpublished manuscript, Oregon Research Institute, Eugene, Ore., 1969.

Wright, H. F. Observational child study. In P. H. Mussen (Ed.), *Handbook of research in child development.* New York: Wiley, 1969.

Yarrow, M. R., Campbell, J. D., & Burton, R. V. *Child rearing: An inquiry into research and methods.* San Francisco: Jossey-Bass, 1968.

THE FAMILY TRAINING PROGRAM MANUAL: THE HOME CHIP SYSTEM

EDWARD R. CHRISTOPHERSEN
SUSAN RAINEY BARNARD
JAMES D. BARNARD
University of Kansas

This manual describes a program that has been developed for working with childhood behavior problems. The procedures have been used with school-age children, in families with from one to six children, with parents' educations ranging from less than high school to postgraduate, and with income levels ranging from poverty to upper-income professional.

The range of problem behavior has extended from minor, everyday difficulties like getting children to bed at night and getting them to keep their rooms neat, to moderate problems like hitting, tantrums, hyperactivity, and backtalking. However, our experience is not sufficient to make any recommendations regarding the use of the program with such severe behavior problems as drug addiction.

This program, at least at first, requires dedicated and highly motivated parents who are willing to put forth the effort necessary to teach their children more appropriate ways of behaving. The program also requires that the children be supervised by someone during the majority of their day. We train parents to be teachers. They cannot teach their children if they are not with them.

INTRODUCTION

The Home Chip System is designed to provide a maximum amount of instruction and feedback to your child through you. Instruction, feedback, and consequences will serve as the means or tools with which you will be able to train your child in new desirable behaviors or eliminate already present undesirable behaviors. The system's effectiveness in changing behaviors will depend upon your thoroughness. It will not operate by itself. Its success will depend upon the degree to which you actively observe and reward or punish the behaviors you see present in your home.

HOW THE SYSTEM WORKS

The system is based upon two simple yet thoroughly effective principles. Behavior that is immediately followed by a good rewarding consequence or event will continue to occur. Behavior that is followed by a nonrewarding or punishing consequence or event will cease to occur or will occur less often.

POKER CHIPS

Chips will serve as those rewarding or punishing events that *must immediately* follow your child's behavior. They will always be available for you to give and take. Chips must be given meaning or value for you to use them effectively. Like money, chips themselves have no value. It is only through their power to purchase necessary and enjoyable goods or activities that they gain meaning and become useful.

MAKING CHIPS POWERFUL

For chips to be used as effective consequences for behavior, earning chips (like earning money) must be rewarding for your child; your child must feel like he or she has indeed gained something. Losing chips (like losing money) must be unpleasant or punishing for your child; your child must feel like he or she has lost something.

Chips will become meaningful for your child as he or she uses them to buy the "privileges" of having or doing that which he or she desires. Privileges are those items or activities that are usually available in your home or community, that your child enjoys and can purchase with his or her chips.

EXPLANATION OF PRIVILEGES

Privileges can be anything that your child likes to do. For example, snacks, playing with friends, playing with toys or games, and shopping with Mom all might be considered privileges by some children. The privilege to have snacks, for instance, permits your child to have snacks when they are available and he or she has paid for them (given you the chips). Snacks might be available in the afternoon or before bed. You should decide what constitutes a snack (e.g., one scoop of ice cream, or two cookies, or one bottle of pop) and the times they can be available.

For the chips to be of value, your child must be required to spend them for his or her privileges. Privileges must be available as often as possible when your child has the chips. Unless the chips are worth something, they will not be effective in changing your child's behavior.

EXAMPLE OF A CHIP SYSTEM

The following list of behaviors is an example of what a chip system looks like. Both social and maintenance behaviors for your chip system will be taken from the list you fill out.

Chips Gained or Lost (Some Examples)

Making bed	+2	−2
Picking up bedroom	+2	−2
Brushing teeth	+2	−2
Picking up toys	+2	−2
Picking up clothes	+5	−2
Dressing yourself	+2	−2
Saying please and thank you	+1	

These behaviors are those which, if completed, result in a chip gain, but, if not completed, result in a chip loss. For example, if your child brushed his or her teeth, 2 chips would be gained but if he or she failed to brush his or her teeth, 2 chips would be lost. *Remember*—it is more important to give chips than it is to take chips away.

There will also be some things which will only earn chips, such as "being good," "helping," or "playing quietly." These are the behaviors which you must be aware of and reward consistently, since that is the type of behavior which you would like to see more of every day.

Chips Lost (Some Examples)

Throwing things	−2
Jumping on furniture	−2
Backtalking	−2
Tantrums	−3
Coming downstairs after bedtime	−2
Interrupting	−4
Running in the house	−2

The behaviors under "chips lost" are those which you would like your child to stop doing. For this system to be effective, you must take the chips away immediately *every* time one of these behaviors occurs.

Privileges (Some Examples and Their Value)

Watching television	5 chips per ½ hr.
Playing outside	5 chips
Snacks	5 per snack
Going to friends	10 chips
Riding bike	5 chips

The "privileges" listed on your home chip system will be those which you and your child recorded on your list. However, the list may not always be complete. You will need to be aware of what your child is doing for fun and add these activities to the list whenever necessary. Most of the things that children do naturally in their spare time are things that they enjoy, and can thus be viewed as privileges and added to the list of privileges.

Examples of Extra Jobs

Setting the table
Sweeping porch
Picking up trash in yard
Dusting
Emptying ash trays
Wiping off table
Folding wash cloths

There are many small jobs around the house that your child is capable of doing. It is important that your child share the responsibilities of the house. This is also an excellent time for you to interact with and teach your child.

A list of jobs, made up by you, will help you to have jobs available when your child needs the chips or wants to help. You can make up such a list and attach it to the front of your refrigerator door with a couple of small magnets.

HOW TO GIVE AND TAKE AWAY CHIPS

Both giving and taking away chips should be pleasant. There are several things that you and your child need to do whenever there is a chip exchange.

Rules for Parents

When giving chips,

1. Be near your child and able to touch him or her (not 20 feet or two rooms away).
2. *Look* at your child and *smile.*
3. Use a *pleasant* voice tone.
4. Make sure your child is *facing* you and *looking* at you.
5. *Praise your child*—"Hey, that's great. You're really doing a nice job. That's really helping me." *Reward your child* with chips—"Here's 2 chips for being so good."
6. Describe the appropriate behavior for your child so he or she knows exactly what behavior he or she is being praised and rewarded for.
7. Hug your child occasionally—kids love it!
8. Have your child acknowledge you—such as, "Thanks, Mom" or "O.K."

When taking away chips,

1. Be near your child and able to touch him or her.
2. *Look* at your child and *smile*.
3. Use a pleasant voice tone. (*Note*: Your child should not be able to tell whether you're going to give or take away chips by the tone of your voice or your facial expression.)
4. Make sure your child is *facing* you and *looking* at you.
5. Explain what was inappropriate (see section on instructions).
6. Be sympathetic. "I know it's hard to lose chips, but that's the rule."
7. Give your child the chip fine.
8. Make sure your child gets the chips appropriately (see next section).
9. Prompting the appropriate responses will sometimes be necessary; for example, "Come on, give me a smile—That's right."
10. If a chip loss is taken very well by your child, it is a good idea to give him or her back a chip or two.
11. If your child is too mad or upset to give you the chips, don't force the issue. Place your child in time out (to cool off) and get the chips.

Rules for Children

When getting chips,

1. You should be *facing your parents, looking at them,* and *smiling.*
2. You should acknowledge the chips by saying "O.K.," "Thanks," or something else pleasant.
3. The chips should be put in the specified container. (Any chips left lying around are lost.)

When losing chips,

1. You should face your parents, look at them, and smile (not frown.)
2. You should acknowledge the chip loss with "O.K." or "All right," "I'll get the chips," etc. (You must keep looking at them and be pleasant.)
3. You should give the chips to your parents pleasantly.

PRACTICING

One situation that is frequently encountered by families on the chip system is the case where a child has done something but hasn't done it very well.

This is an excellent time to teach your child how to do it correctly by having him or her *practice* doing it correctly.

Practicing can be done with both social and maintenance (jobs) behaviors.

Practicing with a Social Behavior

If your child becomes unpleasant and backtalks when he or she loses points, the following rules would be useful in teaching your child the appropriate response.

Backtalk (Social Example)	Rule
1. "You came quickly when I called and I really appreciate that."	Praise a related behavior.
2. "But the rule is that you don't backtalk after a chip loss. I'll have to take off 2 more for backtalking."	Describe fully the inappropriate or inadequate behavior.
3. "Remember—you're supposed to look at me, be pleasant, and say 'O.K., Mom,' in a nice tone of voice."	Describe the appropriate behavior.
4. "This way we'll get along better at home and it will help you take criticism better at school too."	Give a reason for the appropriate behavior.
5. "Do you understand what you're supposed to do?"	Request acknowledgment.
6. "Say it pleasantly and give me a big smile—like this [parent says "O.K." and smiles]."	Model: Show child how to do it.
7. "Now you try it."	Practice.
8. "That's right, you're looking at me with a pleasant facial expression."	Praise or feedback.
9. "Great—that's how it's done—you practiced very well. You can have the chip back."	Praise and reward.

Practicing with a Maintenance Behavior

When teaching your child how to do a new job correctly or when giving him or her feedback on a job poorly done, *practicing* is essential.

For example, if your child is doing the dishes but when you check he or she is not doing them correctly, the following rules will help you "teach" your child the correct way.

Dishwashing (Maintenance Example)	Rule
1. "You're really working steadily and the table looks really clean. Thanks."	Praise related behavior.
2. "But it looks like you haven't gotten all the food off the plates."	Describe fully the inappropriate or inadequate behavior.
3. "It's important that all the dishes are clean with no stuck food left on the plates."	Describe the appropriate behavior.
4. "Because germs can grown on the dishes, and, besides, the next time you use the plate you will want it to be clean."	Give a reason for the appropriate behavior.

5. "Do you understand?"	Request acknowledgment.
6. "When food is stuck, a good way to get it off is to use the scraper instead of the cloth—like this."	Model: Show child how to do it.
7. "Now you try it."	Practice.
8. "Great, you're doing a much better job getting them clean now."	Praise or feedback.
9. "When you get done, come get me and you will get your chips plus 2 for practicing. You're really doing a good job now."	Praise and reward.

When to Practice

The best time to practice any behavior is during the pleasant times of the day. This teaches your child under pleasant circumstances how to respond when things aren't going quite as well. However, prompting the correct response and practicing the correct response are still important after a rule violation or poorly done job has occurred.

When there has not been a rule violation, you can practice using "make believe" violations and "make believe" time out. This is also a good way for your child to earn chips.

Example:

MOTHER: Jim, let's practice how you're supposed to take a chip loss and you can earn 2 chips.

JIM: Sure.

MOTHER: Jim, would you please take 2 chips off for throwing the ball in the house—remember the rule is that all balls must only be thrown outside.

JIM: Sure, Mom (*with pleasant facial expression and tone of voice*).

MOTHER: That was great! If you can remember to do that the next time you lose chips, I'll give you back half of the chips you lost.

JIM: Gee, thanks, Mom.

CHECKING JOBS

Checking jobs, whether daily or extra, is a vital aspect of this program. It not only helps you teach your child the right way to do things, but provides a good opportunity for you to interact with your child.

The rules for practicing are used whenever a job is checked. If the job has been done correctly the first time, you needn't go through all the steps. Instead, make sure you specifically praise the things done well and give chips.

CHIPS FOR JOBS

The number of chips given for a job should be decided beforehand. That way, you can reward with extra chips a job done especially well and fine poorly done jobs. However, all jobs must be done as specified—a poorly done job is not acceptable and must be done again.

For this reason, it is good to define how a job is done and then write the description on the job list so that you can look at the description whenever a question comes up.

If, the first time, your child asks you to check the table and all the above things have been done, *praise* your child and give him or her the full 4 chips. However, if it is not done correctly, go through the practicing components and tell your child that if he or she corrects the faulty job components, he or she can get half of the chips possible (or 2). Be sympathetic, but firm. Encourage your child to do it right this time so he or she can get the 2 chips. If, when checked again, the job is still not done correctly, it's probably not because the child doesn't know how. Place the child in time out (without loss of privileges) to think about it. After time out, have your child again do the things that weren't done right. Be sure and go through *practicing* each time (see section on the time-out procedure).

If after time out your child cooperates and corrects the job, give chips for correcting the job. If your child will not cooperate, place him or her in time out again. Most children will do what is required of them rather than sit in time out. However, once in a while a child will test both you and the rules. Don't give in to such tests, as it may only make it harder to convince your child that you and the rules are here to stay.

MONITORING YOUR CHILD: 10-MINUTE RULE

It is important that you be aware of what your child is doing. Periodic checks should be made so that you can reward (give chips and praise) appropriate behavior, such as playing quietly or working on a job, and punish (take away chips) inappropriate behavior, like fighting or getting into things.

This rule does not mean that you must check exactly every 10 minutes. However, the checks should be done at intervals somewhere between 5 and 20 minutes each. This rule should not be used to harrass your child. When you go to see what he or she is doing, you don't need to interrogate; instead, you should look at his or her behavior and either praise and give chips or take away some chips and give the child feedback. If the child is quietly engaged in a privilege such as playing with a game in his or her room with the door closed, you don't need to open the door every 10 minutes to see what he or she is doing.

PUNISHMENT: WHEN THE CHIPS DON'T WORK

There are at least two different occasions when you will need an effective alternative when the loss of chips isn't effective.

One alternative that we have found to be very effective is what we call "time out." "Time out" means the temporary revoking of *all* privileges and social interaction. Traditionally, this has been done by having a child stand in the corner or go to his or her room. We have changed this somewhat. The time out place should be a dull place but not an ugly place (no closets or dark places!). The best places might be a living-room chair, a kitchen chair, or a front step (if the child is outside).

Occasion 1: Time Out When Your Child Has No Chips

In this case, time out is used when your child has lost by misbehaving as many chips as he or she has gained. This may occur at any time during the day. In other words, when your child's chip container is empty, he or she must go to time out.

Time-Out Procedure

SUGGESTION

It will be necessary to practice time out at times when your child is not upset so that it will be easier for him or her when it actually happens. For example, on a pleasant day your child can earn chips for practicing time out.

PROCEDURE

1. Explain to child that he or she has lost all his chips.
2. Take child to selected spot.
3. Tell your child that he or she must stay in this spot for 5 minutes and must be quiet. Do not start the time until your child is quiet, and if at any time there is noise, the time begins when he or she is again quiet. It is wise to use a timer so that both you and the child know when the time is up.
4. When the initial stay in time out is completed, your child then has the choice to either work or stay in the corner. Most children will choose to work.
5. Your child must work until he or she has earned at least 5 chips and may then go about his or her business.

RULES FOR WHEN YOUR CHILD IS IN TIME OUT

1. When a child is in time out, no chips are taken away. Chips can be earned for behaving while in time out.

2. If undesirable behavior occurs while the child is working his or her way out of time out, he or she goes back to time out for the designated time.

3. Social interaction is forbidden when in time out. Instruct other family members to observe this rule and fine the other children each time they interact with anyone in time out.

4. Ignore all inappropriate behavior that may follow after your child is in time out. Inform your child that 5 minutes will start only when he or she is quiet. If the child leaves time out, replace him or her.

Occasion 2: Time Out for an Angry/Upset Child

There will be times when it is obvious that the chips are not working because your child is too mad or upset. A cooling-off period is then necessary.

The following conversation is an example of when this time out should be used.

MOTHER: Jack, you were really good about getting home on time, but you forgot to hang up your coat. Remember, the rule is that we all hang up our coats as soon as we get home. Would you give me 2 chips and then hang it up—O.K.?

JACK: I don't want to do it right now.

MOTHER: I know it's hard sometimes, but we all have to follow the rules. That's backtalk. Remember, you're supposed to say "OK, Mom," and then go do it. Why don't you give me 2 more chips for backtalk and we'll try it again.

JACK: I'm not going to.

MOTHER: Right now, you're a little mad so you will have to go to time out and cool off. If you do it the right way, I'll give you 2 chips. That's right—I'll get the 4 chips for you. You're really being quiet, that's great. I'll set the timer now.

HINTS FOR PARENTS

1. Nothing good is free. For chips to be powerful and useful as consequences for behavior, it is absolutely necessary that *all* privileges be purchased with chips.

2. If it bugs you, it's bad. If your child does something that annoys you, it probably annoys other adults too. Explain this to your child, set a chip consequence, fine this behavior and reward a more appropriate one. Thus, any behavior that bothers you should probably be modified. You should *define it, instruct your child,* and *provide feedback.*

3. Babysitters. It is absolutely necessary that you have someone you can call on short notice. There will undoubtedly be a time when before a family outing one of your children has no chips to pay for the outing. Since it's not fair to make the rest of the family stay home, you need someone to stay with your child or somewhere to take him or her. If you allow your child to participate in a privilege that he or she can't purchase, you are only *weakening* the whole system.

4. Don't be discouraged when a behavior doesn't change overnight. It usually means that you aren't being consistent enough and are letting things go by too often, or the pay-off (privilege) isn't big enough. You have to be consistent both with taking away chips and giving chips. Don't get discouraged.

5. Prompting. This is very helpful for teaching your child new skills and for avoiding a show of temper. Prompt the right response before you tell the child what he or she did wrong. Example: "Sally, I'm going to tell you something which might make you a little angry but if you keep looking at me, stay pleasant, and take it well, you'll earn an extra 5 chips." Try it—it works.

6. Sympathy. When chip fines are given, remember that you can express your sympathy with your child's unfortunate situation at the same time you are firm in applying the chip losses. Reassure the child who is receiving a lot of chip fines that when you take away chips it doesn't mean that you are mad; it only means that he or she is behaving in a manner that is unacceptable to you.

7. No nagging. Don't try to use unenforceable threats, warnings, emotional pleading, or anger as methods of changing behavior. The data indicate that these do not work. Also, nagging, tantrums, and anger by a parent make life very unpleasant for the whole family. Firm but unemotional and even sympathetic feedback seems to work the best.

8. Chips and praise go together. Chips are not powerful just because they are chips. They must be made powerful. THAT IS THE SECRET TO THE EFFEC-TIVENESS OF YOUR CHIP SYSTEM. To make chips powerful, they must be the *only* way that the child can get his or her privileges. When you give chips, also *give praise.* And, if it is worth a few words of praise, it couldn't hurt to give a few chips.

PHASING OUT THE CHIP SYSTEM

The prime criterion that should be used for deciding when to phase out the chip system is your child's overall behavior. This does not mean that your child must be "perfect" before the chips are taken out. Rather, when your child's behavior has been satisfactory to you *over a period of time,* it is a good time to begin phasing out the chips. You should check with your therapist before attempting this phase-out!

Trial Days

While you are still using the chips on a daily basis, trial days off the chip system may be initiated. The following steps should be followed for any trial day.

1. Explain to your child that you would like to try a day off the chip system.
2. Stress that if things go well, you'll have another trial day the next day, too.
3. Explain that the child must follow the rules just as if he or she were on the system.

4. Explain what will happen if the rules are not followed.
   a. Time out will be used for misbehavior.
   b. If time out is used more than two times for the same behavior, the next day cannot be a trial day.
   c. The chips may be started again at any time during the day.
5. Prompting the right response from your child can be very effective in obtaining cooperation. For example:

MOTHER: Jimmy, before I tell you what I saw, I want you to remember that today is a trial day and I'm sure you'll want to take what I say the right way and be pleasant and say "O.K." Do you understand?

JIMMY: Yes, I understand.

MOTHER: I was watching you and Jane play with your toys. You were really nice to share with her, but when you started playing on the swings, I saw you push Jane off one of the swings, which is against the rules, right?

JIMMY: Right.

MOTHER: Usually you lose chips for that, but since we're not doing that today, let's say that you'll have to wait 15 minutes before playing on the swings again.

JIMMY: O.K., Mom.

It is important for parents to remember that all trial days will not be successful and that it may take some time before the chips can be completely phased out. However, chips can always be used again whether it's been 1 day off the system or 4 weeks. After your child once knows how you want him or her to behave, it is up to you to follow through when a rule is broken.

When your child is on the chip system, breaking a rule should result in a chip loss. When he or she is off the system, breaking a rule should result in time out. If these procedures are not followed by you, then your child will not follow the rules.

Praise for desirable behavior is also a must whether on or off the system. If being good doesn't have a reward (attention, praise, or extra privileges), the desired behavior will not occur as often.

When phasing out the chip system, all the procedures for practicing, checking jobs, and time out should still be followed consistently but with praise rather than chips.

ACKNOWLEDGMENTS

The above is © 1977 by the authors and is reprinted with their permission. The authors were primarily supported during the preparation of this manual by Grant HDO 3144 from the National Institutes of Child and Human Development to the Bureau of Child Research at the University of Kansas. Special thanks are given to Michael Rapoff for his suggestions for revisions of this manual.

INDEX

Italicized page numbers indicate material in figures or tables.